Marketing Massage:
From First Job to Dream Practice
Second Edition

Marketing Massage:

From First Job to Dream Practice

Second Edition

Monica Roseberry

THOMSON

DELMAR LEARNING

Australia Brazil Canada Mexico Singapore Spain United Kingdom United States

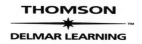

THOMSON
™
DELMAR LEARNING

Marketing Massage: From First Job To Dream Practice, Second Edition
by Monica Roseberry

Vice President, Health Care Business Unit:
William Brottmiller

Director of Learning Solutions:
Matthew Kane

Acquisitions Editor:
Kalen Conerly

Product Manager:
Darcy Scelsi

Editorial Assistant:
Molly Belmont

Marketing Director:
Jennifer McAvey

Marketing Coordinator:
Christopher Manion

Production Director:
Carolyn Miller

Production Manager:
Barbara A. Bullock

Content Project Manager:
Thomas Heffernan

Cover Photography:
Yanik Chauvin
www.touchphotography.com

Library of Congress Cataloging-in-Publication Data

Roseberry, Monica.
  Marketing massage: from first job to dream practice/Monica Roseberry—2nd ed.
    p. cm.
  ISBN 1-4180-3214-X
  1. Massage—Practice.   I. Title.
  RA780.5.R674 2007
  615.8'220688—dc22
                              2006035799

NOTICE TO THE READER

Dedication

To Jeannine Karafotas, without whom this book would not be possible.

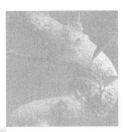

Contents

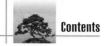

Chapter Two

Marketing Yourself in an Interview / 47

SECTION TWO

MARKETING TO BUILD YOUR DREAM PRACTICE: BARE-BONES ATTRIBUTES, SKILLS, AND TOOLS / 89

Chapter Three

Marketing Attributes / 91

Chapter Four

Skills at the Soul of Success / 129

Chapter Five

The Only Marketing Tools You Really Need / 185

SECTION THREE

MUSCLE MARKETING: REACHING, REBOOKING, AND REFERRALS / 223

Chapter Six

Reaching Skills / 225

Chapter Seven

Reaching Tools / 281

Chapter Eight

Rebooking Skills and Tools / 349

Chapter Nine

Referral Skills and Tools / 413

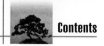

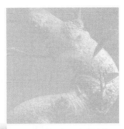

 Preface

WHO THIS BOOK IS FOR

This book is written for anyone who wants to use fast, effective, safe, proactive, low-cost/no-cost **marketing** to build a long-term career in massage. Whether you are a massage student still in school, a recent graduate looking for a first job, a part-time therapist trying to go full time, or you're tired of just getting by financially and want to grow your practice, this book is for you. If you are an experienced therapist moving to a new area, and you need to start a practice from scratch, this book can take months off of your rebuilding process.

If you are changing the emphasis of your practice to a new bodywork modality that will draw from a different market than you are familiar with, or if you want to make the leap from employee status to owning your own practice, this book will give you the marketing tools to help make your dream a reality. Or, if you are an employer working with your massage staff to grow your office, clinic, spa, or business, the content covered in this book can help you reach your goals. Whatever your situation, if you would rather spend your time working on clients than doing traditional marketing, this book is definitely for you!

MARKETING MASSAGE TODAY

Massage is growing at an unprecedented rate and is enjoying a surge in popularity among people from every walk of life. No longer just a luxury for the rich and famous, massage is making its way into the mainstream culture, and businesses and prospective clients everywhere are searching for professional massage therapists to help them with a host of needs. The current state of the profession is exciting, and for those of us who have worked for years to improve the stature, legitimacy, and acceptance of massage, it is gratifying to see the public embracing massage so eagerly.

However, massage is still an emerging profession, and we have much work ahead of us in continuing to define our profession and educate the public about who we are and what we do. Massage has undergone continuous transformation over many centuries in many countries, revealing the fascinating and ever-changing cycles of how humans deal with their bodies and feel about touch. Massage emerges today with practitioners facing opportunities and obstacles unique to this time, place, and profession. Marketing massage in our current environment will take skills practiced by our forerunners in ancient Rome, Greece, Europe, and Asia, but it also will take reaching and serving clients with methods totally unique to our current circumstances. No other service industry faces such tremendous advantages or challenges as does modern-day massage, and understanding how to market during this time can mean the difference between failure and success.

HOW THIS BOOK GOT STARTED

To have a successful career in the current environment of massage, you need to know two things: what successful massage professionals across the country have in common so you can learn from them, and what unsuccessful massage professionals have in common so you can avoid the mistakes that have cost countless practitioners their dreams. Discovering what it takes to succeed in this profession has been my passion, both for my own practice as well as for the thousands of students I have taught.

As a former instructor and Dean of Faculty at the National Holistic Institute in California, one of the largest massage schools in the country, I saw firsthand the difficulties that my students faced in building a practice. To help them, I developed and taught much of a 100-hour business program designed to assure their success. However, even after delivering such an extensive training, I still faced the pain of talking to former students who were not able to make a living with massage, and I knew there was something more, something different than traditional business development skills, that they needed to know.

In my desire to help my graduates succeed, I created seminars on marketing, the one business skill I felt was most important, and most lacking, in their training. However, despite the success of those seminars, deep in my heart I still felt there was something unthought-of and unsaid that cut to the core of true success in the field of massage. I decided to broaden my search and began calling industry leaders, massage school owners, and teachers across the country, hoping to expand my perspective on what was nagging at me about marketing massage. Despite all of that research, I was still unsatisfied and felt I had not found what really mattered when building a long-term practice.

Finally, in the summer of 1999, I went on the ultimate quest for answers about marketing massage. I got a trailer, hitched it up to my truck, and drove 15,988 miles through 24 states over the span of five months, doing field research and conducting countless interviews with massage professionals, massage school owners, employers, and the general public in search of what it takes to truly market massage.

What I learned, especially from the general public, shocked, amazed, pleased, and dismayed me, and eventually forced me to totally reconsider what I believed about marketing. More than anything, I was surprised because, during my search, here's what I found: successful professionals with only a simple business card for advertising; skilled therapists whose primary marketing was wearing a T-shirt that mentioned massage; and person after person who could not tell me how they had marketed their way to a full practice beyond "just talking to everybody." From the mountain peaks of Idaho to the shores of Georgia, I came across therapists who had done little of what experts would consider to be marketing, yet their practices were thriving.

On the other hand, I also met therapists who had all of what I considered the right marketing ingredients, but who weren't making it financially. One woman in particular blew away my last shred of preconceived notions as she was closing up shop in spite of her fancy office with a receptionist, professionally designed cards and brochures, coupons, impressive Web site, and a medical referral and insurance reimbursement setup. I was stunned! Could marketing massage be so basic yet so critical? I realized I'd have to reconsider my ideas from scratch and create a new way of thinking about marketing that was more consistent with my field research.

The book you hold in your hands is the result of my years of searching for how to market massage. After 22 years in private practice, thousands of hours of teaching and writing classes, and hundreds of hours of research, personal interviews, thinking, and rethinking to find real solutions for the real problems that massage therapists and bodyworkers face in starting and building their careers, I think what I have learned can help you. For you as a massage student or professional aiming to make a living with massage, I hope what follows will start you on your way and keep you on the road to helping yourself while helping others.

HOW TO USE THIS BOOK

The lessons I have gathered are recorded in three sections within this book. The first section, "Marketing Yourself to an Employer," covers the tools and skills needed to get hired as an employee. A large number of massage careers are launched by experience gained from working for someone else. In addition, many therapists enjoy full- or part-time work in a variety of settings over the course of their careers. While the majority of this book is about how to market to build a private practice, this first section is vital for those who plan to land a job working in a spa, clinic, medical setting, chiropractor's office, on-site business, or other employment opportunity.

The second section, "Marketing to Build Your Dream Practice," covers the **bare-bones** fundamentals of basic marketing to start a private practice. This section starts with the personal and professional **attributes** that are at the heart of marketing massage. Combining these attributes with key marketing skills and tools addressed in this section should give many professionals the foundation on which to build a flourishing practice. The formula for the second section is simple: Marketing Attributes + Skills + Tools = Success.

Please be forewarned, however, before reading the second section. My goal is to help you become a successful therapist with as many clients as you want, for as many years as you choose to practice. Not everything I say may be comfortable, politically correct, or to everyone's liking. Some of the material may seem simplistic and mundane, or even strongly opinionated, but after interviewing hundreds of people who have received professional massages or hired therapists as employees, I realize that I can take nothing for granted. I apologize up front if these basic but crucial skills of communication and human interaction seem obvious. However, after listening to an onslaught of horror stories about unprofessional behavior by purportedly professional therapists, I would be remiss if I did not do whatever possible to make an impact on my readers about what is bottom-line necessary to make it in this field. Every venture, whether learning a martial art, playing basketball, or building a massage practice, requires practice and mastery of the fundamentals. In this section, you will learn what those fundamentals are.

The third section, "Muscle Marketing," adds meat to the bones of the second section, and is designed to take practitioners to the next step in building a private practice. It covers what virtually every successful practitioner has in common, or what I call the "Three Rs" of marketing. The Three Rs thoroughly cover numerous ways to reach new clients, rebook those clients, and get personal **referrals** from them. The **muscle marketing** content builds on the bare-bones material, adding advanced skills, tools, and concepts designed to help practitioners grow a practice quickly, survive in a highly competitive market, or reach a very select clientele. However, I have found from my research that advanced marketing skills and tools are useless if the basic attributes are not in place, so master the attributes in the second section before you spend your time, energy, and money on the more advanced marketing in the later chapters.

These three sections will help you succeed in your massage career. Whether you are seeking your first job, starting out with a small practice, or building up to a thriving enterprise, read the chapters based on your needs and follow the action steps at the end of each chapter, because knowledge is not sufficient for success: action is.

As you will discover as you read this book, it is not a typical textbook. Having trained thousands of massage students in business classes, I know that you don't want to be lectured at or talked down to. So, I approached this book as more of a conversation. You and I are both on our own paths in our respective journeys in life, and for the brief stretch of time that you are reading this book, we share the path together. What I want to say to you during this time is what I have learned about what works and doesn't work when trying to be a successful massage professional or bodyworker. I wish you the best on your journey!

ABOUT THE AUTHOR

Monica Roseberry, MA, is a speaker, teacher, and international best-selling author, and has been a massage therapist in the San Francisco Bay Area since 1984. A self-described "touch activist," she has reached thousands of massage therapists with the intention of helping each one succeed, driven by her belief that massage and bodywork professionals can change the culture of touch in America, one massage at a time. Ms. Roseberry has written for numerous massage and spa journals, was an Item Writer for the National Certification Exam for Therapeutic Massage and Bodywork, and is the primary massage author for The Body Shop, International. She holds a Master of Arts in Kinesiology, and lives in Walnut Creek, California.

ACKNOWLEDGMENTS

This book would not have been possible without the help and support of numerous people. Special acknowledgment and undying gratitude go to Jeannine Karafotas for her unflagging love and support; to Vav and Tatay for more than I can ever repay; to Susan Koenig, who gave me a true love for massage; to Carol Carpenter Ayala, who fostered my love of the business of massage; and many thanks to the many school directors, teachers, therapists, and countless interviewees who gave me their time and told me their stories that made this book unfold.

Putting together a book is a team effort, and I have been privileged to work with the people at Thomson Delmar Learning, especially the extraordinary Kalen Conerly and Molly Belmont, who made the second edition experience a pleasure. Heartfelt thanks go to copyeditor Chris Downey for making amazing improvements; and to Neha Khattar Malhotra, Antima Gupta and the staff at ICC Macmillan Inc. for shepherding this book through its final stages. Thank you all for helping me and believing in this book and the value of massage.

To contact the author, call 1-925-906-8806, or go to her Web site, http://www.MonicaRoseberry.com.

A NOTE ABOUT THE ARTWORK

Bonsai trees are my favorite symbol for a successful massage practice. They both take love, care, and nurturing over many years, and though both are naturally limited in size, they can still flourish, change, and grow more fascinating with time and intention.

Marketing Yourself to an Employer

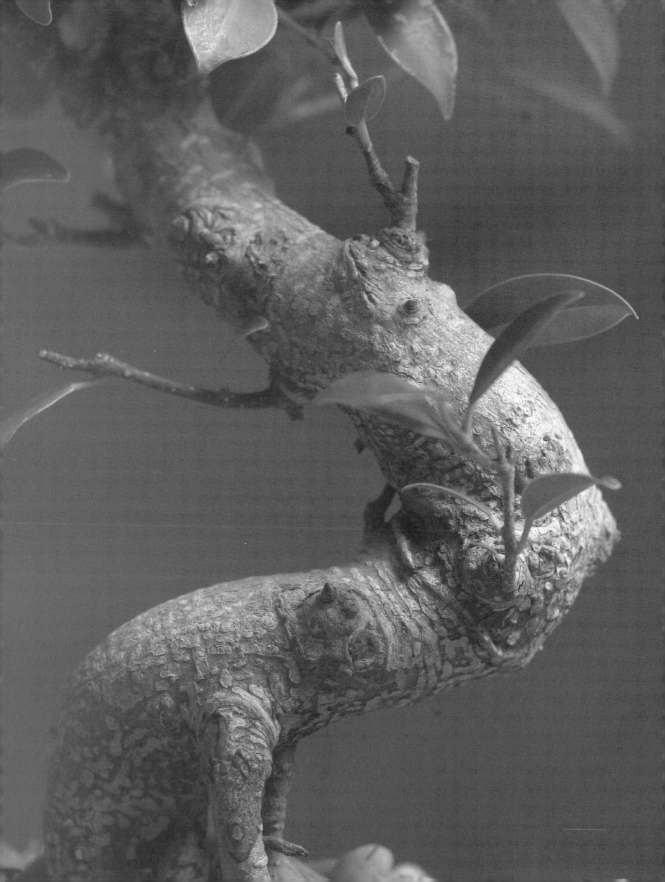

1 | Marketing Yourself With a Resume

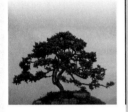

CHAPTER OBJECTIVES

After reading this chapter, you should be able to:

- Identify common employment options for massage therapy positions.
- Discuss four ways of applying for a job.
- Conduct background research on industries and businesses to customize a resume.
- Create a resume tailored for the job position you want.
- Write clear resume objectives.
- Summarize the highlights of your background effectively.
- Choose the most relevant information about your experience and education.
- Format and send electronic and printed resumes.
- Write an attention-getting cover letter.

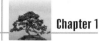
MARKETING YOURSELF WITH A RESUME

Marketing your services as a massage therapist or bodyworker has changed a great deal in the last few years. Until recently, most massage professionals had one primary work option: to start a private practice from scratch and work for themselves their whole career. Fortunately, massage therapists have many more options today, including working as an employee in a wide variety of settings, from hands-on practitioner to team leader, manager, or director.

Your path to marketing your services can be as unique and special as you are. You can graduate from massage school and get a job, gain experience, learn new skills, and then start your own practice. You can start with clients on your own, and then supplement your income and enjoy social interaction with a massage job, and spend your career with a happy mix of both. You can even be an experienced entrepreneur who wants a change or a challenge and opt to work for someone else, using either a new or advanced skill, or you could work in management. Wherever you are on your path, this first section of the book is designed for massage therapists who want to market themselves to an employer.

Marketing yourself to an employer involves three main tasks:

1. Finding the right employer for you

2. Creating a resume and cover letter tailored for the position you want

3. Conducting an interview that will get you the job

This chapter covers how to find the right employer for you and how to write a resume and cover letter that will get you an interview for the job you want. The next chapter provides a thorough, step-by-step overview of the unique circumstances of the massage interview process, guiding you through the verbal and hands-on components from beginning to end, and helping you avoid common interview mistakes.

FINDING THE RIGHT EMPLOYER FOR YOU

Massage therapists have an incredible opportunity to work in a wide variety of environments and with a broad range of people. Unlike most other service professionals, we can take our hands-on skills and apply them in settings ranging from beachfront resorts to world-class hospitals, to senior centers, to sports teams. As you plan your career path in massage, you have many options open to you. However, as you decide what jobs you will apply for, you will need to narrow those options so you can focus your time and energy on a job that is best suited to you.

Step 1: Know Yourself

How do you know what environment will work best for you? You have to get to know yourself. Are you fun or serious, intense or laid-back? Do you like to do one thing really well, or do you like to try many things and always keep learning something new? Do you like being quiet and enjoy solitude, or do you like a lot of activity, talking, and interaction? Can you focus for a long time, or do you have a short attention span and like change? Which part of massage work do you enjoy most—helping people with stress, helping people in pain, or working with high-level athletes? And what kind of clients would you like to work with? You can go from doing the lightest energy work with premature babies to the deepest elbow work on a 300-pound football player. You can move from office to office doing chair massage in a busy downtown high-rise or work barefoot on a beach under a cabana.

You also need to know what goals you have. What lessons do you want to learn? In what ways do you want to grow? What skills do you want to develop? And how much money do you want to make? You may have a long-term career path in mind with a plan of action laid out, or you may just want to try many things and then make up your mind. You may want work that is secure and predictable, or you may need a lot of variety to keep you from getting bored. The beauty of being a massage professional is that you can be who you are and find a place that works for you.

Step 2: Know Employment Options

The second step in finding the right employer for you is knowing what kinds of employment options are currently available for massage therapists. Quite happily, this category is growing rapidly, and more and more businesses are recognizing the value of providing massage for their customers or employees. The following list includes the most common types of employers that hire massage therapists as staff members. This list grows incredibly for self-employed massage therapists who provide massage services for businesses while working for themselves, but then, that's what the second section of this book is for! As you review this list, think about who you are and imagine what kind of clients you would work on, what type of work you would do, what kind of manager and coworkers you might have, and how it would feel to work in these different environments.

Types of Employers

Spas—**club spa, cruise ship spa, day spa, destination spa, medical spa, mineral springs spa, resort/hotel spa**

Beauty salons

Health clubs

Gyms

Golf and tennis clubs

Sports teams

Chiropractors

Medical offices

Clinics

Hospitals/hospices

On-site—offices, airports, mobile teams, corporations, conventions, events

Other—Create your own position in a business that doesn't currently offer massage

Step 3: Target the Best Employment Option for You

Once you have a general idea of what type of work setting or clientele would best suit you, you need to find specific businesses to which you can send your resume. There are four ways you can apply for a job. These are:

✳ Applying to businesses that are currently hiring

✳ Applying to businesses that offer massage but are not currently hiring

❋ Applying to businesses that don't currently offer massage but will create a new position since you asked them to

❋ Posting your resume online and seeing who contacts you

Let's look at each of these application options a little closer.

Applying to Businesses That Are Currently Hiring

Traditionally, employees seeking work look for open positions and research who is hiring by going through "help wanted" ads and newspaper classifieds, searching the Internet, or talking to people they know. As a massage therapist, you can look for open positions listed on massage school Web sites, job boards, or newsletters, and in professional journals or association Web sites for the industry in which you are interested. For example, the International SPA Association (ISPA) has a Web site, found at http://www.experienceispa.com, that lists open spa positions in its job bank. If you have a specific company in mind, look on the Internet and see if they have open jobs listed on their Web site. Other Web sites and connections for job openings are listed in the "Resources" section of this book. For the most current listings, go to any online search engine and type in search terms like "spa massage jobs" or "chiropractic massage jobs," and go from there.

When you apply to a business that is currently hiring, your resume and cover letter should be easier to write because the job description will be clear, the contact information will be spelled out, and your main task will be to convince the reader that you are the right person for the job. Since the employer has put out the word that they are looking for a new massage therapist, you can just send in your resume and cover letter directly to whomever the ad tells you to.

If possible, though, you can improve the odds of getting an interview by having an inside contact help you. For example, if you want to work at a local day spa and have a friend who works or gets massage there, you can ask her if she will alert the hiring manager to look out for your resume. You should also ask if you can use her as a reference in phone calls or in your cover letter. Managers like to reduce their risks on making bad hiring decisions. If people who know the manager tell him or her that they are willing to lend their name and reputation in support of you, it can help get you to the interview stage. Send out an e-mail to people on your address list, and call your friends,

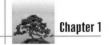

classmates, colleagues, fellow association members, and school (especially the placement director) to see if anyone can get you an inside contact.

Applying to Businesses That Offer Massage but Are Not Currently Hiring

Many businesses that employ massage therapists don't put out "help wanted" ads because they get so many resumes sent to them—they just keep them on file for when they get a job opening. If you really want to work for a particular business, don't wait for them to list a job opening; just send in your resume and cover letter. Make sure you have done your research and know the name of the person who does the hiring so that your resume goes to the right place. Your cover letter will also need to be carefully tailored to that employer, because you will need to convince them to make a place for you or put you on their list for future hiring. Since the manager isn't in the hiring mode, you will be sending an unsolicited resume, known as a **blind pitch,** and it has to be very well done to get their attention off their other tasks.

Conversely, you can do a generic blind pitch to dozens of employers and just send a resume and cover letter that inform potential employers of your background experience and education. For example, if you want to work at a resort spa in California, you can pick up a spa magazine or do a Web search, get the names and addresses of the resorts, and send all of them your resume. To determine what you should focus on in your resume, you can research a number of spas similar to your generic market, see what they are looking for in their job descriptions or even what they offer on their spa menus, and write a resume that would work for them in general.

If you haven't gotten a response within a week of mailing out your resume, call to make sure your resume was received. If you are told that no positions are open, ask when would be a better time to apply. Ask if they have a seasonal flux or a list to call for future openings, and ask if they will hold your resume on file for future consideration.

Applying to Businesses That Don't Currently Offer Massage but Are Creating a New Position

This is a wonderful category for job applications because it is where the massage industry will experience significant growth. There are literally thousands of beauty salons, chiropractic offices, physical therapy clinics, sports teams, corporations, hospitals, gyms, and more that do not currently have a massage therapist on staff or in-house. However, as these businesses see their competitors taking away their business, getting more customers, or getting better employees because they offer massage, they may be ready for an enterprising massage therapist to knock on their door and offer to help them establish massage as one of their regular services.

One very effective success strategy to get a job in a crowded market is to "zig when everybody else zags." With this strategy, if a lot of other massage therapists are applying for jobs in businesses that already offer massage, you can create your own opportunity with no competition by creating a massage job where there isn't one.

In this scenario, your resume and cover letter will need to convince the employer to consider the benefits and profitability of offering massage to their customers or employees. You can tell them that you will help them create and set up an in-house therapist position. If the employer is hesitant, offer to work on the owners, managers, and staff, so that they trust you. Beyond that, if you have really great skills and trust your abilities, you can even offer them a no-risk trial where you work for free for a set time to demonstrate the value of your work. You are the one taking the risk, not them, and it could pay off handsomely for everyone. For employers interested but without the right facilities, you can ask to be a referral for clients outside the office.

To make the most of this category, examine your own background or interests and look at the world with eyes that see opportunities where no one else is looking. Who out there needs touch, massage, stress relief, pain reduction, performance enhancement, or body awareness? What are your dreams, and how can you create a position that would be perfect for you? Do you want to help people going through drug or alcohol rehabilitation, give children in orphanages a loving touch, help dancers at a ballet company, or relax the tight shoulders of factory employees doing repetitive work on an assembly line? Are other massage therapists already working in those settings? Probably not. This gives you the opportunity to capitalize on all the favorable press that massage has received over the last few years and create a job where there never used to be one.

Even settings like movie production studios or software companies, where self-employed massage therapists have occasionally worked, may now be open to creating permanent employee positions because they have seen the benefits of massage firsthand. How will you know if they will hire you? ASK! They can say no, but if you can present a good case for the benefits you offer and how these will profit or support their facility, give it a try. It may be easier to get in the door if you work for yourself and are not an employee, but you can start there.

Posting Your Resume online and Seeing Who Calls You

Given the wide world of massage and how many employers are desperately seeking quality therapists, putting your resume online on a job search Web site can open doors you didn't even know existed. Since you won't know who will be looking at your resume, you will not be able to customize it the way you would for a specific employer. However, we will cover what a typical employer is looking for so that you will have a resume that still catches their attention. In a later section called "Keywords," we will discuss the specifics of how to submit a **scannable resume** that has the right search words most employers will be using to find your resume online. Companies like Monster.com and HotJobs.com are searched by a worldwide audience, and if you want to look beyond your own neighborhood for work opportunities, this could be a great option for you.

GETTING READY TO WRITE YOUR RESUME

Now that you have a better idea of who you are, where you will fit, and what kinds of opportunities are out there, it is time to write a resume that will attract the right employer to you. Your next step is to do research on the industry in which you want to work. If you have particular businesses and positions in mind, you will also need to research those specifically, so you can customize your resume for them.

Researching an Industry

The best place to start researching an industry is through professional journals, newsletters, and consumer magazines that specialize in the topic. You can look in bookstores, libraries, or online for all the periodicals that serve that particular industry. All it takes is a couple of copies to get a pretty clear idea of the industry trends, needs, problems, issues, and even common complaints from employers. Look at the ads, the regular features, and the columns, and familiarize yourself with what your future employer is dealing with. Pay close attention to industry jargon and common buzzwords, especially if you are going to post your resume online, since these will be the words the employer is scanning for. Look for announcements about upcoming conventions and conferences, and note what the theme is and what the speakers will be talking about. Often these announcements list Web sites that tell you more, so check them out, too.

Professional industry associations are the other great source for insider information. Look up associations on the Internet and search for data that can help you get inside the mind of your prospective employer. Is the industry growing, downsizing, specializing, or consolidating? How much are consumers spending, and on what services? As you gather this data, think about how you can address the employer's current issues in your resume, cover letter, and interview.

Researching a Business

Every business has its own challenges and needs, along with a unique corporate culture, work environment, client base, specialized services, and competitors. By understanding these factors, you can further customize your resume for your target business. You can do off-site research by calling and asking them to send you written materials, as if you were a prospective customer. They may have brochures, service menus, price lists, and other literature that can tell you volumes about the business. You can do an Internet search by typing in the business name or the name of the owner. (See Figure 1–1.)

Other massage therapists can provide information, as well. Join online massage chat rooms, go on massage bulletin boards and post a question, or talk to colleagues, classmates, teachers, your massage school placement director, or local massage association members. On-site visits will tell you the most, and you can ask for an informational interview or, best of all, visit the business as an anonymous paying client and see what it's like from the inside.

Researching a Position

The factor that will most shape your resume will be the job description for the position you are seeking. As much as possible, find out what your regular tasks would be. What are the most commonly requested massage and bodywork tasks; what specialized treatments will you need to perform; and what

Figure 1–1 | Research companies online and find out who is hiring massage practitioners.

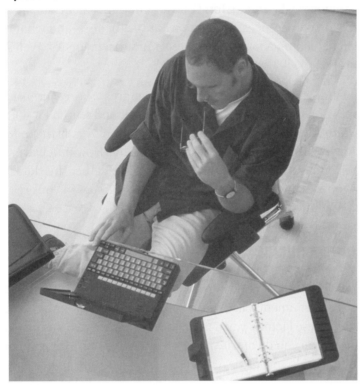

equipment will you use? Will you also perform non-massage tasks, such as answering the phones or working in the retail sales area? Even if you can't get all the details, if you have done your industry research, you can make an educated guess about what your position will entail. If all you know is that there is a "help wanted" ad posted in the health-food store for a job at a local day spa, get a copy of *DAYSPA* magazine and read through it so you understand what a typical day spa offers.

Getting Contact Information

Finally, your most important research will be to gather the contact information of your target employers. Gather the addresses, phone numbers, names, and titles of those who are in charge of hiring, and, above all, make sure you get everything spelled correctly.

CREATING A RESUME AND COVER LETTER TAILORED FOR THE POSITION YOU WANT

Now that you know yourself and your ideal job, have targeted an employer, and have done your research about that employer, it is time to tell them in the few pages of your resume and cover letter who you are and how you will fit into their team.

While you have much to tell an employer, remember that a resume has one primary function: to create enough interest in you to get an interview. That's it! Since many managers often deal with stacks of resumes, yours has to capture their attention, tell them at a glance that it is worth reading more carefully, and, once they read it, to then contact you for an interview.

To get a sense of what the employer goes through when facing a pile of resumes, think about how you feel when you are watching TV and channel surfing for something good to watch, or when you are searching the Internet for a particular topic. If you're like a lot of people, you've got your finger on the remote or mouse, and you give the show or Web site a few seconds to interest you; otherwise, you move on. Your decision to stay or go is based on a whole lot of little details, reviewed both consciously and subconsciously. Employers scanning resumes for the right person are often flipping through them with the same speed and attention span as a channel surfer, waiting for something to leap out and make them stop in their tracks with the sense that they have found exactly what they are looking for.

Getting employers to pick your resume out of the pile will depend on how your resume looks and what it says. Let's start with what your resume should say.

Resume Content

Having graded hundreds of resumes during my days of teaching resume writing, I know firsthand what an amazing and diverse group of people come into the massage profession. Some people have strong backgrounds in traditional medicine, alternative health, or massage. Some have advanced degrees, unique talents in art or acting, or are getting out of the corporate rat race. Others are new mothers wanting a well-paying, part-time job with flexible hours so they can raise their kids. Increasingly, many are straight out of high school and have very little experience other than just loving to massage their families and friends.

Whatever your story, background, set of skills, past experience, education, and job goals are, your resume will need to be customized to highlight your strengths, downplay your limitations, and otherwise show you in your best light. If your strength is in your background, you will spend the bulk of your resume demonstrating how your past experience will help you be successful in the future. If your experience is limited, then you will need to highlight your education and how you performed as a student to indicate how well you will perform as an employee in the future. If you don't have a strong base of experience, and you don't even have a strong education, then you will need to highlight aspects of your background, skill set, and personality that will still make employers consider themselves fortunate to have found you.

My favorite example of this last category comes from my days working for a sailing club. Our office manager was moving, and we were interviewing people to take over the position of running the administrative side of the club. One woman in particular caught my attention, as she apologized repeatedly during the interview for being a stay-at-home mom who was returning to the workforce and didn't have any recent job experience. Then I found out that she had raised five boys! If she had known how to write a resume the way you're going to learn to, she would not have apologized but would have proudly emphasized that she had 20+ years of experience with all the skills the position required, including: time management, budgeting, multitasking, handling interpersonal conflicts, enforcing rules, communicating effectively, picking up and delivering items, negotiating deals, and so forth. She had dozens of other skills, abilities, and qualities that were directly transferable from raising five boys to running our office and club, especially since most of our members were male. She was perfect for the job, but she didn't know how to say it. We won't let that happen to you!

While there are many ways to write a resume, the style we are going to use here has been carefully chosen because it makes your resume a powerful marketing tool that grabs the reader's attention faster than more traditional and non-customized resumes. We will be using the standard sections an employer would expect in a resume, but with additions that will get you noticed. The hard part is knowing the most important information about yourself to include. By doing your research and knowing what an employer is looking for, you can narrow down the list of your many skills and abilities to show you have just what they want, and that you can help them with their needs.

THE COMMON ELEMENTS OF A RESUME

We are going to cover the common elements of a resume and go into detail on each section so that you craft the right resume for the job you want. Like a 30-second commercial, your resume must introduce you rapidly, keep the reader's attention, explain how you are different than other candidates, and make them want to get you in for an interview.

The main sections of a resume include the following sections:

- Contact Information
- Objective
- Summary of Qualifications
- Professional Experience
- Education

These can be followed by the optional sections:

- Special Skills/Relevant Information
- References Available Upon Request

Contact Section

The first part of any resume tells how the employer can get in touch with you to ask questions or schedule an interview. In this section, you need to include your:

- Name (and title initials, if applicable)
- Address
- Phone
- E-mail address
- Web site (if you have one)

This section is pretty straightforward, but here are a few tips to consider. First, how you show your name graphically (boldfaced or italic fonts, sizes of letters, capitalization, etc.) sets the tone for the rest of the resume. Your name is where you make a personal statement, and it can be conservative, big and bold, or expressive; just make sure it's legible. Your goal is to make sure the way you show your name is considered appropriate but interesting by the kind of manager reviewing the resume. Your name starts the resume, and it should be in a larger type than the rest of the text.

When employers are interested in contacting you, they want to do so quickly, so make your contact information easy to find at the top of the page. Most employers use phone or e-mail to contact you, so choose or obtain a new e-mail address that is professional. If your current e-mail address has words in it that aren't going to sit well with an employer, don't use it. Also, don't use work-related e-mail addresses, since it is not a good sign to an employer that you are using work time and facilities to find a new job. The same goes for listing phone numbers. Do not use a work phone as your main contact number.

Objective

The objective section of the resume consists of a short statement of purpose, and it is where you do your most important marketing. Traditional or generic resumes don't use objectives, but they are missing a great opportunity to market, as long as the objective is focused on the needs of the employer, not on the needs of the applicant. The objective tells the reader why you wrote the resume and what job you are interested in, and it emphasizes how you will benefit the company by taking the position.

For example, if you want to work at a spa doing massage, a simple objective could be, "To serve the customers of XYZ Spa by providing excellent massage therapy services." If this were a day spa and you knew its needs well, because you had done your research, you could have an even better objective, such as, "To provide outstanding massage therapy and customer service for the clients of XYZ Spa so that they return for regular treatments." If you want to work in a medical setting, such as a chiropractor's office, an objective could be, "To assist Dr. X's patients by providing massage therapy that optimally prepares them for adjustments." If you want to work at a health club or gym, an objective could be, "To advance the health, well-being, and loyalty of XYZ's members by providing massage therapy that enables them to fully benefit from their membership."

While employers fully realize that the main reason most people want jobs is to be able to pay their bills, no employer wants to hear that. They want to know that you understand their problems and needs; if you can help them with theirs, they will help you with yours. The more clear you are in the objective that you understand their unique needs and can help them with your services, the more excited they will be to hire you. Here are some other objectives as examples:

- To help the athletes of the XYZ sports team prevent injuries, speed recovery, and improve performance by providing ongoing pre-event, post-event, and maintenance sports massage.

- To assist the members of XYZ Tennis Club by providing therapeutic and sports massage that will reduce players' risk of injury, speed recovery from practice and workouts, and prepare them for peak performance mentally and physically.

- To help XYZ Spa retain and rebook regular massage clientele by providing outstanding massage and customer service. (See Figure 1–2.)

- To help reduce absenteeism and prevent repetitive movement injuries by providing regular desk massage for the employees of XYZ Corporation.

- To improve morale, reduce stress, and increase productivity of the employees of XYZ Corporation by providing weekly chair-massage sessions.

- To increase the success and profitability of XYZ Spa by providing excellent massages and spa treatments for its customers.

- To support the success of XYZ Spa by providing management, leadership, and organizational skills tailored to the unique needs of the massage therapy department.

Figure 1-2 | What skills can you offer to a business?

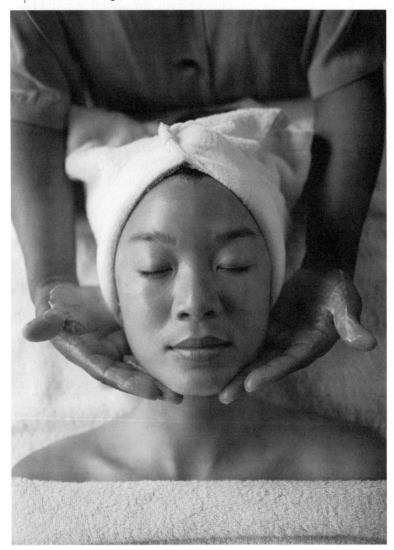

EXERCISE: WRITING AN OBJECTIVE

Your objective is one of the most important marketing aspects of your resume. Imagine the perfect job for you, and then think about how you can write an objective specifically for that job. Write out a number of objectives until you have one you like. Then imagine an employer reading it and ask yourself if your objective would make them want to call you up for an interview. If you are in a group, read your objective aloud to the others and get their feedback.

_____

_____

_____

_____

_____

_____

_____

Summary of Qualifications

Following the impact of the objective, your next big impression will be created by your summary of qualifications. This is a section of three or more bullet points that summarizes the most important highlights of your qualifications. Like the sound-bites at the beginning of a TV news program that highlight the upcoming stories so you stay tuned, your summary is designed to keep the reader from "changing the channel" and moving on to the next resume.

A standard qualifications summary might look something like this:

- Certified Massage Therapist with 1,000-hour training
- Experienced practitioner in Reiki, acupressure, Swedish, and deep tissue
- Attentive listener with strong interpersonal communication skills
- Responsible professional with commitment to providing outstanding customer service

These lines are pretty generic because they address the basic needs that every employer has: they need you to be educated, know specific massage modalities, have good communication skills, and be a professional. To set you apart from other resumes, though, you need to also highlight aspects of yourself that are unique to you while still being desirable to the employer.

One way to choose your "highlight reel" is to go back to your research on the specific needs of the business, and then make sure that your summary of qualifications lets them know you have something special that they want. For example, if you want a job at a tennis club and you specialize in working with tennis players, you should state the basics, such as that you are trained in sports massage or have experience working with athletes. However, if you also add that you are an avid tennis player and understand the mentality of tennis players, you will be a much more appealing candidate for the job, since you bring an insight to the clients that other applicants may not have. Your bullet point could say something like, "Avid tennis player with personal experience of mental, emotional, and physical demands of the game."

Similarly, if you want to work at a sports rehabilitation clinic for injured athletes and you have personally experienced sports injuries, you could state that you have a strong understanding of the clients' needs because you have used sports rehabilitation yourself. Your bullet point could say, "Direct experience with extensive sports rehabilitation and personal understanding of motivation strategies needed for injury recovery." Or, if you want to work with an orthopedic doctor or physical therapy clinic, and you survived an accident and went through major rehabilitation yourself, you could use a similar point to emphasize your ability to help patients work through pain and not give up, since you know what it's like. These highlights are the "extras" on top of the ordinary, and they are what make you "extraordinary" to the employer.

Another way to select the elements for your summary of qualifications is to directly address common problems you have discovered in your research. For example, if you were applying at XYZ Day Spa, and you knew that they were having difficulties with therapists coming to work late, you could impress the manager with qualifications that show you are punctual. Your bullet point line could say something like, "Strong sense of responsibility with proven track record of punctuality." Even if your track record is that you showed up to every class or clinic on time, that past behavior indicates your future potential. When you get to the section of the resume on education, you can clarify that point by saying that you had perfect attendance at school and were never late for classes or clinics. Of course, this has to be true for you to claim it! Punctuality is a crucial part of what employers want; if you learn how to show up on time for school or work, you can use it as a way to separate yourself from other applicants.

Similarly, if the spa is having difficulty finding therapists with current state licenses or who have passed the National Certification Exam, put those points right at the top of your summary. At a glance, tell them your best points so they will keep reading!

Once you've chosen the elements that will best market you in the summary, you need to distill them into bullet-point language. Start each point with strong, positive descriptive words or action verbs. You want your reader to imagine you in action, engaging with their clients, taking charge of situations, handling issues, solving problems, and otherwise making their business more successful.

Here are some bullet points starting with descriptive words:

- Extensive knowledge of anatomy and physiology
- Strong background in multiple massage modalities
- Proven track record of **rebooking** 80 percent of first-time clients
- Positive team player who gets along with wide variety of personalities
- Fast and willing learner able to quickly master new techniques
- Motivated self-starter who thrives in fast-paced clinic environment
- Results-oriented specialist trained in advanced medical massage techniques

You could just start these points with the noun, like *knowledge* of anatomy, or *background* in massage, but that would be boring and dry. Your job is to accentuate your ability in subtle ways, and the descriptor words give you the opportunity to shine.

Here are some bullet points starting with action verbs:

- Organized and led year-long study group with 15 classmates
- Coordinated 20-member volunteer massage team for Leukemia Foundation fundraiser
- Built solid customer base in two years
- Administered an average of five massages a day in prior position
- Managed full-time job while earning 3.5 GPA in massage school

✳ Attended 100 hours of advanced training in therapeutic modalities

✳ Increased profits for XYZ Spa by $2,000/month with cost-cutting suggestions

However you choose to write your summary of qualifications, it is best to start each line with the same type of word, whether it is a descriptive adjective or an action verb. Mixing these together makes it confusing to read. You want to use a consistent choice of wording, known as **parallel structure,** and keep your bullet points sounding the same. To best accomplish this, imagine that you are completing a sentence that starts the same way every time. With descriptive words, pretend that the start of your sentence is, "You should hire me because I have . . . X" (an extensive background, a proven track record, a 1,000-hour education); or "I am . . . X" (a motivated learner, a strong leader, a flexible team-player).

With action verbs, pretend the start of your sentence is, "You should hire me because I did . . . X" (managed a business, completed specialized training, graduated top of my class, volunteered at 10 sports massage events). The best way to test your structure is to read it out loud and listen for whether it sounds smooth and flowing. If it's choppy sounding, rewrite it until it has a nice rhythm to it.

Notice in the second set of bullet points that each one was quantified. Your qualifications are more believable and make more impact if you can prove your statement with measurable factors and numbers. If you have a track record of making money, cutting costs, reaching goals in a short amount of time, or other impressive and quantifiable data, put it here.

Professional Experience or Work History

Once you have your summary of qualifications, the following information is prioritized in an order that shows your best points first. Depending on your massage background, your professional experience could be the next item on your resume. If you have a lot of hands-on experience, put this section before the education section. Remember, you may only have a few moments to capture your reader's attention, so put your strongest points first.

The professional experience section is traditionally written in reverse chronological order. This means that you list your most recent experience first and work backward. If you have a lot of experience, you can list all your relevant past jobs and give a little bit of information about each. The traditional basics are the name of the company you worked for, your job title, the city and state, and the dates that you worked there. While this is standard, it's pretty boring and doesn't really tell the employer much about why they should hire you. Marketing with your resume means highlighting your strengths and past experiences that will mean the most to your reader. Don't waste your space with trivia like employment location, street addresses, or bosses' names, especially if you have to fill out an application that will repeat the same information; instead, use your space wisely by giving more details about the jobs, and choose the details that best show your potential and have the most in common with your target job.

What should you highlight in your few words? Explain what your job responsibilities were, what accomplishments you achieved, and what commendations and promotions you received. Write your experience and accomplishments in bullets, since this is eye-catching and much more readable than paragraph style. It also lets you cut out unnecessary words. With bullet points, the reader can gather the data in bite-sized chunks, remember them, and then move on to the next piece of information. If you have a long list that would take up too many lines, use a bullet-style list.

Let's look at how to show your skills and potential, even if your only experience is doing your clinic hours in school. Your professional experience section could look like this:

XYZ Massage School: Student Clinician, Anytown, CA, 2006.

Responsibilities included: calling clients to confirm appointments; answering phones to assist customers; conducting client intakes and recording health histories; conducting new client evaluations; providing customized massage sessions based on client needs; accepting payment through cash, check, and credit card; processing and filing client paperwork; operating industrial laundry machines; restocking supplies and setting up massage stations between clients; staying within 50-minute session time; performing three massages back-to-back per shift.

If you can do each of those tasks and do them well, you have just told the employer that you are capable of handling pretty much any entry-level massage job. By spelling out each skill you have practiced, you help them imagine you doing the kind of job they are hiring for, and that is good marketing. Obviously, if you have some strong work experience that can better demonstrate your character and abilities, don't take a lot of space writing about doing laundry or answering phones; only use this level of detail if you don't have a lot else to say.

Your professional experience section can also include nonpaid positions, such as volunteer work, sitting on committees or boards, and professional association work. One of the best ways to get experience without having much background is to do volunteer work. In addition, it shows initiative and the ability to work well with others, be a team player, demonstrate dedication and loyalty, and practice leadership—all characteristics that employers want.

Certificates and licenses are also listed in this section. This is where you would list, for instance, that you are "Nationally Certified in Therapeutic Massage and Bodywork (NCTMB)" by taking the National Certification Exam, or that you have a state license to practice massage or other licensed services, such as cosmetology. The title that you earn from your school, or a certificate that you get in an advanced modality or specialty, such as aromatherapy, is listed in the education section of the resume.

Finally, professional memberships in associations or organizations round out this section. Many massage therapists join associations such as the American Massage Therapy Association (AMTA) or Associated Bodywork & Massage Professionals (ABMP) to get access to professional liability insurance and other benefits. Both offer opportunities to get involved and make a difference in the profession, as do other associations (see the "Resources" section). If you take on roles of leadership or get involved in projects, include them in your resume.

Education

If you are a recent massage school graduate, and you don't have a lot of work experience in massage or other professions, put your education section before the professional experience section since this will be your area of strength to highlight after the summary of qualifications. Depending on how much other education you have, this section can be very detailed about your massage school experience or it can just give the basics. Your goal in this section is to again demonstrate that you have good potential in the future based on your track record in the past. Therefore, choose points to include here that tell the employer that you are willing and able to grow, learn, and excel, no matter where you are.

Typically the education section is written in reverse chronological order, with the most recent school listed first. With each line, list your:

* School name
* Area of concentration
* Degree or certification
* Date graduated or will graduate
* GPA (optional, and only if above 3.5)

Beyond these basics, you can include:

* Honors/awards/scholarships
* Activities
* Specific classes or specialties, and number of hours of each topic relevant to the job

Here again, if you have little to say but still want a good-looking resume, list your classes so the employer knows what you've been trained in. Since massage schools across the country offer widely varying programs, it can really help the employer to know how much anatomy and physiology training you've received, how many hours of clinic, internship, or externship you've had (if any), how many hours were dedicated to specific modalities, and if you've followed any particular interest track, such as spa treatments, Eastern techniques, or medical massage. As we will discuss in the upcoming interview chapter, many people in charge of hiring massage employees are new at evaluating the qualifications of massage therapists, so spelling out the primary segments of your education can help them understand your skills better.

Specialized Training/Continuing Education

One of the traits that smart employers look for when they are trying to figure out how you will behave in the future is whether you go above and beyond what you have to do in school just to get by. One way to show that you are willing to go the extra step and do more than the bare minimum is to take continuing education classes and attend professional conferences. An employer looking through a stack of resumes from therapists all listing pretty much the same educational background will stop and take notice of those who demonstrate the drive to learn beyond their certification program. Even while you are in school, if you can attend a conference, take a specialty seminar, or even start and lead a study group in school, you can put this in your education section and stand out from the crowd.

Employers in medical or therapeutic settings will especially be looking for training in advanced modalities that are usually taught by specialists in seminars designed for people who have already graduated from their basic training program. How do you find out about those specialties? Do your research! Read professional journals, such as *Massage Magazine*, *Massage Therapy Journal*, *Massage & Bodywork*, and *Massage Today*, many of which feature online articles, and keep up with the latest techniques that are attractive to employers.

Special Skills/Relevant Information

Your resume can be quite complete with the elements we have covered. However, you may have additional and relevant skills, talents, and abilities that are not part of your school or work experience, and you think they will make the employer even more interested in you. Based on your research, think about who you are, what you know, or what you have done that would help the employer believe you are well suited for the position.

For example, if you want to work for a large chain of resort spas that have facilities all over the world, you could include special skills such as fluency in a foreign language, a background of extensive travel, and a stated willingness to relocate.

You can also point to having a similar background to the clientele you would serve. For example: you overcame years of chronic pain and now want to help others in a pain clinic; you were a former all-star athlete now looking to work in a sports therapy clinic; you have 15 years of background in meditation and want to work at a retreat center; you have trained extensively in yoga and want to do massage in a yoga center, and so forth.

The special skills section can also be your most important section after your summary of qualifications and doesn't have to be kept near the bottom of your resume. One reason to move this section higher is to highlight the massage skills you have, even if you don't have a lot of experience or education. This section could simply consist of bullet points of your best modalities to inform the reader right up front that your skills are more important than your work history or education. If you are fresh out of school and have no work experience, or are highly expert and want to emphasize your expertise, list your skills and massage techniques and move them higher up the page.

References Available Upon Request

Either at the bottom of your resume or on your cover letter, write in the phrase: "References available upon request." Many employers basically want someone else to vouch that you are a decent, upstanding citizen and will be a good employee. So who should be on your reference list? Think of people who can speak well of any aspect of your work experience, education, volunteer work, abilities, personality, or other things that matter to the employer. If possible, pick people who have strong credentials, important titles, and other qualifications that indicate they are someone to whom an employer should listen.

For example, when I applied to graduate school and had to provide a reference list, of all the people I know who could vouch for me, I chose my friend Ted because he had been a graduate-level college professor. When the dean of my department called him to talk about me, they could relate as peers, and my dean knew he was getting the kind of information about me he could trust.

Once you pick your people, ask them if they will be references for you. If they say yes, ask what contact number you can use. Then tell them about the jobs you are applying for so they can speak well of you using the most pertinent information. When you send out your resumes, send them one, too, so they are well prepared and reminded to be ready for an employer to contact them.

On the actual reference page, type out each reference's name, title, phone number, e-mail, address, and relationship to you. You can also include further details that show the caliber of people you know, or point out qualifications that will impress the reader.

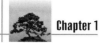

Keywords

In today's tech-savvy world, there is one more element you will need in your resume if you are dealing with electronic applications. This is the keywords element. Many companies now use computer-scanning software to electronically review resumes for specific buzzwords and industry terms used in a specific job. If those keywords aren't in the resume, the program eliminates the resume without ever passing it on to a human being. Some people type in a long list of keywords in hopes of increasing their odds of having their resume kept, but this looks strange, takes up precious space, and isn't always appreciated by employers. If you want to include a keyword list, put it at the very top of your scannable electronic resume and type in the words, separated by periods. For example, if you were posting your resume online for a spa company to find you, a keyword list could be something like: Massage Therapy. Spa Massage. Spa Treatments. Body Treatments. Swedish Massage. Deep Tissue Massage. Reiki. Thai Massage., and so on.

The best way to make sure your resume gets kept is to include the keywords in your text as part of a description of your past experience. How do know what the keywords are? They are the same exact words used in the job posting or description for the job you want. If you don't have a specific job in mind, research job descriptions from similar businesses and use the keywords they use. If the job description is looking for a person who can do "body treatments" and "spa massage" or "reflexology," use these exact words in your resume content. When you write up your professional experience or education highlights, make sure you include these words as an important part of your background.

WRITING YOUR RESUME

Once you have gathered your thoughts and information for your objective, summary of qualifications, professional experience, education, and other parts, write up a first draft. Don't worry about how it looks or if everything is perfect. Just get everything down on paper. Once that is done, you can move from the gathering stage to the refining stage. Your goal at this point is to turn this diamond in the rough into a polished gem that shows off your many facets.

The first step of refining is to get your information down to a maximum of two pages, and preferably to one. Opinions differ on this point, but remember, the goal of the resume is to get an interview, not a job, so save the noncritical details for the interview. Language here is key. Cut out all extraneous, dull, or useless words, such as "I," "me," "my," "a," "an," and "the," and turn the details of your life into interesting, active, descriptive terms. Your job is to essentially edit the movie of your life, including your experience, education, skills, and personality, down to a fascinating snapshot. Your details need to be tightly written, well composed, and succinct. Each line should take your reader straight to the point, and every word should count. This is a lot easier said than done! Expect to go through many rewrites and new versions as you further distill your information.

Editing Your Resume

Once you have your draft really polished, put it aside for a day or two and then come back to it with fresh eyes. Your subconscious mind will most likely have thought of something else to add, reword, or change, so give it time to work. Sometimes even your dreams can help you figure out what to say. As you edit your resume, think of your ideal employer in his or her office, holding your resume and trying to picture who you are and how you will fit into the spa, clinic, office, cruise ship, sports team, or wherever you are applying. Read from their point of view and think about what would thrill them to finally see on a resume. Then rewrite some more, and finesse every little detail. Your resume has to be flawless, with perfect spelling and punctuation. Practice reading it aloud, and edit it to make it sound good. Get out your dictionary and check your spelling, and do not rely on your computer's spell checker to get things right. Many words sound the same but have different spellings and meanings, so make sure your message is clear and accurate.

The most common mistakes to watch for are inconsistencies. These can include a breakdown of the parallel structure in phrasing, style choices, and punctuation. Similarly, there can be inconsistencies between past and present tense. If you are writing about jobs that you used to have, write about them in the past tense. If you still have the job, write about it in the present tense. The look or style of each section also needs to be consistent. If you underline the title of your last job, make sure that you underline the title of every job, and so on. The same goes for punctuation. While the rules for how to punctuate a resume vary, what matters is that you choose one style and stick with it. For example, if you put a colon after the name of the last company you worked for, make sure that you put a colon after the names of all the other companies you list.

Finally, have at least five people review your resume. It is far better to have those who know and love you critique it and correct mistakes, or say that it feels unfocused, than to have an employer think the same and decide not to interview you. Swallow your pride, if that is an issue for you, and let others look it over before you send it out. If that is too hard to face, ask a friend to pass your resume out for review, and let him or her gather the critiques and make the changes for you. Whatever it takes to make it perfect, do it.

For further details on writing, consult a style manual, look at books on resume writing, or hire a professional resume writer to do it for you. For $300 to $600, you can hire a professional to do the work for you, and the more high profile or higher paying the position you are seeking, the more you should consider this option. To find a professional resume writer, try these options:

- Professional Association of Resume Writers and Career Coaches: http://www.parw.com

- Professional Resume Writing and Research Association: http://www.prwra.com

- National Resume Writers' Association: http://www.nrwaweb.com

For the most recent rules and styles of resume writing, which change frequently, go on the Internet and type in search words like "resume writing" or "scannable resume," and see what comes up. There are dozens of Web sites dedicated to helping you write the perfect resume. They will give you sample resumes, cover letters, thank-you letters, and follow-up letters, and they can sell you very inexpensive software for resume templates and distribution services. You are not alone in this process, so get help from every source you can.

SAMPLE RESUME

I could write dozens of sample resumes that would be different based on all the combinations of factors we have covered so far. However, I am only going to create a few to put the whole package together, and I strongly urge you to look at the many samples that are included in other books or online Web sites dedicated solely to resume writing.

The first sample is my fantasy resume I wanted to write a number of years ago, and it's just a fun exercise to give you an example of this marketing-oriented style of resume. (See Figure 1–3.) This is an e-mail–formatted, scannable resume that has no commands in it, such as boldface text, underlining, centering, or bullet points, since these often get messed up during transition over the Internet. This resume uses a one-page, stripped-to-the-bone style that has one purpose: to get the reader interested enough to e-mail me back. I have

Figure 1–3 | An example of a scannable resume written in plain text for online submission.

> scannable resumes look boring, but use them for online submissions

> put all words on the left margin

> don't use bolds or italics, but use all capitals to make the words stand out

> no bullet points

> with a lot of experience, list only highlights with a few details

> spell out an acronym the first time it is used

> tell more about yourself if it will grab the interest of the reader

Monica Roseberry, MA HHPE
XXXX Street, Walnut Creek, CA 94597
925-906-8806
mroseberry@earthlink.net
www.MonicaRoseberry.com

OBJECTIVE
To help prevent injury, relieve pain, improve productivity, and reduce stress for the cast and crew on the New Zealand set of Xena: Warrior Princess, by providing therapeutic and relaxation massage.

SUMMARY OF QUALIFICATIONS
Nationally Certified Sports Massage Therapist since 1987
Proven professional with strong track record helping world-class athletes
Experienced therapist able to address range of needs with multiple massage modalities
Easy-going and friendly team player able to get along with wide variety of people
Flexible personality able to adapt to any situation and provide massage in any setting

PROFESSIONAL EXPERIENCE
Professional Massage Therapist in private practice in San Francisco area, 1984 to Present
Sports Massage Therapist for NBA Golden State Warriors, and Olympic and amateur athletes
Teacher of 4,000+ massage students and Dean of Faculty at one of the largest US massage schools
Speaker in US, Asia, and Europe on massage, stress management, and spa topics
International bestselling author of four massage books by publishers Thomson Delmar Learning;
Simon & Schuster; Barnes & Noble; and The Body Shop, International
Contributing Editor to professional massage and spa journals and consumer magazines

PROFESSIONAL AFFILIATIONS
American Massage Therapy Association (AMTA) and National Sports Massage Team Member since 1987; awarded AMTA California Community Service Award in 2003; National Certification Board for Therapeutic Massage and Bodywork; passed National Certification Exam (NCE) in 1992 and 1995; served as Test Item Writer for NCE in 1993

EDUCATION
Master of Arts in Kinesiology: Saint Mary's College of California, Moraga, CA, 2003-2006
Holistic Health Practitioner and Educator: 1,000-hour training; included 500-hour Certified Massage Therapist training; National Holistic Institute, Oakland, CA, 1984-1986
Bachelor of Arts in Communication Studies: Emphasis in Public Relations and Advertising; Minor in Journalism; California State University, Sacramento, 1982-1984
Continuing Education: Trained in numerous advanced bodywork modalities including The BodyTalk System; Quantum Touch; Reiki; BrainGym; Bowen, and more

RELEVANT INFORMATION
Have traveled extensively internationally and lived abroad in Asia and Europe for 12+ years

References available upon request

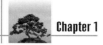
thought about what concerns, fears, and needs the reader has, and I have tried to address those in my objective and summary of qualifications. Then I use my professional experience and education section to prove that I am capable and qualified to meet the stated objective. The details in this are true about me, and this would be the kind of resume I would write for this situation.

This second resume is a more visually appealing piece designed for being printed and mailed. (See Figure 1–4.) It is a fictitious resume for a recent

Figure 1–4 | **An example of a resume for a therapist with minimal hands-on experience.**

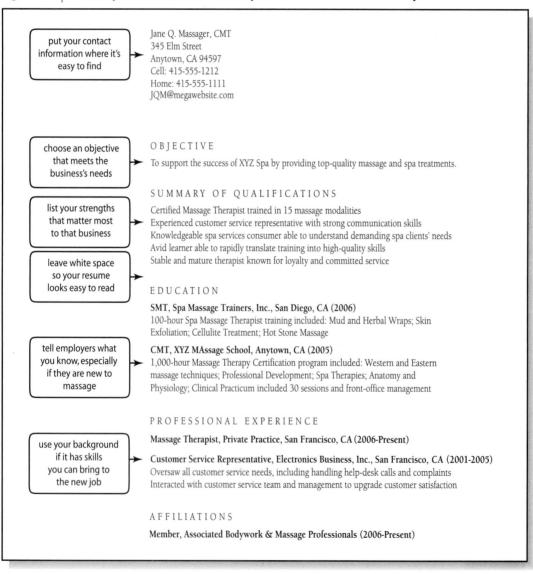

put your contact information where it's easy to find

Jane Q. Massager, CMT
345 Elm Street
Anytown, CA 94597
Cell: 415-555-1212
Home: 415-555-1111
JQM@megawebsite.com

choose an objective that meets the business's needs

OBJECTIVE

To support the success of XYZ Spa by providing top-quality massage and spa treatments.

SUMMARY OF QUALIFICATIONS

list your strengths that matter most to that business

Certified Massage Therapist trained in 15 massage modalities
Experienced customer service representative with strong communication skills
Knowledgeable spa services consumer able to understand demanding spa clients' needs
Avid learner able to rapidly translate training into high-quality skills
Stable and mature therapist known for loyalty and committed service

leave white space so your resume looks easy to read

EDUCATION

SMT, Spa Massage Trainers, Inc., San Diego, CA (2006)
100-hour Spa Massage Therapist training included: Mud and Herbal Wraps; Skin Exfoliation; Cellulite Treatment; Hot Stone Massage

tell employers what you know, especially if they are new to massage

CMT, XYZ MAssage School, Anytown, CA (2005)
1,000-hour Massage Therapy Certification program included: Western and Eastern massage techniques; Professional Development; Spa Therapies; Anatomy and Physiology; Clinical Practicum included 30 sessions and front-office management

PROFESSIONAL EXPERIENCE

use your background if it has skills you can bring to the new job

Massage Therapist, Private Practice, San Francisco, CA (2006-Present)

Customer Service Representative, Electronics Business, Inc., San Francisco, CA (2001-2005)
Oversaw all customer service needs, including handling help-desk calls and complaints
Interacted with customer service team and management to upgrade customer satisfaction

AFFILIATIONS

Member, Associated Bodywork & Massage Professionals (2006-Present)

massage school graduate applying for a position with a spa. Notice as you read it how, even with very little experience, the therapist comes across as competent and qualified.

FORMATTING AND SENDING YOUR RESUME

In the not-too-distant past, sending your resume out was pretty simple. You got a nice envelope, wrote the employer's name and address on it, licked your stamp, and mailed it off. If you were really fancy, you'd hire a courier to deliver it in person to make a big statement of how serious you were about the position.

Today, resumes need to be customized depending on how the employer wants one sent. Many employers want a resume sent by e-mail, while some prefer post mail or fax. This means you may have to create multiple versions of your resume in a variety of formats so you can get your information to the right place in the right way.

Formatting E-mail or Scannable Resumes

For e-mailed or scannable resumes, or anything that goes online, you must make your text "scanner friendly" and remove all formatting (such as centered titles), and eliminate enhancements (such as boldface text or underlining). Keep everything aligned to the left and don't center anything. Use hard returns instead of word wraps to keep your lines divided in the place you want. To create a number of spaces, use the space bar, not the tab key. Don't use dashes, dots, boldface, italics, underlines, special characters, bullets, or even apostrophes, if you can avoid them. Don't even use graphics or tables. These commands often get translated incorrectly or get reformatted if your receiver is using a different computer platform (Mac or PC) or service provider (Hotmail, Yahoo!, AOL, Earthlink, etc.). To set your sections apart visually, put section headers in all capital letters. You can type up your resume in this plain style, and then copy and paste it into an e-mail without it getting messed up or having strange characters magically replace your content. To make extra sure your e-mailed resume gets through, you can send it in ASCII (American Standard Code for Information Exchange) so all computers can read it. To make an ASCII file, type up your resume and then save the document as "text only" under the Save or Save As commands.

Do not send your resume as an attachment unless the employer specifically asks you to. Even if you do send an attached document, also send a copy-and-paste version in plain text (ASCII) in case they can't open the attachment. Because of the prevalence of computer viruses, many employers don't open attachments, or their scanning software strips out all attachments automatically. You can say something like, "I am pasting in a plain text version of my resume and attaching one as well."

Make sure your name is on each page of your scannable resume, and that all pages are numbered. For example, I would write at the top of a second page: "Roseberry—Page 2 of 2." Scanning computers can separate pages, and the best page of your resume can accidentally get forwarded by itself to the employer without them being able to figure out who you are.

Formatting Paper Resumes

Paper resumes can be a work of art, and you should go to the library or bookstore to look at resume writing books for samples of how to lay out a stunning masterpiece on paper. There are also hundreds of resume samples online. Visually, you want your resume appealing to the eyes, and kinesthetically, you want it to feel good in the hands. A busy manager flipping through a pile of resumes will create a "yes" pile and a "no" pile. If the first process of elimination is based solely on how good the piece of paper looks, which happens more than you'd think, keep yourself in the "yes" pile with a sharp-looking presentation. And, since I have been asked this question a lot, no, you cannot send in a handwritten resume; it has to be typed. Period.

Here are a few simple rules for making a good-looking paper resume.

❉ Leave a lot of white space. Don't fill in every inch of the page or it will look like too much work to read.

❉ Have margins of 1 to 1.5 inches. Don't make margins too big, or it looks like you don't have enough to say, and don't make them too small, because it just gets crowded and overwhelming. Managers are human, too, and they can be tired, lazy, overworked, or irritable. You want your resume to look like it will be a nice, easy, informative read.

❉ Set apart your sections with clear titles (experience, education, etc.), and leave two to three spaces between your sections.

✳ Choose a style and be consistent with it. Make sure all capitalization, boldface, punctuation, spacing, underlining, and other style choices are used the same way in each new section. Ask the people who review your resume to watch for consistency in your style choices as well as your content.

✳ Pick one font, and only one. While it is fun to think you finally get to use the 853 fonts that came with your computer program, resist the urge. Resumes that look like ransom notes are the mark of an amateur. The most common professional fonts are Times New Roman and Arial, and they should be used at an 11-point size minimum. Though they may look more conservative than other more fun and expressive fonts, wait until you get the interview to show more character. If you just can't stand those fonts, pick one that is easy to read, doesn't have curlicues, and still looks professional. Busy managers won't spend their time trying to decipher cursive or highly stylized fonts, so don't use them. For variety, use the same font in different sizes, and use boldface, italics, or underlining to give it good visual appeal.

Printing Your Resume

How your resume feels is important in conveying the best presentation possible. High-quality bond paper of 20 lbs. or more gives a strong, positive impression. Colors like white, off white, or ivory are recommended, mainly because they look professional, but most importantly because your reader can easily copy and fax them to others. Oftentimes hiring decisions are made by committee, and your resume will be scanned, faxed, or photocopied and passed around a table while the group discusses the candidates for the position. Colored paper, even gray or pastel, will come out looking murky or unreadable when copied or scanned, which isn't quite the impression you want to make. So, while you may want your resume to stand out in a crowd, colored paper is not the way to do it. The same rule goes for ink color; black copies best, so stick with it. For American employers, use 8.5×11-inch paper, which is the standard letter size.

If you have a high-quality printer at home or available through work, school, or a friend, use it. Otherwise, get copies made at a professional printer. You can bring with you a disk or USB mass storage device with your document saved on it, or e-mail yourself a copy and download it at the printer's computer.

Bring good paper or buy it there, and get your originals printed. Make a number of additional copies as well, so that when you go to your interview you can bring copies with you. It may sound like a lot of effort, but it is worth it for a job you really want.

Mailing Your Resume

For hard-copy paper resumes, your first introduction will be your envelope, so make sure it looks good. To make your best presentation, use a large envelope so you don't have to fold your pages. If you think your resume will be scanned to pass along to others, don't fold it; bent paper is difficult to lay flat on scanner beds, and shadows from the folds can confuse the software that is trying to read it. Handwritten envelopes are fine, but make your handwriting neat and legible. For the final visual touch, put your stamp on straight. Sloppy writing, words that cover the whole surface, and crooked stamps tell the receiver that details don't matter to you, which isn't the way you want to be perceived. Most important, triple-check that you have the correct spelling for names and addresses. If you received a letter with your name spelled incorrectly, would you want to open it? Remember, you have one chance to make a good first impression, so be a perfectionist, pay attention to every detail, and then be ready for your phone to ring!

EXERCISE: WRITE YOUR RESUME

A resume is an important marketing tool, whether you are applying for a job or building a private practice. Using what this chapter has covered, write a resume for the kind of job you want. If you already have a target employer in mind, use this exercise to write your first draft.

COVER LETTERS

The second tool you can use to market yourself to a prospective employer is a cover letter, which accompanies your resume. The purpose of a cover letter is to get that potential employer to read your resume, much like the purpose of your resume is to get an interview. (See Figure 1–5.)

Figure 1–5 | **A cover letter for a therapist with minimal hands-on experience.**

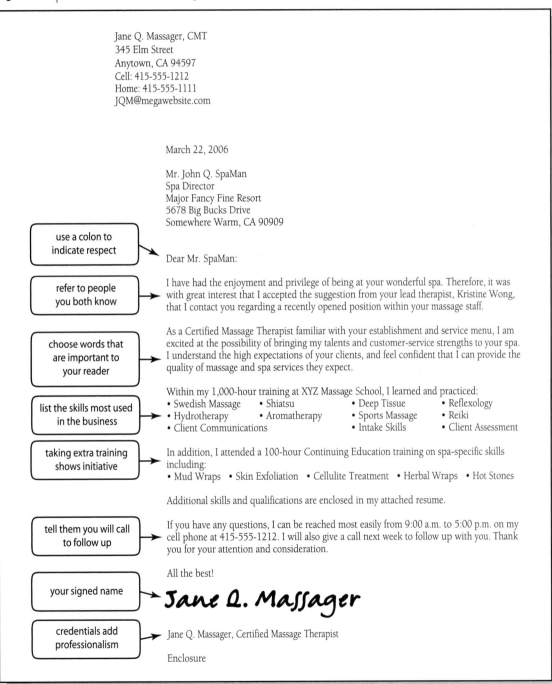

Jane Q. Massager, CMT
345 Elm Street
Anytown, CA 94597
Cell: 415-555-1212
Home: 415-555-1111
JQM@megawebsite.com

March 22, 2006

Mr. John Q. SpaMan
Spa Director
Major Fancy Fine Resort
5678 Big Bucks Drive
Somewhere Warm, CA 90909

use a colon to indicate respect →

Dear Mr. SpaMan:

refer to people you both know →

I have had the enjoyment and privilege of being at your wonderful spa. Therefore, it was with great interest that I accepted the suggestion from your lead therapist, Kristine Wong, that I contact you regarding a recently opened position within your massage staff.

choose words that are important to your reader →

As a Certified Massage Therapist familiar with your establishment and service menu, I am excited at the possibility of bringing my talents and customer-service strengths to your spa. I understand the high expectations of your clients, and feel confident that I can provide the quality of massage and spa services they expect.

Within my 1,000-hour training at XYZ Massage School, I learned and practiced:

list the skills most used in the business →

- Swedish Massage
- Shiatsu
- Deep Tissue
- Reflexology
- Hydrotherapy
- Aromatherapy
- Sports Massage
- Reiki
- Client Communications
- Intake Skills
- Client Assessment

taking extra training shows initiative →

In addition, I attended a 100-hour Continuing Education training on spa-specific skills including:

- Mud Wraps • Skin Exfoliation • Cellulite Treatment • Herbal Wraps • Hot Stones

Additional skills and qualifications are enclosed in my attached resume.

tell them you will call to follow up →

If you have any questions, I can be reached most easily from 9:00 a.m. to 5:00 p.m. on my cell phone at 415-555-1212. I will also give a call next week to follow up with you. Thank you for your attention and consideration.

All the best!

your signed name →

Jane Q. Massager

credentials add professionalism →

Jane Q. Massager, Certified Massage Therapist

Enclosure

Your job as a marketer is to write a letter that looks great, is targeted to your employer, is clear and to the point, and makes your reader excited to see what your resume has to say. It should take a minute or two to read, and it should never be more than one page. Your letter should be a strong demonstration of your personality, not dry and boring. Be professional and polite, but include a bit of enthusiasm and personality, giving readers a breath of fresh air if all they have received have been stuffy application letters.

COVER LETTER CONTENT

Your cover letter should have the following elements:

- Your name and contact information
- The name and title of the person doing the hiring
- The name and address of the business
- Date
- Formal greeting
- Opening paragraph
- Explanatory section
- Next-step paragraph
- Closing line
- Signature
- Typed name

If you know the name and title of the person in charge of hiring for the position you want, include it at the top of your letter. This information is not always made available, especially with very brief help-wanted ads. Take the time to find out who that individual is, either by researching online or calling and asking the name of the person in charge of hiring for that position.

Formal Greeting

Open your letter with a greeting. If you know the person's name, simply say: Dear Mr., Ms., or Dr., followed by the person's last name. Do not just use his or her first name. Follow the name with a colon, not a comma. The colon indicates respect and formality, while a comma is more informal. If you only know the title, use it in the greeting (e.g., "To the Spa Director at XYZ Spa"). In the worst-case scenario, if you just can't get the person's name or title, use the generic phrase, "To Whom it May Concern."

Opening Paragraph

The opening paragraph must capture and keep the reader's attention. It explains why you are writing and makes reference to the position you seek. Be interesting in this first paragraph. Don't start with boring sentences like, "Enclosed, please find my resume." Instead, personalize it by saying you saw their ad, admire their company, want to follow up on a phone conversation you had, or that one of their clients or employees suggested that you apply for a position there. Indicate your interest in a job opening, even if one was not advertised.

If you have gone to this business as a paying customer and have developed a **rapport** with a staff member who has given you permission to use his or her name, this is the place to do so. This process, called name dropping, tells the reader that you both know the same person, and it gives you an advantage over other applicants because it raises a level of trust about you.

Explanatory Section

In the explanatory section, use short sentences and bullet points to tell the employer how you are qualified for the job. Think from the reader's point of view. They are reading your letter with the hope that they will find the right person for the job, and they want you to tell them how you can help their business be more successful. Show that you have done your research, and explain how you can help them specifically. Exhibit your knowledge of the field as a whole, and their business in particular. You want to come across as capable and competent, not desperate and certainly not arrogant, and show them that you have much to offer them. Emphasize your skills and, if possible, quantify your accomplishments in numbers and dollars. This is the place to give a few highlights that are strong selling points about you and will make them want to read your resume. Whatever you do, don't exaggerate your abilities and skills or use superlative terms such as "best," "great," or "extraordinary." You can use bullet points in your letter, which break up big blocks of text and clearly point out the details you most want the employer to see.

Next-Step Paragraph

In the final paragraph, talk about the next step. Invite the reader to contact you for an interview, and provide the best way to reach you and the best time to talk. Also inform them that you will be following up within a week with a phone call.

Closing

Your closing is a simple courtesy phrase. Common ones are "Sincerely," "Regards," or an upbeat "All the best!"

Below the closing, give yourself four rows of space and write your signature in the space with a dark, high-quality pen. Then, below that, type your name.

Here is another example of a resume and cover letter, so that you can see other ways to write them and consider other elements to include. (See Figure 1–6.)

Printing Your Cover Letter

Print your cover letter on the same high-quality paper stock as your resume, and enclose it with your resume in the large envelope. Keep a copy for yourself, and write on it when you sent it and when you will make your follow-up call. Then make sure to mark in your calendar when you need to make your calls!

EXERCISE: WRITE YOUR COVER LETTER

Based on your resume and target employer, write a one-page cover letter that will make the reader excited to look at your resume.

Follow Up

About a week after you mail out your packet, call and confirm that it has arrived. Some employers clearly state in their "help wanted" ad not to call them; if that is the case, follow their instructions and don't call. If possible, find out when a decision will be made about who will be interviewed and when the interviews will be conducted. Record the name of the person you talk to and any other information you gather from the call. Be polite and

Figure 1–6 | A second sample resume and cover letter.

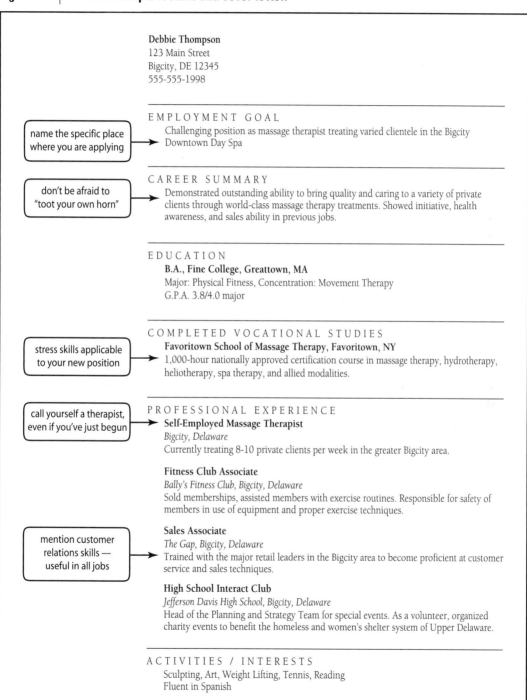

Debbie Thompson
123 Main Street
Bigcity, DE 12345
555-555-1998

EMPLOYMENT GOAL

> *name the specific place where you are applying*

Challenging position as massage therapist treating varied clientele in the Bigcity Downtown Day Spa

CAREER SUMMARY

> *don't be afraid to "toot your own horn"*

Demonstrated outstanding ability to bring quality and caring to a variety of private clients through world-class massage therapy treatments. Showed initiative, health awareness, and sales ability in previous jobs.

EDUCATION

B.A., Fine College, Greattown, MA
Major: Physical Fitness, Concentration: Movement Therapy
G.P.A. 3.8/4.0 major

COMPLETED VOCATIONAL STUDIES

> *stress skills applicable to your new position*

Favoritown School of Massage Therapy, Favoritown, NY
1,000-hour nationally approved certification course in massage therapy, hydrotherapy, heliotherapy, spa therapy, and allied modalities.

PROFESSIONAL EXPERIENCE

> *call yourself a therapist, even if you've just begun*

Self-Employed Massage Therapist
Bigcity, Delaware
Currently treating 8-10 private clients per week in the greater Bigcity area.

Fitness Club Associate
Bally's Fitness Club, Bigcity, Delaware
Sold memberships, assisted members with exercise routines. Responsible for safety of members in use of equipment and proper exercise techniques.

> *mention customer relations skills — useful in all jobs*

Sales Associate
The Gap, Bigcity, Delaware
Trained with the major retail leaders in the Bigcity area to become proficient at customer service and sales techniques.

High School Interact Club
Jefferson Davis High School, Bigcity, Delaware
Head of the Planning and Strategy Team for special events. As a volunteer, organized charity events to benefit the homeless and women's shelter system of Upper Delaware.

ACTIVITIES / INTERESTS
Sculpting, Art, Weight Lifting, Tennis, Reading
Fluent in Spanish

(CONTINUES)

Figure 1–6 | **(continued).**

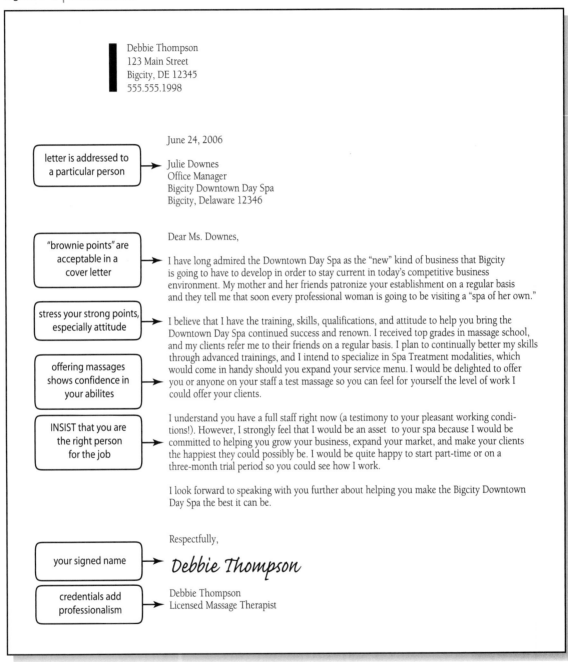

Debbie Thompson
123 Main Street
Bigcity, DE 12345
555.555.1998

June 24, 2006

letter is addressed to a particular person →

Julie Downes
Office Manager
Bigcity Downtown Day Spa
Bigcity, Delaware 12346

Dear Ms. Downes,

"brownie points" are acceptable in a cover letter →

I have long admired the Downtown Day Spa as the "new" kind of business that Bigcity is going to have to develop in order to stay current in today's competitive business environment. My mother and her friends patronize your establishment on a regular basis and they tell me that soon every professional woman is going to be visiting a "spa of her own."

stress your strong points, especially attitude →

offering massages shows confidence in your abilites →

I believe that I have the training, skills, qualifications, and attitude to help you bring the Downtown Day Spa continued success and renown. I received top grades in massage school, and my clients refer me to their friends on a regular basis. I plan to continually better my skills through advanced trainings, and I intend to specialize in Spa Treatment modalities, which would come in handy should you expand your service menu. I would be delighted to offer you or anyone on your staff a test massage so you can feel for yourself the level of work I could offer your clients.

INSIST that you are the right person for the job →

I understand you have a full staff right now (a testimony to your pleasant working conditions!). However, I strongly feel that I would be an asset to your spa because I would be committed to helping you grow your business, expand your market, and make your clients the happiest they could possibly be. I would be quite happy to start part-time or on a three-month trial period so you could see how I work.

I look forward to speaking with you further about helping you make the Bigcity Downtown Day Spa the best it can be.

Respectfully,

your signed name →

Debbie Thompson

credentials add professionalism →

Debbie Thompson
Licensed Massage Therapist

respectful; the people answering the phone are often gatekeepers to the person doing the interviewing, and they can be key in the hiring process. They may not be able to answer your questions at that point, so ask when you can call back at a later date for clarification. If you do find out that you are on the candidate list, and when you will be interviewed, what can you expect next? Go to the next chapter and find out!

CHAPTER 1   SUMMARY

Employment opportunities for massage therapists are growing every day, and the way you can take advantage of those opportunities is to grab the attention of employers with a great resume and cover letter. This chapter has given you the big-picture overview and minutest details of how to present your best self within the specific structures of a resume and cover letter. You have so much to offer people with your skilled touch and caring hands, and a well-crafted resume helps you notify potential employers of who you are and how you can help them and their customers with your massage.

CHAPTER 1   ACTION STEPS

Based on the information in this chapter, do the following to market yourself to an employer:

- Think about who you are and what kind of work environment will best suit you.

- Consider your employment options and choose one right for you.

- Look for open positions or create one yourself.

- Research the industry, company, and position in which you are interested.

- Create an objective for the position you want.

- Select the highlights of your background for your summary of qualifications.

- Write out the relevant points of your education and professional experience.

✳ Write, edit, and hand out your resume for other people to review.

✳ Write, edit, and hand out your cover letter for other people to review.

✳ Contact people to be your references.

✳ Send your resume and cover letter to your chosen employers.

✳ Follow up with a phone call within a week.

CHAPTER 1   KNOWLEDGE CHECK

Check your understanding of the chapter by reviewing these questions and answers.

Q: List three types of employers.
A: Spas, beauty salons, cruise ships, health clubs, gyms, and so forth.

Q: True or False? If there are no job openings, you shouldn't send a resume.
A: False.

Q: List two ways to research an industry.
A: Read industry journals or magazines; look up the professional associations online.

Q: True or False? You can do good research by getting a massage where you want to work.
A: True.

Q: List three of the sections commonly used in a resume.
A: Contact information, objective, summary of qualifications, professional experience, education, and relevant skills.

Q: List three mistakes you must be careful of in a resume.
A: Errors in spelling, grammar, and punctuation; and inconsistencies in structure, style, and wording.

Q: What are three ways you can send a resume?
A: Post mail, e-mail, and fax.

Q: True or False? To make sure your resume stands out, you should use colored paper.
A: False.

Q: True or False? A cover letter has to be one page only.
A: True.

Q: True or False? In your cover letter you should say you are the best therapist and they would be sorry if they didn't hire you.
A: False.

Q: True or False? You should always make follow-up phone calls, even if the employer says not to call.
A: False.

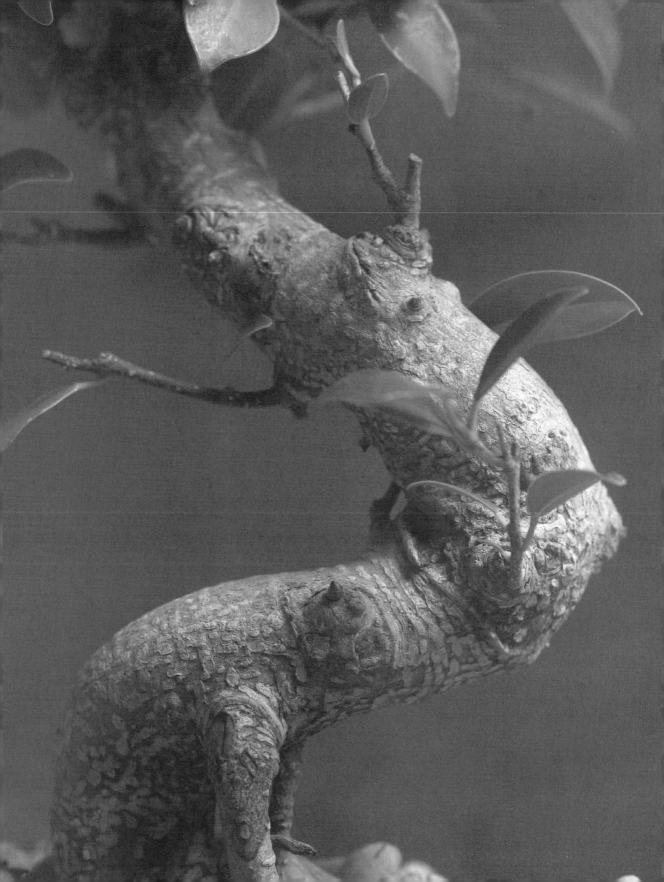

2 Marketing Yourself in an Interview

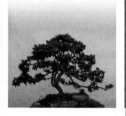

CHAPTER OBJECTIVES

After reading this chapter, you should be able to:

❋ Discuss what employers value most in employees.

❋ Describe the elements of a **partner mentality**.

❋ Describe the three stages of an interview.

❋ List what you need to bring with you to an interview.

❋ Anticipate common questions that interviewers ask.

❋ Create questions that you should ask an interviewer.

❋ Describe what interviewers evaluate during a **hands-on interview**.

❋ Discuss common elements of a **compensation package**.

MARKETING YOURSELF TO AN EMPLOYER IN AN INTERVIEW

The next step in marketing yourself to an employer is the mutual getting-to-know-you process of interviews. Designed especially for massage therapists applying for their first job in massage, this chapter will take you step by step through the interview process. Based on my many conversations and interviews with massage employers and employees, I am including not only what you need to know about verbal and hands-on interviews, but also what common mistakes you must avoid. These include mistakes that can keep you from getting a job you want or, on the other hand, from taking a job that is not right for you. Even if you have prior experience with job interviews, this chapter will cover the needs and issues unique to the massage profession. And, if you have a private practice and are looking to add more variety or stability to your work with a new job, this chapter will help prepare you for the many differences between working for yourself and working for others.

WHAT EMPLOYERS LOOK FOR IN EMPLOYEES

Interviewing has three stages: before, during, and after the interview, and we will cover each stage thoroughly so you can best market yourself to get the job you want. However, before we get to the nuts-and-bolts information about interviews, I want to go over what employers will be looking for throughout your encounters together. We are covering these points here so that, as you read and think about how to prepare for each stage of the interview process, you can imagine yourself communicating verbally and nonverbally in ways that show you are the kind of person they want to hire. While interviewers in spas, clinics, chiropractic offices, and elsewhere will have different requirements about such things as what modalities you know, there are other factors, such as personality and attitude, to which every employer is paying attention.

Of all the elements I have heard or read about that make a massage therapist desirable to an employer, a positive attitude and good potential, or aptitude, top the list. One top spa director and consultant, Peggy Wynne Borgman, CEO of Preston Wynne, Inc., told me: "We hire for aptitude and attitude, instead of experience. We can train skills, but we can't train attitude." How does an employer determine your attitude? By how you talk about your last job, your home life, your massage school, other people, and life in general.

For example, if all of someone's stories end with the point that other people are to blame for such things as bad grades at school, getting fired from a job, or being late because of traffic, he or she has just demonstrated an attitude of being a helpless victim who takes no responsibility for his or her life. Bosses listening to a litany of complaints or excuses won't care how good a person's hands-on skills are; all they know is that this person will eventually be an excuse-giver and blamer in their business, and they will end the interview quickly.

I bring up this issue since many employers I have interviewed are frustrated by how much "whining" and how many helpless attitudes they get from their massage staffs. In particular, I recall a moment when I was one of three massage school directors invited to a round-table discussion with 16 spa managers, to help us better prepare our students to work in spas. One woman captured the managers' feelings when she looked at us and begged, "Just tell them to stop whining! Stop whining!" Imagine, then, someone being in an interview with her and complaining about how the room was too cold, or the smell of the new carpet in her office was offensive, or that the overhead fluorescent lights were causing a headache. Even if all those things were true, I suspect that would end the interview with this spa manager pretty quickly!

Employers are looking for people who take responsibility, who can be resourceful when things go wrong, and who can be flexible when situations suddenly change or aren't ideal. They want employees who can be realistic, professional, and customer oriented, not stuck on how things should be in a perfect world that revolves around them. They want people who can communicate effectively and clearly, get along with other employees, and be team players. Again, many complaints I have heard, especially from spa directors, are about massage staff infighting, backstabbing, accusations of favoritism, and unwillingness to do non-massage tasks, like laundry or scheduling appointments, because it's "beneath" the massage therapists.

Of the many descriptions I have heard of the ideal job candidate, my favorite comes from a conversation with Peggy Francis, the spa director at Napa Valley's famed Auberge du Soleil resort. She described looking for an employee "who had a desire to serve people and the capacity to genuinely care." She wants therapists who can come in to the job as a "full person with an open heart, and can back it up with great massage." In her interviews, she looks for well-rounded people who can have interesting conversations with high-level clientele, who will represent the spa with

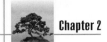

professionalism and enthusiasm, and who are willing to do what it takes to help the business succeed.

What Employers Value Most

Here is a list of other factors employers look for during their interviews. They want a massage therapist who is

- Confident
- Goal-oriented
- Decisive
- Loyal
- Honest
- Friendly
- Punctual
- Attentive
- Mature
- Stable
- Dependable
- Focused on the job at hand
- Has a sense of humor
- Professional in appearance
- Willing to learn new skills
- Planning to stay a while
- Fulfilled by doing massage
- Thinks massage is fun

EXERCISE: IF YOU WERE AN EMPLOYER

Imagine you are the owner of a business similar to one for which you would like to work. Take a few minutes and make your own list of what factors you would most value in an applicant who wanted to work for you. If you are with a group, share with them what you think is important in your hiring decision.

_____

_____

_____

_____

_____

_____

All of these traits matter for two reasons. One, so you know what really matters to employers, so you can highlight these traits about yourself during your interview; and two, so that even if you don't have a lot of experience or specialized training, you can still go to interviews with confidence if you have a lot of these characteristics. In fact, I interviewed a number of employers who actually prefer to hire therapists straight out of school so they can train them in how they want them to work. These employers look for good people who will be good employees, and experience isn't important at all.

The Partner Mentality

Another way to make sure you present yourself well and demonstrate your attitude and potential is to approach the job with the mindset that you are not just going to be an employee; you are going to be a "partner" in the business. This doesn't mean you will be a financial partner; it means you will approach every task and person as if you had a personal stake in the success and reputation of the business.

Why should you have a partner mentality? Because it will put you head and shoulders above the whiners and people with self-centered, "me-first" entitlement attitudes, which are unfortunately all too common today. A partner mentality will help you get the job, keep the job, and get raises and promotions faster. Most important, if you want to start your own practice or open your own spa or clinic someday, you will already have an ownership mentality and skill set honed and practiced. A first job is often a first step toward building a dream practice, and your odds of future success will be greatly increased with a partner mentality.

THE PARTNER MENTALITY

With a partner mentality, you would be:

- ✳ Interested in the profitability and success of the business
- ✳ Knowledgeable about the corporate mission, and have ideas on how to fulfill that mission
- ✳ Management friendly, and not stuck in an "us versus them" mentality with owners or bosses
- ✳ Allied to all employees, treating everyone with respect
- ✳ Willing to do whatever is needed, even if it's not in your job description
- ✳ Focused on helping meet the needs every business has, which are:

Getting new customers in the door

Keeping current customers happy and coming back

Leading customers to book more frequent visits or more expensive services

Getting word-of-mouth referrals from satisfied customers

Keeping costs down

Saving time and being more efficient

Making enough profit to justify keeping the doors open

EXERCISE: MIDWEEK SALES BRAINSTORM

Imagine you are working for a day spa, and there are very few clients coming in during the middle of the week. Since you have a partner mentality, you want to help bring business in the door. Write down five ideas you would suggest to your manager that could bring in customers on a slow day. If you are in a group, share your answers and gather a list you can all use in future jobs or in your own practices.

_____

_____

_____

Confidence in Spa Interviews

If you are interested in working at a spa, you should know not only what matters to the employer, but also what matters to the client. According to the 2004 *Consumer Trends Report* from the International SPA Association, what the consumers of spas want are not just all the high-end services and exotic treatments, but the more "bread and butter" services, namely, basic massage. According to the report, "As spas tend toward expansion, centralization, and nationalization, the consumers are looking increasingly toward human interaction, personalization, and customization." In addition, most spa-goers are "infrequent day spa users interested in indulgence, an escape, or perhaps specific benefits (i.e., relieve a headache, soften tight shoulders, de-stress, etc.)." Therefore, you don't have to feel a lack of confidence going into your interview if you don't know a lot of advanced spa treatments. First, the demand for them isn't that high, and second, the spa will probably have special or signature treatments they will train you in themselves. If you are good with people, have good hands, are a fast and willing learner, and can get along with coworkers and management, you will be an interviewer's dream come true.

So, now that you have a better idea of what employers are looking for during an interview, let's get you ready for the phone to ring!

BEFORE THE INTERVIEW

Once your resume has been sent to one or more prospective employers, be ready to be contacted. Whether you are reached by phone, mail, or e-mail, someone wants to know more about you and how you can help their business succeed. You must be prepared ahead of time with everything you need for that moment of contact, especially if it's a phone call. First, answer the phone as if any call could be your future boss on the line. The most simple and professional greeting is to give your name. I answer the phone by saying, "This is Monica." This lets callers know they have reached me and have not gotten a wrong number or somebody else. By putting the caller at ease immediately, you start off your initial phone interview well.

Second, in addition to a professional, in-person answer, have an outgoing message that markets you well. On your message machine or answering service, make sure to include your name with a brief and courteous message. A simple message that covers all the points could be something like this: "Hello! You've reached the message machine for Monica Roseberry. I'm sorry I missed your call, but if you leave your name and number and a good time to call you back, I'll be happy to return your call as soon as possible." This message is upbeat, clear, tells the caller what to do and what to expect, and puts the word "happy" into the mix. Do employers want to hire people who are happy? Of course they do!

EXERCISE: CREATE AN OUTGOING MESSAGE FOR A POTENTIAL EMPLOYER

Imagine that you have sent out a number of resumes to employers for whom you would really like to work. You are waiting for them to call you, but since you can't always answer the phone, you know they might get your answering machine or voice mail. Take a few minutes and write out a short but professional message that would represent you well to a potential employer. Make sure to include your name; instructions for what to do (leave a message, call your cell phone, page you); and what to expect from your return call (I'll call back as soon as possible, I will return calls after 11:00 a.m. tomorrow morning, I'll be out of town until Friday, etc.). If you are in a group, practice your outgoing message with three other people and revise it until it sounds just right.

_____

_____

_____

_____

_____

In order to be prepared for a phone interview, go through this chapter, think about its contents, and have your questions and answers thought through, written out, and by the phone. Then, if an employer calls and wants to conduct an on-the-spot **screening interview**, you will be ready. If you have multiple resumes out to different employers, have your files (which we'll cover later) by the phone, so you can quickly and easily flip to the pages that can tell you more about the person with whom you are speaking.

In addition, have blank paper and a pen handy so you can take notes as you talk. Listen especially for their instructions on what the next step of the interview process requires, and write down everything that you have to do for an in-person interview. This is crucial because busy interviewers don't want to waste time dealing with people who aren't right for the job. To help them speed up the elimination process, they often create simple but specific rules to follow for the interview. For example, you may be told to bring to the interview another copy of your resume, a reference list, or letters of recommendation. If, on the day of the interview, you show up without the item they asked you to bring, expect to be shown the door without any further conversation.

If you do well in the initial phone interview, you will be invited to go to the next level. Be ready for anything. You may have to go through a number of interviews, including meeting with a screener from the human resources department, going out to lunch for an informal-style review, or going through a group or committee interview in a big conference room. You could be asked to do a long-distance videophone interview, an in-office, one-on-one interview, or even a series of interviews in one day or over a number of days. Some employers also require that you take a standardized personality profile test, and most employers will ask you to do one or more massages on a variety of people.

Once you know you have the interview, do some research, unless you already did it before you sent out your resume. Research the business online, and call and ask for literature as if you were a prospective client. If you live close by, visit the facilities as an anonymous paying client to get a real feel for the atmosphere and working conditions. To get a sense of the kinds of clients and employees they have, tour the common areas. If you can't easily get in the building, sit in the parking lot and watch the people coming in and out of the facility. Would you enjoy working with them? In your last task as a junior detective, pay attention, if you can, to what employees are wearing so you will have a good idea of how to dress for your hands-on interview.

You can ask your family and friends if anyone knows an employee, client, or someone else who can tell you more about the business as an insider. You'd be surprised by how often someone knows someone who knows an employee or client of the business in which you're interested. Nothing impresses an

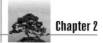

employer more than an interviewee who has done some research, so gather brochures, print out Web sites, get a massage, and otherwise show you are serious about the company to which you are applying.

THE DAY OF THE INTERVIEW

Your big day is now here! How do you best handle it? First, you should eat well so if the interview goes over many hours, you won't have a blood-sugar crash in the middle of it. Second, you need to get dressed. How you should dress may be told to you in the phone interview. You could be told to dress ready to do a massage, or told that a hands-on evaluation will be conducted on a different day. If you have only a verbal, formal interview, dress your best. Unless you have to do a massage, the basic rule in interviews is to dress a little bit better than your interviewer. At the very least, dress as well as what you imagine the massage staff wears to work, which is usually a polo shirt and khaki or dark slacks.

If you don't already have good interview clothes, go out and get some that will present you as a professional. Why? Not only will it help you get the job, but the better you look, the more people will think they should pay you. A massage therapist showing up in wrinkled drawstring pants and sandals sends a message that he or she isn't a polished professional, and this subconsciously tells the employer they can offer a lower starting wage. A massage therapist showing up in a suit says he or she knows business and means business, and that person will be treated more as a peer and possibly offered a better wage.

Once you are dressed, gather together your interview kit. If you wear a suit, bring a change of clothes in case you have to do a massage. In a folder, bring with you at least three copies of your resume, a list of questions you want to ask, other details about yourself that you want to talk more about, answers to questions you are anticipating, and any research you have done on the business. (See Figure 2–1.) Imagine what an interviewer would think if you pulled up a printed-out page of their Web site and asked a question about their mission statement, five-year goals for the business, or demographics of their clientele. If all they had faced so far were interviews with therapists whose only questions were about pay, benefits, and vacation, they would probably put a big star at the top of your resume.

In your folder, also bring a list of references, letters of recommendation, a copy of your application, and a few business cards, if you have them.

Figure 2–1 | **Prepare your interview kit the night before so you are ready the next day.**

Check List for Interview

❑ Clothes for test massage

❑ Shoes and socks for massage

❑ Watch

❑ 3 copies of resume

❑ List of references

❑ Letters of recommendation

❑ Copy of application (if there is one)

❑ Pen

❑ Calendar

❑ List of questions you want to ask

❑ List of details about yourself beyond what's on your resume

❑ Answers to common interview questions

❑ Research data about their business

❑ Business cards

❑ Copy of school transcript (if recent graduate)

❑ Positive evaluations or letters about your work

❑ Anything the interviewer asked you to bring

❑ Map and driving directions, phone number of interviewer

If you're a recent massage school graduate, bring a copy of your transcript. If you have positive evaluations from your hands-on tests in school, or from the school's massage clinic, internship, or externship program, bring them too. Any written evidence you can gather that lets people speak about your abilities can show an interviewer that others think highly of your skills. Even if you never pull these pieces of paper out during the interview, these items can give you confidence because you know they are there, and, during an interview, confidence is invaluable. Finally, pack your calendar and a pen so that when you are asked back for a second interview or, even better, asked when you can start the job, you can pull out your calendar and give an answer right there.

Getting to the Interview

Once you are dressed and packed, it's time to leave. However, before you can get to an in-person interview, you have to know where you are going. If you have been invited to do an interview but don't know exactly where to go, you can call later and ask a receptionist for directions, do an Internet printout on mapping sites such as http://www.mapquest.com, or look on a map yourself. To be on the safe side, do all three, since some people give bad directions and the Web site map may not be totally accurate. If you are late, no excuse will be good enough. If possible, do a test-drive beforehand, at the same day and time as your interview, to make sure you know where to go and how long it takes to get there.

On the day of the interview, get there at least 15 minutes early. Give yourself time to find a parking place, go to the bathroom, check your appearance, and otherwise prepare to look your best. Take the time to get rid of all distractions so you can focus: finish your coffee or tea, throw out chewing gum, turn off your cell phone, turn off the iPod or MP3 player, close up the PDA, and leave water bottles in the car. You want to arrive at the interview unplugged and empty-handed, except for your file and calendar, ready for anything. If you have a lot of stress, get there earlier, walk around, breathe, visualize, meditate, review your question and answer pages, and otherwise get "present" to the moment.

In addition, make sure you have nothing else scheduled soon after the interview. The process could take many hours, and you don't want to be anxious to leave by a specific time or have to interrupt a conversation to make a call to cancel something else.

Waiting for the Interviewer

An interview often starts with a lot of sitting around in a waiting area. Be prepared for the interviewer to be late; he or she may be testing you to see how you handle stress. Handle the wait smoothly and calmly. Be patient and polite, and don't fidget, pace, or repeatedly ask the receptionist where the interviewer is. Bring something to read, review your preparation notes, and observe what the other people in the business are like and how they act.

If you can see clients, pay attention and imagine yourself working with them. Think about what their needs would be and how you would best serve them. Then keep them in mind as your interviewer asks questions. For example, if you are interviewing for a job in a doctor's office, notice the age and condition of the patients in the waiting room. If most of them are frail and elderly, let that shape your answers during the interview. If you are asked to describe your style of bodywork, you don't want to go on about all the big, muscular athletes you used to have as sports massage clients. You want to craft your answer to let the interviewer know you can be gentle yet effective, and list the modalities you know that would best serve their patients.

If you are in a room with other people, such as receptionists, don't talk with them too much. Don't nervously chatter or make small talk unless they start a conversation or ask you a question. Be a professional, and be respectful of others' work and time. They may also be a secret part of the interview process, so don't confide in them about your nervousness, ask what the boss is really like, or say anything you don't want reported back to the employer.

While you are waiting, look around and notice anything of interest you can comment on later when the walking-to-the-office small talk happens. Look around for a pretty picture, an exquisite rug, an interesting photograph, a bouquet of flowers, a general feeling of well-being, or anything you can make positive remarks about as you have your first "icebreaker" conversation with your interviewer. Above all, take the opportunity to pick up on the "vibe" of the place, and imagine how you would feel working there.

First Contact with the Interviewer

When your interviewer comes out to greet you, stand up tall, make good, direct, steady eye contact, reach out to shake his or her hand, give it a nice, firm,

Figure 2–2 | To make your best impression, stand up tall, make steady eye contact, and smile at the interviewer.

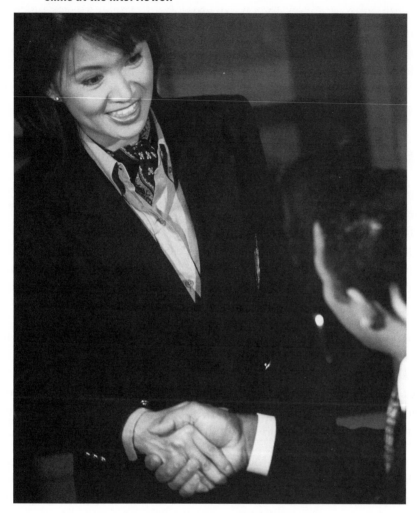

glad-to-meet-you shake, and smile a warm, friendly smile. (See Figure 2–2.) This is where your first impression is set, so make it a good one. Expect that the interviewer will call you by your name. If your name is mispronounced, don't make a big deal out of it. Just say it correctly and go on with your greeting. My name gets mispronounced often, and if this happened to me, I would just say, "I'm Monica Roseberry, and I'm very pleased to meet you."

Listen carefully in this initial greeting for how the interviewer gives his or her name. If you are only given a first name, then feel free to use it. However, if the interviewer gives you his or her full name, with or without a title, then stay with a more formal address and call them Mr., Ms., or Dr. So-and-so, until you are told otherwise. Showing respect for a person's name and status is important. You don't want to make the mistake of sounding too familiar with the interviewer. Since boundary issues are prevalent in the massage field, interviewers may be looking for how you address them as an indication of your ability to handle professional boundaries.

Getting to the Office

Between the initial greeting and the formal interview is a crucial stage for which you must be prepared. This is the breaking-the-ice stage, and it usually consists of some form of small talk conducted while standing in the front office or walking to the area for the formal interview. This stage is where you create your next impression, and it puts down the foundation for your interview. Expect some common conversation starters such as, "How was your drive here?" or "I'm sorry to keep you waiting," or "How was the traffic?" Always, always, your answer should be upbeat and short. Simply answer, "It was no problem getting here," or "The traffic was fine," or "I enjoyed seeing what kind of clients you have while I was waiting." Then you can add something to further build your relationship, such as, "I loved the flowers out front," or "What a beautiful location," or anything else to show you are positive and present. If it would feel forced to you, don't do this, but it expresses to an employer that you are a positive and observant person.

Once in the Office

The next step of the process usually takes you to an office or area where the formal interview will be conducted. Once in that room, stand still and wait to follow instructions about where to sit. When a chair has been indicated, sit down politely, sit upright, lean toward the interviewer, and otherwise show a professional respect and interest. Keep both feet on the floor and don't lean on the desk, slump into a couch, or slouch over on the arm of a chair. In other words, show a sense of readiness and confidence with your body language. (See Figure 2–3.) As the interview goes on, you can get more comfortable, but still sit more properly than you would just sitting around at home. I know this point may seem obvious, but I'll never forget an employer calling me to say that one of my students he had interviewed had walked into the office, taken off her shoes, and then plopped down cross-legged on the floor to start the interview. Do you think she got the job?

Figure 2-3 | During the interview, sit in a way that is professional and on-purpose.

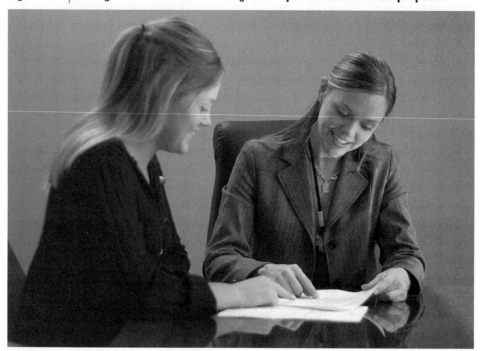

THE VERBAL INTERVIEW

The verbal interview, which usually comes before the hands-on evaluation, has a number of components for which you need to be prepared. While the order of them is unpredictable, expect to:

- Review your resume
- Answer questions you are asked
- Ask questions yourself
- Discuss the next step of the interview process

Reviewing Your Resume

As we covered in the last chapter, a resume should at least have a job objective, summary of qualifications, and information about your professional experience and education. During the review of your resume, pull out your own copy, along with your notes about anything else to add that wasn't included in the copy you sent. Since resumes should generally be kept to one page, there is likely more that you want to say about yourself, and this is the time and place to do so.

Answering Questions in an Interview

Much of your interview will consist of answering questions based on your resume. Give answers that fully inform the interviewer without going too long or too short. Listen carefully to the question, and only answer that question. If the question is vague, respond with your own question to get clarification. For example, if the interviewer says, "Tell me about yourself," answer with something like, "Would you like me to focus on my work experience?" Be concise and clear, and don't start with information that is irrelevant, such as where you grew up, or that you're a mother of two, or a Libra. Try to get them to narrow down an open question, but if they won't, respond with points that you know are relevant to the position.

Since who you are as a person often matters as much as your skills, show your best self as you answer questions. Be interesting, real, passionate, and enthusiastic. Boring answers, monotone responses, or stiff presentations will make the interviewer worry that you will be boring and stiff with clients, or that you just don't have the personality to fit with the staff. When you talk, be personable and animated, yet still appropriate for the interview setting. Above all, don't use foul language. If you do, you won't get hired.

When you are asked about school, prior employers, why you left your last job, or anything about other people, NEVER say anything negative. Smart employers know that what went wrong in someone's last job may say more about the person than about the previous employer. If a person has a string of stories about other bosses who made his or her life miserable, coworkers who were mean, events that were unfair, and so on, that person unwittingly warns the interviewer that he or she will bring trouble with them to the new job. The saying "Wherever you go, there you are" is especially pertinent to interviewers because they know people often behave the same old way, even in a new setting. Therefore, don't bad-mouth your school, teachers, classmates, family, other therapists, bosses, or anyone else, because interviewers will think that someday you will do the same to them.

When you are asked open-ended questions, if possible, use stories and not just facts to illustrate good points about yourself. If the employer is conducting many interviews and is getting a lot of the same kinds of answers, what will separate you from the others are good, evocative stories that demonstrate your skills and abilities. Stories are easier to remember than facts, so develop and practice a few good stories to illustrate your finer points.

For example, if you are asked about how you would describe good customer service, tell a story. It could be about a client you really helped, customers you took care of in a non-massage job, or, if you have no work background, refer to a great service experience you received that you would like to emulate. A showstopping story could be about how you came to their spa or clinic and got a massage from one of their employees, and how you would love to be able to have the opportunity to provide that level of service yourself if you worked there. If you are asked why you went to massage school, have an inspiring story ready that tells a lot about who you really are and why you are in this profession.

Handling Difficult Questions

You should expect some questions that might make you feel uncomfortable. Sometimes the interviewer does this on purpose, to see how you handle stressful situations. Sometimes they just really want to know whether or not you are qualified for the job or will fit well in their work environment or corporate culture. Therefore, as you market yourself in an interview, expect that objections or concerns will come up. Treat these as opportunities to further educate the interviewer.

Objections could be about your level of experience, amount of training, what massage school you went to, appearance (such as piercings or tattoos), and more. Whatever you do, don't get upset or defensive. Take a breath and calmly ask the interviewer to clarify the objection or concern. Ask him or her to be more specific or give you an example. Then listen carefully, and once you are sure you understand the concern, either address it directly or respond indirectly by emphasizing a strength you have that can overcome the weakness.

For example, if the concern is that you don't have a lot of professional massage experience, address it with a direct response by saying something like, "I know I don't have much professional experience, but I have been massaging family and friends informally for years, and they were the ones who encouraged me to go to massage school. I have also done more than

30 sessions at my school's massage clinic, and I got really good evaluations, which I brought with me if you'd like to see them. If you let me give you a massage, I think you will find I can offer your guests a really great experience."

An indirect response could be, "I understand you are concerned about my lack of experience, but I am a fast learner and am committed to ongoing training. As you can see in my resume, I have taken a number of continuing education classes beyond my certification program, and I have worked hard to advance my skill level. If you let me give you a massage, I think you will find my skills could be quite helpful to your clinic patients."

In both of these cases, you acknowledge the concern, move past it, ask to get to the hands-on stage of the interview, and talk about how you can help their customers. Notice that you don't talk just about yourself. Your final emphasis when responding to any concern should be about being able to serve their customers.

EXERCISE: CONCERN ABOUT LACK OF EXPERIENCE

Imagine you are in an interview and the interviewer is scanning your resume when he suddenly stops, frowns, and then looks at you and says, "I see you have just graduated from massage school, and that you have no formal job experience. I'm worried about bringing an inexperienced therapist onto our staff. Tell me why I should hire you with no experience." Write out three or four sentences of what you would say to address this concern so that you build the interviewer's confidence in your skills. If you are in a group, get into pairs and role-play being both the interviewer and interviewee. Practice different answers until you have one that is polished and convincing.

_____

_____

_____

_____

_____

_____

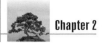

Background Checks

If you are interviewing with a fairly large spa, clinic, hospital, or business, anticipate that the employer will run a background check on you. If you know your records contain things like a drunken driving arrest, bankruptcy, or bad credit (which many employers are now checking), be ready with an answer that tells them how you have learned from your mistakes and what you have done to correct them. If you have some black marks on your record, make as positive an interpretation or "spin" as you can and describe those tough times as learning experiences, growth opportunities, or challenges you've overcome. Emphasize the bright future ahead that you are striving for, or tell about how you went to massage school so you could help others get through some of the hard times you once faced. I was often amazed and moved by my students who had overcome enormous obstacles and difficulties in their past, and I felt privileged to be a part of their getting a fresh start. While your past may matter to some employers, it is your future potential that will interest most of them.

What an Employer Does Not Need to Know About You

Employers have the right to fairly evaluate your skills and abilities, and to check your background. However, there are very specific boundaries over which American employers can't step. These include questions about your age, marital status, sexual orientation, religious beliefs, race, number of children, and anything else that would let them discriminate against you illegally. If an interviewer asks questions about these topics, you need to politely decline to answer. Many new managers have no knowledge of the laws regarding hiring, and you can simply say something like, "I appreciate your interest in that topic. May I ask why you wish to know that? I believe that may be an illegal question, but I would be happy to answer other questions for you."

Helping an Inexperienced Interviewer

This last point brings up an issue you may face, which is being evaluated by an inexperienced interviewer. In the past, massage therapists mostly worked for themselves, and only in the last few years has there been a sudden and enormous demand for massage employees. What this means for you is that many employers are new to hiring therapists, and there just aren't enough managers who know what to look for in a qualified job applicant. I recall talking with a spa director from a well-known resort area in Mexico who witnessed the explosion in the number of resort spas and the fallout of not being able to find qualified managers for all of them. As she described in one story, a nearby resort desperately turned to a saleswoman in the time-share department and made her the spa director. Imagine what it was like for her the first time she had to interview a new massage therapist for a job.

The lack of interviewers experienced in hiring massage therapists is widespread. Within the spa industry in the United States, which is still very young, many managers are inexperienced because, just a few years ago, there weren't that many spas in which to get experience. Alternatively, there are spa directors with hiring experience, but they have been brought over from managing other arenas of the hospitality industry and are unfamiliar with massage as well.

In the same way, many beauty salons that have recently converted into day spas are owned or managed by hairstylists or aestheticians who have little or no background in massage. Inexperience in hiring massage therapists is also common among chiropractic offices and medical clinics. Having a massage therapist on staff is a new idea for many, and you may be in the first round of interviews they conduct. Chiropractic colleges and medical schools rarely give doctors training on even the basics of hiring staff or how to bring a massage therapist into their practice.

If you realize during your interview that the person scanning your resume doesn't know how to evaluate what they are reading, and doesn't know Shiatsu from Swedish, you may need to help him or her (and yourself) out a bit. For example, you can give longer answers to the questions and, in the process, fit in more information on topics the interviewer may not know to ask you about. Or, you can say something like, "I would love to take a moment and tell you more about the kinds of massage I do. There are so many styles of bodywork that they are hard to keep track of, but I want to tell you about the styles I know that I think can help your customers."

While there are many experienced and qualified managers out there, you need to be prepared for those who are new to interviewing massage therapists. In the "Questions" sections below, we will cover key points that need to be discussed so your interviewer can clearly understand the value of your skills and abilities. That said, do not, under any circumstances, question out loud the ability of the interviewer to evaluate your skills. You may both know the interviewer is new at this, but if you dare say it out loud, don't expect to be hired. Even if you wonder where in the world the interviewer is going with questions, just follow his or her lead, and politely and respectfully answer all questions.

Common Questions Interviewers Ask

There are a number of questions you may get asked in an interview. Go through possible questions, answer them in your mind, write out your answers, and practice rehearsing them in mock interviews. You can ask a friend, family member, classmate, teacher, colleague, or someone you know who has conducted interviews to ask you the questions and give you feedback on your answers. Practice your answers in a mirror, or even videotape yourself so you can see how you come across to others. The more you practice and visualize, the more comfortable and confident you will be in the real interview.

COMMON QUESTIONS INTERVIEWERS ASK

Why did you become a massage therapist?

How did you choose your massage school?

Tell me about your massage school experience.

What were your favorite classes, and why?

Describe your style of bodywork.

What is your philosophy in bodywork?

How do you take care of yourself in order to stay working in massage?

Why did you decide to get a massage job instead of starting a private practice?

What are your strengths?

What are your weaknesses?

What are your goals for the next 3, 5, 10 years?

What do you really want to do in life?

What are your long-term career goals?

How would you describe yourself?

(continues)

How would others, like your teachers, classmates, friends, and family, describe you?

Why should I hire you?

Why do you think you are qualified for this position?

Why did you decide to apply for a job with this company?

What do you know about this company?

What motivates you?

How well do you work as a team member?

How do you handle criticism?

How do you handle stress?

Tell me about your last job.

Tell me about the best and worst manager you've ever had.

What were the people like that you worked with in other jobs?

If you have a job, what do you think of your current supervisor?

Why are you leaving your current job?

What would you change about your current job?

What is your compensation or pay at your current job?

What compensation would you require to start for our company?

Are you willing to sell retail products?

How do you feel about doing tasks such as laundry or answering phones?

Are you willing to train in new treatments or techniques?

EXERCISE: ANSWERING COMMON INTERVIEW QUESTIONS

If you are in a large group, separate into groups of four, pick two of the common interview questions, and practice answering them in front of your group. Practice looking at all members of your "interview panel" and giving good eye contact as you talk, to get used to group interviews. Switch roles as interviewers and interviewees until all four have had a turn in each role.

QUESTIONS YOU CAN ASK AN EMPLOYER

During an interview, there should come a moment when the interviewer stops and says, "Do you have any questions for me?" At this point, you need to ask the questions that will help you decide whether or not this would be the right job for you. Here are some sample questions to consider:

What would you consider to be the traits of an ideal candidate for this job?

What would a typical workday and workweek be like here?

Please tell me more about the job.

Please tell me a bit about your current employees.

How are schedules set and shifts assigned?

What are the opportunities for advancement, and how is that determined?

How do you measure employee performance, and how often are evaluations?

Is there a probation period?

What is your orientation process?

Is there mentoring from senior employees?

How long do people stay here as employees?

What is the management philosophy and corporate culture like?

Please tell me a bit about your clientele.

Are new clients given an intake with a full health history?

Can I refuse to work on clients with contraindications?

Please tell me a bit about the products you use for treatments.

Will I have the ability to control the temperature and music in the massage room?

How many massages should I expect to do every day?

What kind of massages are clients requesting most?

What other kinds of treatments besides massage will I need to perform?

What non-massage tasks will be expected of me?

What is the length of a session, and how are breaks between them scheduled?

Are the massage tables easily adjustable to different heights?

While there are many more questions to ask, notice that none are listed about moving into management. One of the mistakes many overly confident new therapists make is to presume they will be moving quickly into management positions. Of all the things that put off the employers I interviewed, the presumption of a fast and easy transition into a management position topped the list for many of them. Even if it is your ultimate goal, do not say that your long-term plan is to replace the manager interviewing you, and certainly don't talk about how you are going to open your own spa or clinic soon. You may think you are sounding properly ambitious and goal-oriented, but to the interviewer you are sounding arrogant, ignorant, and not worth investing in, since you plan to leave the position as soon as you can. Your first task is to get the massage job and then excel in it, so make that the emphasis of your stated goals.

Questions Specifically for Spas

If you are interviewing for a position in a spa, you need to fully understand what is expected of you within the entire scope of the job. Some spas just keep the therapists busy with massages and treatments, while others rotate therapists into non-massage tasks like laundry, turning rooms, and cleaning equipment such as hydrotherapy tubs or hot stone roasters. You also may be asked to answer the phones, make follow-up calls to clients, go to staff meetings, watch product demonstrations by manufacturers' representatives, attend trainings, and do promotional activities such as chair massages or foot reflexology in other parts of the spa to encourage business.

While some of this might seem like drudge work, one of the reasons spas do this is to keep therapists from getting injured by doing massages back-to-back all day long. Since they want to keep you around for your shift but don't want you to get hurt, they will usually pay you to stay on the premises and do other functions that give your body and hands a rest.

Another way that spas keep therapists from overuse injuries is to have them perform spa services such as herbal, seaweed, or mud wraps, exfoliation scrubs, aromatherapy services, or other body treatments. These don't require an intensive use of the hands, and they often cost more and are therefore more profitable to the spa. You may also be asked to administer hydrotherapy treatments or even perform a massage in your bathing suit while the client lies under a continuous spray of water.

While some therapists negatively view these spa treatments as being worthless "rub and scrub" or not being "real" massage, keep an open mind and a good attitude if you are asked to train in and perform these services as part of the job you want. These treatments can be very beneficial to health and well-being, and besides, doing massage all day, every day, can be tiring and painful. Many spas have learned the hard way that having their therapists do too many massages in a row results in injuries and prematurely ended careers. This leads to very high workers' compensation insurance, adding tens of thousands of dollars to spas' costs and wiping out their profit margins. If you really don't want to learn or do these services, find out during this time of the interview if they are a required part of the job. Then make an informed decision about whether or not to continue with the interview process.

One other question you should get answered during the interview is what will be required of you in terms of retail sales. Some spas don't want or ask their therapists to sell retail products, some give a commission fee for sales, and some pay less for your massage services or let you go if you don't meet a set sales quota. You need to be clear about what dollar amounts are expected of you, if any, what products you will be asked to sell, how you will be trained to sell, and what happens if you don't meet your quotas.

This topic has been a thorny one for many people, and it should be discussed clearly and openly in the interview. On the one hand, many massage therapists feel uncomfortable, pushy, anxious, and even unethical talking with clients about buying anything, from relaxation CDs to eye pillows, skin care creams, or aromatherapy candles. On the other hand, most spas would go out of business if they didn't have a large volume of retail sales. While aestheticians and hairstylists have few problems or concerns with selling products, massage therapists often do, and so do many massage clients, especially if retail sales conversations occur during their session.

What seems to make the biggest difference in this subject is how the therapist feels about the products available for sale. Therapists genuinely excited about the benefits of a product can't keep quiet about it and will really want their clients to know how much using the product at home can help them. They naturally educate clients about how a product is benefiting them during the course of the session, and it never feels like selling because it isn't; it's just sharing something you feel strongly about. In addition, when the massage staff sees that they can help their clients by making sure they aren't using things such as petroleum-based skin creams usually bought at the drug or department store, they not only promote good products that work well, but they also keep clients from buying stuff that is potentially harmful to them. In your interview, ask what product lines you might be expected to sell, and then look them up online later to see if you can get engaged or excited by them.

I have given seminars and written about this topic to help bridge the gap between what spas need and how massage therapists feel about selling products, but there is more work to be done on this subject. If you are fine with selling home-care products that spa-goers can take with them to use in between sessions to maintain the benefits of your services, then let your interviewer know this early into your time together. If you have some concerns, talk it out. Finally, if you are offered and accept the job knowing that product sales are part of the package, please, please don't complain about it later.

EXERCISE: ASKING AN INTERVIEWER QUESTIONS

Imagine you are in an interview and are asked if you have any questions. Write down a list of at least five questions you most want to ask. Then rank them in order of how much you really need to know the answer in order to help you decide if this is the right job for you. Put a star by the points that are the "deal breaker" issues so you will be sure to ask them in an interview. In front of a mirror or with a partner, practice asking your most important questions in a calm, professional manner.

_____

_____

_____

_____

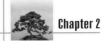

The Next Step of the Interview

At the end of the verbal interview, a number of things can happen. You can be told right then and there that you have the job, or that you don't. I have heard stories of massage therapists finishing the interview, being hired on the spot, getting handed the business's polo shirt, and being told to get ready to do a massage! You can be asked to return for another verbal interview or to move on to a test massage, either right then or on another day.

GIVING A TEST MASSAGE

Most employers want to feel a massage from you to make sure you have the kind of touch, technique, tableside manner, and professionalism that will keep their customers happy and coming back for more. Be prepared to give a massage to the interviewer, the owner of the business, the lead massage therapist, or others trained to evaluate your hands-on skills. You may give only one massage, or you may give multiple massages. Some employers may want you to come back on a different day for the hands-on evaluation, and some will want the session to follow your verbal interview. A number of employers do it the other way around and have the hands-on evaluation before they conduct any verbal interview. When you are contacted to come in for an interview, make sure to find out if and when the massage evaluation will be conducted.

What You Are Evaluated On in a Test Massage

During your massage, you will be judged on many factors. These can include:

Punctual arrival and being prepared to work

Proper attire for massage

Proper hygiene, including washed hands, brushed teeth, no perfume, and no smoking smell

Efficient and neat room setup

Ability to treat the tester as a first-time client

Figure 2–4 | **In your test massage, demonstrate your knowledge of visual, palpatory, and verbal evaluation skills.**

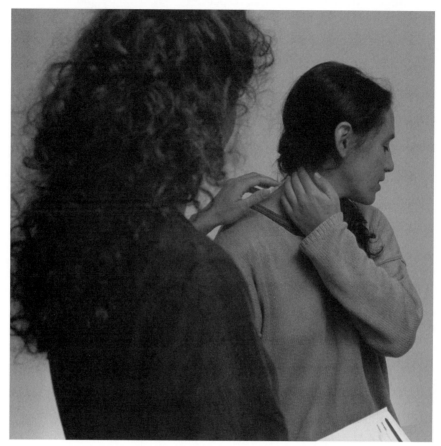

Good listening and documentation skills during the intake and health history

Ability to understand and work with contraindications and preferences

Visual, palpatory, and verbal evaluation skills (See Figure 2–4.)

Client-friendly communication skills, including small talk and giving instructions such as how to disrobe, take off jewelry, where to put clothes, how to get on table, position self on table, and so forth

Introduction of hands and touch

Grounding and breathing

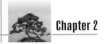

Draping skills

Manners, courtesy, politeness, respect

Boundary skills, including not talking much or until talked to during the session

Quality and application of touch

Good use of hands, including not overusing thumbs

Flow, rhythm, maintaining contact

Smooth beginnings, endings, and transitions of strokes

Ability to "connect" and be present with the client

Ability to do what was asked during intake

Comfortable and smooth with a **verbal check-in**

Ability to adjust work based on verbal or physical feedback

Ability to answer questions about what you are doing and why

Positive overall attitude and energy

Proper body mechanics and posture

Knowledge of a variety of techniques

Knowledge of anatomy

Ability to finish service in time allotted

Ability to create a sense of completion and closure

Post-Massage Stage

It is up to the reviewer how long you will work in the hands-on evaluation. Presume you will need to demonstrate a full session, or two or three. In busy spas or clinics, the ability to do one massage right after the other is crucial. If you have to do multiple massages, your ability to turn the room around, prepare for the next session, and maintain quality work over time will be closely watched. After your massage, leave quietly and wait for the interviewer to emerge.

Spa specialist Steve Capellini, in his book *Massage Therapy Career Guide for Hands-On Success* (see the "Resources" section), describes his experience of receiving hundreds of test massages from job applicants. According to Steve, despite how nervous you may feel, you should not ask how you did. An experienced interviewer will anticipate that you are nervous, and will know that under the pressure you may not have done your best work. In addition, know that while you may feel a lot of pressure to do well in the massage, so does the interviewer. The interviewer is a human being with needs, concerns, fears, and responsibilities, and doesn't want to make a mistake and hire someone who doesn't fit with the staff or won't satisfy the clients. They want you to do well as much as you want to!

Ending the Interview

At the end of your time together, the interviewer will usually make some concluding remarks, start gathering papers, and otherwise give cues that this part of the process is over. Wait to be told what to expect next, such as that you will be called back for another interview with other people, or by when a decision will be made. However, if the interview is ending and you aren't told anything, be proactive about what will happen next. Don't be passive and leave the interview wondering what to expect. Ask for when you will hear from them either way. Ask what the next step is in the hiring process, and if you can call back for follow-up.

If you want to leave with some idea of whether or not you will get the job, you can ask a simple question, such as, "Is there a match between my qualifications and what you are looking for?" You may get a positive answer, but there may be more the interviewer has to do, such as check your references, before any offer can be made. Don't be impatient at this point! Employers often have to do background checks and verify your resume information before they can make a formal offer, so don't expect that you will be hired at the end of the interview.

You really know the session is over when the interviewer stands up to escort you out. Stand up tall, smile, shake hands, and thank the interviewer for his or her time and consideration. If you still want the job at this point, let the interviewer know by saying something like, "I have enjoyed meeting you and hope I get the opportunity to work for you." Then walk out with your head high and smile at everyone you pass on the way out. Even if you think the interview went badly, act as if it went well. So many people have told me stories of interviews that seemed like one disaster after another, only to be called later and offered the job.

AFTER THE INTERVIEW

As you will find with virtually any job, there are benefits and drawbacks to each one. Some places may pay well but have inconsistent bookings, or the wages may be lower than you'd hoped but you will have a predictable paycheck and steady work. Some places may have unfriendly management but customers and coworkers you would really enjoy, while other places may have a really cool boss but clients who aren't your type.

Do You Still Want the Job?

This is the time when your priorities must be thoroughly reexamined and you must decide if the job is right for you. Will this job help you reach future goals, learn new skills that can get you better or higher paying work, and give you a place to grow and discover yourself? Will you fit well there with staff, clients, owners, and management? In other words, is the job what you thought it was, and do you still want it?

Or, should you keep looking? This is the time to trust your intuition and follow your gut. Many new therapists take the first job offered without really thinking about whether or not it is truly right for them. It can be intimidating to interview in a bustling clinic or spa, and it is common to be overly impressed by the surroundings, but tune in to your heart and soul, compare the resonance of the business with yours, and ask if this is a place where you can be happy and prosper.

Post-Interview Thank-You Letter

When you get home from the interview, immediately sit down and write a thank-you note to your interviewer. In the note, thank the interviewer for his or her time and consideration of you as a candidate. If you still want the job, express your continuing interest in the position, and reaffirm your ability to do the job well. Send your note either by mail or e-mail, though a card or paper letter has more power to it than an e-mail does. What matters most is the speed of getting the thank-you note out, so do it within 24 hours of the interview. Even if you decide you don't want the job, send a thank-you note anyway and say the position isn't right for you at this time. This leaves the door open for you at a future date, and it keeps your reputation good as a professional.

Follow-up Contact

At the end of the interview, you should ask when a hiring decision will be made and what to expect in terms of notification. If you did not get this information, you can call or e-mail later with **follow-up contact** to inquire about when a decision will be made. While you may be anxious or want to demonstrate how much you want the job, don't harass the employer with a lot of calls or e-mails. If a week passes, or the decision date comes and goes and you haven't heard anything, absolutely call to ask how the hiring process is proceeding. The interviewer may have had a family emergency, gotten transferred, or some such unexpected thing, and no decision has yet been made. Sometimes decisions can take many weeks, so be patient, but do stay in touch occasionally to keep your name in front of them.

Keeping Track of Multiple Opportunities

Applying for multiple jobs at the same time is a common practice. You may be busy and running from one interview to another, but that can be a good thing. First, you learn what options are available and what different businesses and managers are like, and you can get a better sense of where you would fit well. Having multiple options open can be stressful, and weighing the pros and cons of each job can make your head spin. However, you increase your odds of getting a job within the time frame that you need one, and, if a number of businesses offer you a job, you have better leverage to get a higher wage.

Multiple options require good record keeping and tracking the progress of each job opportunity. To stay organized, keep handy the files you brought with you to each interview. In each file, keep a copy of the resume you used, what job or position you applied for, the job description, and the contact information, including business name, address, hiring manager, or department. Add to this file notes from your interview such as what you discussed, who you met or massaged, what the follow-up process would be, the date of the interview, and any other details you may want to refer to quickly. If you get called back for another interview, or to be offered the job, you will be able to rapidly remind yourself about that particular job.

Handling "No"

The opportunity to interview with someone does not guarantee you will get the job. It is not uncommon for well-known spas, for example, to get 50 or more applications for one opening. This means 49 people will be told they didn't get the job. If you are told that someone else was given the position, it may hurt a bit, but don't let it stop you from your job search. More often than not, I hear people say that, in retrospect, they are glad they didn't get a job because they found one better suited for them later on. Some people have even felt themselves divinely protected from what could have turned into a bad situation, and though they were initially upset at not getting a job, they realized later it was for the best.

If you don't get a job you interviewed for, use your experience to make your next interview better. I have talked to a number of people who have deliberately interviewed for jobs they didn't really want just so they could get the practice before interviewing for the job they did want! Interviewing is a skill, and you may need more practice before you get it right or find the right place for you.

Handling "Yes"

I know, I know. You've been reading this whole chapter wondering when we were going to get to the important stuff, the stuff about money. Well, here it is, near the end of the chapter, and it's here for a number of reasons. First, money may not even be discussed in your first interview. In some cases, only when the employer has interviewed other candidates and knows they want to hire you will money be brought up. Second, people who want to skip all the points we've covered so far and just "cut to the chase" often upset or put off interviewers. If you bring up money prematurely, you may annoy the interviewer to the point that you may not get the job, or you may get offered less than you could have gotten.

Your job is to make them so excited to hire you (with your great attitude, strong aptitude, and wonderful hands-on skills) that they find a way to come up with more money than they might have planned to originally offer. Many jobs have pay scales that depend on your skills, experience, number of clients you bring with you to their facility, number of advanced modalities you know, and more. You want all your good points on the table before a dollar amount is stated. In short, they have to want you first; then they will talk about rewarding you monetarily for the value you will bring to their business.

THE COMPENSATION PACKAGE

In exchange for your services, employers will offer you a compensation package. While these can vary a great deal, a package can include:

* Wages (hourly, salary, commission)
* Benefits
* Training
* Tuition reimbursement for continuing education
* Use of facilities and services such as weight rooms, fitness classes, and health care
* Use of rooms and equipment to do trades with coworkers
* Discounts on products
* Tips
* Paid time off

While not all of these may be offered to you, you can certainly ask for them, especially if they don't cost the employer much money. Benefits such as health insurance and paid time off may not be so easy to get, as employees in many other industries well know. For many therapists, the primary pay will be wages and tips.

Having Appropriate Expectations

It is exciting to be offered a job, but to make sure that the offer stage of the interview process doesn't result in you sitting there in silent shock or, worse, getting angry at the interviewer, I want to let you know that many new massage therapists are surprised and disappointed by what they are offered in their compensation package. Why? Because their expectations are often based on hopes, dreams, and overly optimistic guessing, not on market realities.

What are the market realities that affect your pay? Mainly, costs and the inconsistent frequency of paid appointments. Unlike many massage therapists, who have basic home offices or do outcall practices, employers frequently have astronomical costs and overhead, and they have to keep paying them even if no customers come in. When things get busy, it looks like they are making piles of money, but all too often, once they pay the bills, very little is left. This leaves employers having to reduce their risks and costs by only offering therapists part-time jobs or independent contractor positions, and making no promises of consistent paychecks.

Spas are especially likely to have huge overhead expenses and wide or seasonal swings of paying customers. When magazine stories about the latest resort or destination spa brag about expenditures like $75 million for a renovation, or $100 million to build new facilities, how those spas will eventually recoup their initial costs, much less pay their operating expenses, is unfathomable. It is not surprising, then, that spa services cost so much, but it is surprising to therapists when they find out they will not be making a significant percentage of the price of the services they perform.

In short, be prepared, during the point in the interview when wages come up, that your pay won't come close to what the customer is paying. Also, don't be surprised that employee pay is much lower than what experienced therapists charge in a private practice. Since the business is providing the facilities, clients, equipment, laundry, cleaning services, utilities like heating or air conditioning, hot water, electricity, product, training, benefits, and more, they will, by necessity, need to take a significant portion of the money from each massage or service. Their costs for rent or mortgage, permits, licenses, taxes, advertising, management salaries, consultants, workers' compensation, liability insurance, and other insurance are all "invisible" expenses that add up quickly. In addition, businesses that have seasonal swings will continue to have high overhead expenses even when they have little business coming in, and they must make extra in the high season to be able to pay the bills in the low season. Perhaps more than anything, businesses shoulder the risk of failure. By taking the risks on the downside, businesses want the rewards and profits on the upside. So, not only are their costs high, but businesses want a decent profit for the work and risk they have taken. When you start a private practice, you will work hard and take risks as well, and you, too, will want a profit to show for it.

Wage Variances

Unlike many jobs, massage jobs offer pay that can vary under different circumstances. Busy clinics, offices, and spas can often provide a work shift that is booked solid with massage. However, if they rotate you out to other non-massage services to protect your hands, or if they don't have clients for you to work on, they may have a lower pay rate. In spas that have seasonal cycles, it is often difficult for the spa director to keep employees on staff when there aren't many paying clients, and every business has slow days. During the wage discussion part of the interview, you need to make sure you understand what to expect financially if there aren't many customers or if you are doing non-massage functions. You may get paid different fees for different services, get a flat salary that doesn't vary at all, or get a commission-only structure where you get paid only when you do a massage.

Other **wage variances** in your pay can come from bringing in your own clients to the facility. Many employers will give you a better percentage cut or higher pay since they didn't have to spend anything to get a new customer. Some facilities even let therapists see their own private clients in the office without taking any cut, which is a nice added benefit. If you have your own clients and would like to work with them on the job, bring it up during the interview. This is a valuable asset with which you can negotiate. Be careful, though. If you have to sign a contract that says all clients are essentially the property of the business and you can't take them with you when you leave, add a clause that clearly states that your personal clients are not part of the agreement. On the flip side, if you bring a client to a business, and the client uses other services in the business, consider negotiating to get a percentage of the work others do since you were the one who brought in the client.

The unpredictable factor in pay is what you can make from tips. In the interview, ask what the standard tipping procedure is and, if you provide great service with a busy schedule, what you can expect to make in tips. The interviewer may not know or be willing to predict or guarantee what you could make in tips, but see if you can get a general number. In service businesses such as spas or salons, tipping is fairly common. However, in health care clinics, doctor or chiropractic offices, or other medical facilities, tipping is not common. People don't tip physical therapists, X-ray technicians, or nurses when they provide medical services, and if you work in a medical facility, expect to be treated the same as other personnel.

The biggest factor affecting wage variance is the status of your position. Is your position status as an employee, an independent contractor, or a renter? Is it full time, part time, or seasonal? Make sure you know what kind of job you are accepting. If you are an employee, your employer will withhold your income taxes, withhold and pay Social Security and Medicare taxes, and pay unemployment tax on your wages. If you are going to be a full-time employee, your employer may offer benefits, though many don't. If you are going to be an independent contractor, you should expect a higher rate than employees because you will pay your own taxes and probably get no major benefits. If you are offered a position as an independent contractor, you need to learn more about the particulars of this job. In general, an employee is a person who is told by the employer what to do, how to do it, where to do it, and when to do it. With an independent contractor, the employer has the right to control or direct only the result of the work done, and not the means and methods of accomplishing the result.

If you are offered an independent contractor position, go to the library or bookstore, or go online to http://www.irs.gov and read up on the most current laws about what makes this kind of position different from being an employee.

Intangible Benefits

Beyond the monetary value of wages, benefits, training, and more are the many **intangible benefits** that make taking a job a good option for many therapists. First, you get to just show up for work and do massage instead of having to find your own clients. Second, you take virtually no risks and have no major costs. Third, you get a place to develop your skills, discover new talents, learn new techniques, and be supported by coworkers, support staff, and management.

Of all the intangibles, one of the most important is social interaction. (See Figure 2–5.) So often I have heard that the hardest part of a private massage practice is the loneliness, isolation, and boredom brought on by working with

Figure 2-5 | Social interaction is one of the most valuable intangible benefits of working for an employer.

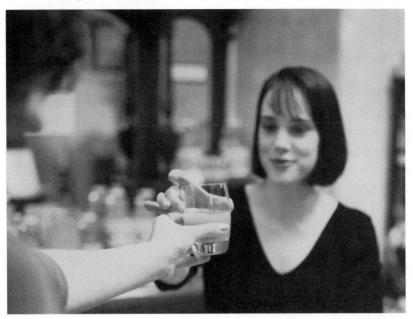

people who are silently relaxing, asleep, or only focused on their own needs. These factors have caused many therapists to end their careers prematurely. In a business setting, coworkers, management, and support staff can provide a social and stimulating environment, which can be invaluable to you on many levels.

Finally, if you are looking for that first job, one of the best benefits of a massage position with an employer is that you get a place to learn about the business of massage while making better money than many jobs on the open market. In addition, even though it may seem that you make a lot less than a therapist in a private practice, you will likely come out ahead financially as an employee, due to a steady stream of clients and no costs to you. Yes, an experienced therapist can charge private clients more and may have a full, busy practice, but it takes time, effort, energy, and money to get to that stage. In order for you to eventually get your dream practice, you now have an opportunity that was virtually unheard of even a few years ago, which is starting your career within the security and protection of a massage job.

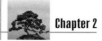
CHAPTER 2   SUMMARY

The first section of this edition was added to help you take full advantage of the many options open to you as a massage employee. You have many paths you can choose, and my goal is to make sure that you have the skills, tools, and understanding to get hired in your first job and get your career under way. If you write a great resume, do well in your interviews, and learn all you can as an employee, your options and opportunities will grow, as will your earnings. You may find that you love working for and with others, and you may spend your massage career primarily as an employee. If or when you decide you want to take the next step toward building your dream practice, please turn the page and let the rest of this book help you succeed in the next stage of your journey.

CHAPTER 2   ACTION STEPS

To prepare yourself for an interview, take the following action steps:

❋ Review the list under "What Employers Value Most," and honestly ask yourself how you compare to the list. If there are factors you need to work on, whether it's learning how to be on time or developing a stronger sense of self-confidence, make a commitment to yourself to improve in these areas.

❋ Prepare your files on each employer you have sent a resume to, and keep them near the phone. In the files, put a copy of the resume and cover letter you sent them, blank paper for taking notes when they call, a list of questions you want to ask, details about yourself that you did not include in your resume, answers to the common questions that employers ask, and research notes on the business.

❋ Prepare your interview kit. Put in it at least three copies of your resume, the list of questions you want to ask, details about yourself that you did not include in your resume, answers to the common questions employers ask, and research notes on the business. Add a list of references, letters of recommendation, a copy of your application, business cards, school grades or transcripts, and positive evaluations from hands-on tests or clinic clients in school, and bring your calendar and a pen. Also include printed driving directions if you are unfamiliar with the location of the interview.

✷ Practice answering the questions in the section "Questions Employers Often Ask." Practice answering them while you look in a mirror, and do mock interviews with other people until your answers come out smoothly and easily.

✷ Practice asking your most important questions for the interviewer. Hone your list of questions down to four or five in case that is all you have time for.

✷ Practice giving timed test massages, and make sure you work on all the points under the section "What You Are Evaluated On in a Test Massage."

✷ Research what employers are paying new therapists in jobs similar to the one for which you are interviewing. Find massage therapist chat rooms on the Internet, ask people about the typical pay scales, and otherwise get an accurate idea of what massage wages are in your area.

✷ If you need to, buy new clothes for the interview. Males and females usually wear the same outfits, which are nice slacks and a short-sleeved polo shirt.

✷ Review your personal and professional goals. With every interview, make sure that the job will help you reach your goals.

CHAPTER 2   KNOWLEDGE CHECK

Check your understanding of the chapter by reviewing these questions and answers.

Q: What are the top two elements that make a massage therapist desirable to an employer?
A: Attitude and aptitude.

Q: What are three factors that employers look for in an applicant during an interview?
A: A massage therapist who is confident, goal-oriented, honest, friendly, punctual, and so on.

Q: What are three needs every business has?
A: Getting new customers, keeping current customers happy, booking more frequent visits, keeping costs down, saving time, making a profit, and so forth.

Q: What are three ways you can research a business?
A: On the Internet, call and ask for literature, visit the facility, observe people in the parking lot, ask contacts for insider information, and so on.

Q: What are three things you can put in your interview kit?
A: Copies of your resume, a list of questions to ask, additional information about you, answers to common interview questions, research papers on the business, clinic or school evaluations, and school grades.

Q: True or False? An interviewer can ask how old you are.
A: False.

Q: True or False? Employers love it when you say your goal is to move quickly into management.
A: False.

Q: What are two ways spas keep massage therapists from getting overuse injuries?
A: Having them do non-massage tasks and perform spa treatments.

Q: When should you send a thank-you note to an interviewer?
A: Within 24 hours of the interview.

Q: What is often listed as the most important intangible benefit of being an employee?
A: Social interaction with the staff.

REFERENCES

Capellini, S. (2006). *Massage therapy career guide for hands-on success* (2nd edition). Albany, NY: Thomson Delmar Learning.

The Hartman Group, Inc., for the International SPA Association. (2004), *ISPA 2004 consumer trends report: Variations & trends on the consumer spa experience:* Bellevue, WA.

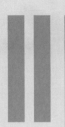

Marketing to Build Your Dream Practice: Bare-Bones Attributes, Skills, and Tools

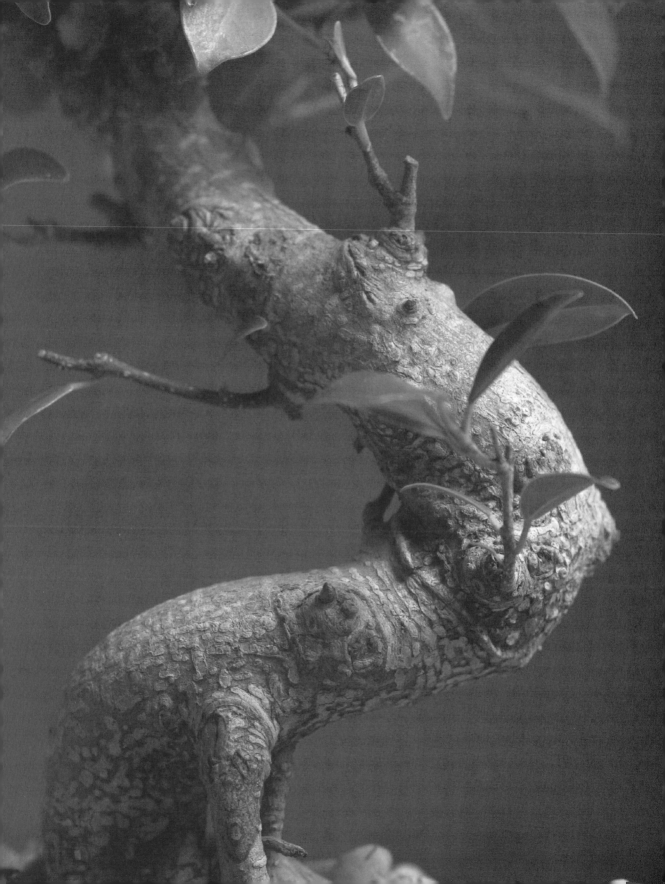

3 Marketing Attributes

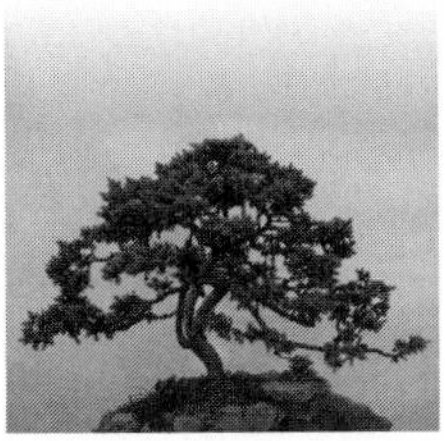

CHAPTER OBJECTIVES

After reading this chapter, you should be able to:

- Identify the four personal and professional attributes of successful massage professionals.
- Identify your personal definition of success.
- Describe the elements of your dream practice.
- Identify common obstacles to success.
- Explain the importance of setting boundaries.

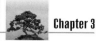

THE DEFINITION OF MARKETING

For massage therapists building a dream practice, the definition of marketing is broad but simple. Marketing is essentially anything you do that affects your ability to get new clients and keep them coming back. Using this broad definition, marketing becomes a way of being, not just a few tips on how to design a business card or build a Web site. Marketing, at its heart, involves representing yourself, your work, and your profession in thousands of tangible and intangible ways. With this definition, marketing can range from your choice of conversation topics during a session to the temperature settings in your massage room, or how you write a **press release** when you open your first office. Marketing can be the message you leave on your telephone answering machine, the television ad you create, or the extra five minutes you spend listening to a lonely client.

Essentially, everything you are and do that affects your success, from your first job to your dream practice, is marketing. Touch professionals have the power in their hands to change the world, and marketing is what it takes to get clients under your hands. As a touch professional, you are going to learn here what it truly takes to get and keep the clients you need to be successful as long as you want to practice the art and science of massage.

THE ATTRIBUTES OF A SUCCESSFUL PROFESSIONAL

The first step in marketing massage is to recognize that massage therapy, unlike some professions, is driven by the personality and attributes of the practitioner. Massage is a personal service profession, but what makes us so different from other service professionals is that most therapists who have Swedish-based practices basically touch naked people as a function of their work. This fact alone separates us from virtually every other service profession, and it is why traditional marketing techniques and books have not been very effective in our field. Because we touch naked people, how we comport ourselves and how we behave make all the difference in the world in our ability to make a living. Plumbers and electricians can be rude or late, interior decorators can be brusque or condescending, Web designers can be surly and unkempt, and landscapers do not have to make conversation as long as they do their jobs well. You, by comparison, need to be on time, respectful, courteous, professionally dressed, and able to communicate at many levels. Even medical professionals who also deal with naked bodies can have poor bedside manner, but patients have little choice because medical care for illnesses or injuries is necessary, not optional like massage.

Compared to most other professionals, massage therapists are often judged and hired by who we are and how we look and behave, not just by our set of bodywork skills. Quite simply, if potential employers or clients do not trust or like us, we will not get the chance to demonstrate our hands-on skills, no matter how good they are.

Therefore, your top priority for marketing is to understand and develop the personal attributes that build trust, and to maintain that trust during every step of the client/therapist relationship. This chapter will identify and detail the key attributes that successful practitioners have in common and that unsuccessful practitioners are missing. In my research, I discovered that if these key attributes were in place, therapists could make a living no matter what their working environment and regardless of their competition, regulatory laws, local economy, or education level. While these attributes may seem more about human nature than traditional marketing, you must understand them to get and keep clients.

MARKETING ATTRIBUTE #1: THE DESIRE TO SERVE

The first and most important attribute is the **desire to serve**. This may sound obvious and simplistic, but it is not. While visiting a fraction of the massage schools that have sprouted up across the country, I have found many filled with students who yearn to serve, mixed in with students lured primarily by dreams of easy money and high per-hour fees. While money is a crucial factor of success, long-term financial rewards are earned through years of work, and they are sustained and motivated through the normal ups and downs of life by the unflagging desire to serve. Clients, whether they can verbalize it or not, know when their massage therapist genuinely cares about them, and they can tell when the therapist is disengaged or disinterested.

Due to the very personal nature of massage, most private practices have been, and will continue to be, successful because of repeat clients and referrals. While other professions may say, in their marketing, that they offer genuine caring, the factor of touch in massage means that your desire to serve (or not) can be felt directly by your clients. Short-term success may be achieved without this attribute, but massage therapists who have achieved long-term success carry in their hearts and hands a genuine desire to help others.

If you want to strengthen your ability to care for others so that you can market more effectively, I'll let you in on a secret: successful massage therapists serve others because it feels good. True service brings them a lifetime of joy and satisfaction. When you help other people feel good, or you relieve their pain, you get to be happy, engaged with life, present, and fulfilled. When given the responsibility of touching other people's lives, and their bodies, you get to grow and learn. These are some of the core factors of human happiness.

Serving others offers a great payoff, but it is also risky. Caring about others opens you up to being hurt. Clients will leave you, and people will turn down your heartfelt offers of serving and caring. You may do your best work, and recipients may seem ungrateful or dismissive. Really, serving others is not for wimps. Having a passion for helping others may not be considered cool in a culture where the "me-first" attitude seems so pervasive, but it is great for succeeding in massage.

Building a successful career demands a foundation of the desire to serve. (See Figure 3–1.) Without that desire, your job or practice will collapse with the tremors that eventually shake every therapist. If you don't have the desire to serve, cut your losses now. Put this book down, rethink your career, and

Figure 3–1 | **The desire to serve others is your key to success.**

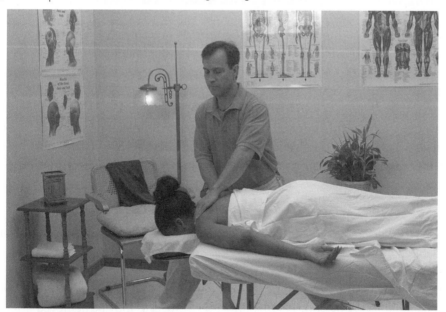

consider other work options. It will save you time, money, and great frustration, because long-term success is not possible in massage without the drive fed by the desire to serve. However, if joy, happiness, financial reward, and personal fulfillment are part of what you envision in your work, keep reading. Explore the adventure of serving others, and you will be richly rewarded in ways that will amaze you.

MARKETING ATTRIBUTE #2: THE COMMITMENT TO SUCCEED

The second most important attribute of long-term therapists is the **commitment to succeed**. This commitment is a much more complex attribute than the desire to serve. While most professionals in this field have a genuine desire to serve, the subject of success can become cloudy. First, every person has his or her own unique definition of success. Second, many people do not know what it truly takes to succeed in massage. Third, many massage therapists have subconscious fears about the consequences of being successful.

The Definition of Success

Before you can take steps toward success, you have to know what success is. What is your definition of success? Do you have a clear and ready answer, or are you not all that sure? Have you made up your own definition, or has it been handed to you by others, such as your parents, teachers, friends, or the media? Is success a feeling you have, or is it based on what money can buy? Is it a big house on the hill, or is it making a contribution to humanity? Is it making the world a better place, or is it raising good children? Or is it all of these? No answer is right or wrong. No answer is "better" than another. Your definition of success can be a powerful motivator for you, and you should not edit it just because someone else has a different definition.

The big secret of success is to make it easy to feel successful. Success breeds success, so start by setting and reaching small, short-term goals, such as setting up your first interview or getting your first paying client. As you get comfortable with and used to success, set bigger goals and build toward long-term dreams. Don't make it too difficult to feel successful, and certainly don't wait to be happy until you have reached some of your long-term goals. Accomplishing small achievements along the way can keep you motivated and feeling good about yourself, which makes a huge difference when you hit the inevitable roadblocks in your career.

Successful work is yours to define as well. If you want a part-time job or to practice a few days a week out of your home while you pursue your acting career, that's fine. If you want to start a day spa, own a chain of massage franchises, or run a retreat center on 100 acres of wilderness with 20 healing arts practitioners from different disciplines, that's great too. If you want to work with dancers, infants, world-class athletes, or homeless people, it is your prerogative to include them in your dream practice. This is your life and your practice that you will need marketing to make real. How are you going to define your own success?

EXERCISE: DEFINING SUCCESS

Think about what success would look or feel like to you. Write down at least five factors that would describe your successful dream practice.

Example: In my dream practice, I will enjoy

   Interesting and enjoyable clients who love getting regular massage

   Being able to help clients with a wide range of needs

   Working in a gorgeous, peaceful setting with a view out the window

   Being able to travel and do massage in other countries

   Making a difference in people's lives

   Making a great living, with money for a home, travel, and investments

_____

_____

_____

_____

_____

_____

What It Takes

Once you have your personal definition of success, you then need to make a commitment to reaching that success. This may sound kind of obvious, but many people confuse hoping and wishing with commitment. If hoping and wishing worked, we would all have ponies, or motorcycles, or be great guitarists in a rock-and-roll band. Hoping and wishing have their place, but they don't get results. Commitment does. Resolve, determination, and doing what it takes will lead you to success.

The commitment to succeed became very clear to me when I interviewed a woman who began her practice in the 1970s. At that time, she did not have a massage table, a car, or a telephone. Most people would consider those items the bare necessities of building a practice, but to get started, she rode her bicycle to her clients' homes, put pillows on the floor, and gave massages for $5.00. When I interviewed this woman in March of 2000, her practice was still going strong. While her life is easier now that she has a table, a car, and a telephone, I know that she can be successful no matter what her circumstances. She knows the secret to success: make your commitment and don't give up. Her commitment to succeed supersedes any excuses, leaving her with what matters: results.

Overcoming Obstacles

The first step in building your commitment to succeed is to work on your ability and willingness to manage and overcome obstacles. These can be external obstacles, such as punitive licensing laws, or internal obstacles, such as the fear of rejection. People end up with one of two outcomes when facing the inevitable obstacles to getting a job or building a practice: good excuses or good results. Successful therapists work through external obstacles such as unfair treatment by authorities, establishments, employers, or building owners. They overcome hostile environments and zoning laws, competitors with major advantages, or being forced to practice without a license because the city in which they work refuses to give business permits to massage therapists. Regardless of their circumstances, successful therapists use their determination to work their way around whomever or whatever gets in their way.

Professionals I spoke with across the country who had long-term practices had also dealt with internal obstacles such as low self-esteem, flagging confidence, fear of the unknown, a sense of inadequacy, and weak boundary skills. Many of them also had grappled with taking money for their caring touch. Issues such as these face almost every massage therapist I have met or taught. While one may not consider confidence or self-esteem part of marketing, a lack of either can make it very difficult to get and keep clients. The commitment to succeed calls for dealing with difficult internal and external barriers of all types: it makes the difference between having a happy and satisfying massage career or just working on a few friends and family members.

The unsuccessful therapists I met complained about everything imaginable. It was as if they believed that anything painful, disruptive, difficult, or inconvenient was a personal affront to them and a valid reason to quit. Whether their friends and family sympathized with their struggles, or they felt self-righteous in blaming the environment, their school, or the ever popular "saturated market" for their lack of clients, their commitment was to defending their excuses, not to doing whatever it took to succeed. Unfortunately, their seemingly valid excuses kept them from achieving their dream of making a living with massage.

It is perfectly normal to feel fear, balk at change, or be resistant to new ideas. However, when these challenges are expressed in the form of complaining or blaming, the commitment to succeed has to kick in; otherwise, they can slow or stop you from reaching your goals. In one memorable example, when I was a massage teacher, a group of students got upset because the school where I worked didn't have a bicycle rack. When a new student who rode a bike wanted a rack, and the school was slow in putting one in, you would have thought the school was on fire given the outpouring of energy and angry letters, even from students who weren't in his class. I had seen this behavior before, especially near graduation time, and all I could do was once again marvel that the normal fear that comes with growth and change could be transformed into misdirected anger over something so trivial. Over and over I saw the same process: just when students were reaching stages of major growth and change, they became obsessed with something minor and backed away from the real issues they needed to face head-on. In this particular instance, some students became so wrapped up in being upset about the inconsequential bike rack that they damaged a significant portion of their learning experience, and very likely harmed their careers.

If you catch yourself getting angry or upset at seeming injustices and obstacles to building your practice, that's normal and okay. It is when you get stuck in anger and frustration that the commitment to succeed and desire to serve must take over and move you past the obstacle. If you have a "bike rack" obstacle that looks like a big deal, but in the broader perspective probably isn't, consider the possibility that it is a distraction technique created by your subconscious mind to protect you from feeling the fears and anxieties that are a natural part of growth and change. Treat those fears with respect, and deal with them. If you don't, you risk the pattern of generating so many excuses and smoke screens that you never get around to the actual work of getting and keeping clients.

Marketing, and all that it represents in taking steps to meet people, tell them about your work, and book an appointment, can sometimes set off internal alarm bells and push buttons of fear and survival. If your commitment is to being safe and comfortable, or to never feeling rejected or afraid, then you cannot grow the amount necessary to run a long-term practice. Growth can be scary, but it can also be exhilarating and life changing. If you want to succeed, push yourself to grow and move past your fears and obstacles. This is part of maturing as a human being, and the process is actually one of the best side benefits of being a massage therapist.

From Fear to Growth

Marketing brings up anxiety and fears for many people. If this is true for you, then you need to learn how to understand and manage those fears in order to succeed. Your first step is to get curious about fear. Humans rarely like admitting they're afraid of something, yet millions of people pay good money to be scared watching horror movies, reading creepy novels, or riding harrowing amusement-park rides. Kids love ghost stories and getting scared about the monsters under their beds. Television shows that cause great fear and anxiety are considered grand entertainment. We do not like to admit that we are afraid of things, but we seem to enjoy the sensations of fear. What is wrong with this picture?

Perhaps fear is a big seller because most people are bored with their safe, predictable lives. Or maybe it is easier to deal with fantastical fears than with real, basic human fears. After all, which is scarier to consider: being attacked

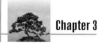

by a giant python in the Amazon jungle, or facing the criticizing voice in your head that tells you you're not good enough or that you're not wanted? Anyone opt for the snake?

Since facing fear is usually a significant part of any success, you need to learn to harness fear. If fear can be stimulating, engaging, and exciting in the movie theater, why not make it that way in your own life? Try approaching fear, not with the intention of eliminating it, but with the intention of using it for your own purposes. If you are experiencing fear, make the most of it and use it to strengthen your commitment to succeed.

Turning Fear into Success

Fear can be transformed into growth and success in countless ways. Here are three very helpful methods:

1. Name and embrace your fears.

2. Visualize what scares you about success, and practice different scenarios with the images until your fear changes.

3. Put your fears into perspective with a personal mission.

The act of naming, acknowledging, and embracing your fears is a huge leap toward success. The first step in the process is to verbalize your fears. These fears may include talking about money, or being afraid your work isn't good enough and won't help people. Once you recognize a fear, don't try to banish it. Instead, do the opposite and embrace it. Thank your fear for protecting you from the harm it imagines will befall you. Then explain to your fear that it will not hurt you to talk to a new client about your rates, or pick up a telephone and call a new referral. It may feel scary, but once you do what you were afraid of, the exhilaration is wonderful and freeing. Your hands may shake for a half hour, but then many people pay $4.00 for a double espresso to get the same feeling.

The next time you face the necessity of repeating this particular stress-causing activity, your brain will remember that you have done it before. You may experience discomfort or anxiety the second time, but most likely you will not have as strong a reaction as the first time, since the behavior will not be totally new. The third time, you may only feel twinges of doubt or fear, and after that, each subsequent act will affect you less.

EXERCISE: MANAGING COMMON FEARS

Reviewing all the fears that can block the path to your dream practice is beyond the scope of this book. However, after listening to my students over the years, I've learned that there are a few fears that seem to show up more frequently than others. Take a moment and look at the following list of common fears that many massage therapists face. See if any ring a bell for you. Even acknowledging a fear is helpful because you can then consider that fear is a possible cause if you suddenly find yourself doing things that undermine your commitment to succeed.

COMMON FEARS

On a scale of 1–10, with 1 being low and 10 being high, rank each common fear by how much it might affect your practice.

____ Fear of failure

____ Fear of success

____ Fear of ridicule or being made fun of

____ Fear of looking foolish

____ Fear of being wrong about your decision to become a massage therapist

____ Fear of becoming successful when other people said you wouldn't be

____ Fear of rejection by people you ask to be your clients

____ Fear of abandonment by your clients

____ Fear of loss of love from those you care about, especially as you grow and change

____ Fear of disappointing yourself or others, especially if you can't help their problems

____ Fear of criticism

____ Fear of making mistakes

____ Fear of not being good enough

____ Fear of not being wanted

____ Other fears _____

Give any fear that scored a number higher than five the respect and attention it is due. Some fears are very old and deep-seated, and take hard work to overcome. Some will vanish as soon as they are named and recognized. Remember, you do not have to eliminate a fear to move forward. Many successful massage therapists pushed toward goals with fears in full and glorious bloom. Do not wait for fear to go away before you build or grow your practice. Push on in the face of it and learn to succeed regardless of what arises.

Visualization

Of the fears we have just covered, some are learned and some are instinctive. It may seem paradoxical, but many pains and fears are actually good for us. They are crucial for our survival, and, in fact, without them most of us would die at a very young age. Pain and fear are deeply wired into our nervous systems to protect us from what can hurt us. However, sometimes that protective mechanism can go too far and tell us that things are dangerous when they aren't. This is especially true of fear of the unknown, which can come up when we face something new or different. To get your first job or build a practice will require doing many things that are new and different, and while some people are engaged with the adventure of it all, others may be paralyzed by fear. To override this protective mechanism, we must somehow notify the nervous system that the new activity in which we are about to engage is not life threatening and does not require the fight-or-flight response to save us.

If you find yourself suddenly needing to wash and wax the car, dust the hall closet, or change the vacuum bag, you may be showing signs of avoidance, one of the favorite methods of coping with fear of the unknown. If that is the case, it may be time to pull out one of our most powerful fear-busting tools: visualization. Quite simply, visualization is using your imagination for a specific reason. Since many fears are based on the unfamiliar, one way to deal with them is to make them familiar and safe in your imagination before you do them in reality. Visualization can let you do a mental walk-through of new experiences before you actually become involved in them. By seeing, feeling, and experiencing situations that are new or frightening to you, you can monitor your own reactions and practice the visualization over and over until all your physical and emotional responses are what you would want them to be in a real setting.

If, for example, you have a businesswoman in mind with whom you would like to work, visualize your first interaction with her. Imagine how you would introduce yourself, what you would say to make her excited about getting massage from you, and how you would respond to a number of different reactions she might have to you. For instance, imagine that you are at a party and someone has just introduced you to her and told her that you do massage. What would you say to her? See her face, hear her words, and notice how you feel as you imagine this scenario. Then imagine that someone has given you this businesswoman's card and told you that she was looking for a massage therapist. See yourself picking up the phone and calling her at her office. How will you start the conversation? How will you introduce yourself? What will you say if you get her voice mail? What will you say if she is busy and can't talk right then? Practice these and other scenarios, and as you end each one, see yourself writing her name down in your appointment book. Then imagine that she has a large circle of friends she would love to refer to you! Imagine your telephone ringing as all her friends call you, eager to get a massage and ready with waiting checkbooks.

It is helpful to practice a number of scenarios, including a worst-case scenario, in which you have different ways of handling or ending a marketing conversation until you can run through it without feeling stress or fear. You even can practice handling a conversation that has started badly and turning it around so that it has a great ending.

The fear of success can be a big one for massage therapists, and while some fears of success are valid, most are not. Typical fears of success include not being able to fulfill others' expectations, feeling like a fraud and having people "discover" that you don't really know what you're talking about, or worrying that your success will come at too high a price. Take your fears out of the shadows and into the light of day. Examine them closely, and you will see that there are ways to handle each of them. If you are afraid of not meeting people's expectations, it may be helpful to realize that your work can often get results where other medical techniques cannot. If you are afraid of not knowing enough, realize that while you may not know everything, you probably know more than enough to help people.

If you are afraid of success, you need to know you are capable of managing it without hurting your body, your relationships, your soul, or anything else you might fear that success could conceivably damage. If you find yourself in a moment of doubt, do a quick visualization. Imagine yourself quickly and effectively handling the situation with confidence, skill, or whatever you need to turn that fear into preparedness. If you are generally anxious, imagine yourself in a quiet and beautiful place where you can be still long enough to figure out what is bothering you. Imagine bringing in a wise person to talk to, perhaps a mentor or teacher. Take advantage of the moment and train your brain for success. Imagine things like seeing yourself healthy and strong, enjoying the love and support of family and friends, helping people, growing your bank account, or whatever motivates you. Visualization is a wonderful tool, and you can use it to move yourself toward success with remarkable speed.

Self-Sabotage

Understanding and planning how you will handle success is important because, in the face of fear and change, many people commit **self-sabotage** on themselves or their careers. It is not uncommon for therapists to feel that they do not deserve success. Some may have been told by parents or teachers that they would never amount to anything, or they may have some unrecognized belief that runs contrary to what they are working toward. For example, if a woman was raised with the strong belief that "the love of money is the root of all evil," but she wants to charge reasonable rates for her massage services, those beliefs can conflict. The result of conflicting beliefs is often odd and contradictory behavior. For example, the woman who associates evil with money may set her rates too low to make a living, give away too many free sessions, or feel so guilty taking money that she makes her paying clients uncomfortable by having a hard time taking their checks.

The commitment to succeed carries with it the task of monitoring yourself and noticing if you are doing things that run counter to what you say you want or will do. If you say you want to get 10 new clients, but then just sit home and watch television all day, question what is going on inside yourself that is keeping you from your goal. I have known therapists who accomplished major breakthroughs toward reaching their goals, but then ruined their practices one way or another. One therapist kept having little accidents, another showed up chronically late until he was fired from a job he worked hard to get, and another kept "forgetting" to show up for appointments. While good excuses could be made for all these cases, they resulted in the ending of a job or practice. That is not the purpose of this book.

I suspect there are more than a few good massage therapists who have ruined their practices because of unrecognized fears and conflicting beliefs. I have heard therapists express concern that financial stability would lead them to become lazy or lose their conscience, that clients leaving them would be too painful, or that success would make them greedy and heartless. Knowing yourself and your beliefs can help you tremendously if you start to recognize that you are overtly or covertly sabotaging your practice. Part of the commitment to succeed involves recognizing and changing self-sabotaging behavior before it hurts you or your practice. Below is a list of classic sabotaging behaviors. If you recognize any of them, take time to think about how they will eventually affect your practice over the long run. Think about the success you want, and then ask yourself if it is possible to build your dream practice while maintaining these behaviors:

- Chronically showing up late (see Figure 3–2)
- Breaking promises
- Accidents and forms of physical injury
- Misplacing or losing things, such as telephone numbers or appointment books
- Procrastination
- Perfectionism
- Getting sidetracked
- Being forgetful about business-related matters
- Chronic avoidance, such as computer games, television, naps, or sleeping late

None of these behaviors is necessarily "wrong." However, accumulated over time and with repetition, these can block your success, so pay attention to them and handle them to empower your commitment to succeed.

Being a Beginner

Most anything in life that is worth doing has a learning or beginning stage. Some people perpetually look for new things to start or learn, while others prefer the security of the familiar. For the growth necessary to run a long-term,

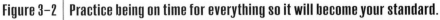
Figure 3–2 | Practice being on time for everything so it will become your standard.

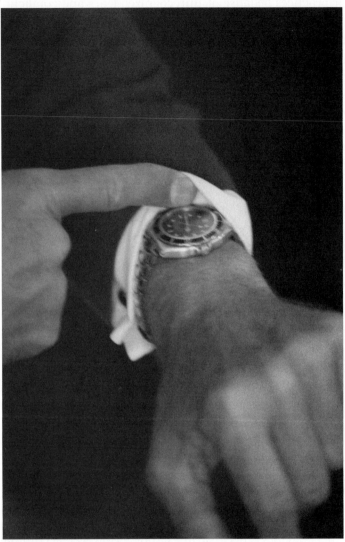

full-time practice, there are going to be times when you will be a beginner. This is when you will need to take action in the face of being uncomfortable or unconfident. While that may not sound difficult, millions of people live lives of boredom, repetition, and stagnation because they cannot handle being challenged or feeling out of control.

It is safer to sit in front of the television with a bucket of ice cream instead of following dreams, and even though it is ultimately dissatisfying and empty, a significant percentage of people will live this way their whole lives. Memories from our past, such as criticisms from childhood, failures in school, teasing, and other traumas associated with being a beginner, can lay dormant and not affect us much until we try something new. Then those memories wake up and warn us to stop whatever we are doing so that we don't cause ourselves pain like we felt before.

It is understandable if you do not like feeling like a beginner, but you should question your reasons. Some people are embarrassed to say, "I don't know," or flinch at the thought of asking anyone for help. The desire to appear intelligent or competent is very powerful, but it can run counter to the commitment to succeed. As a beginner, ask questions, seek out mentors, be willing to make mistakes, and don't let pride and ego get in the way of learning what it takes to become successful.

The Desire to Learn

One of the most consistent factors I have found among massage professionals with more than 20 years of experience is that they have an intense desire to learn new things while striving to master the fundamentals of their work. I have yet to meet a successful therapist who was complacent and felt like there was nothing else worth learning. From my research, I can conclude that the ability to succeed is directly tied to the desire to learn. Seminars, classes, books, magazines, conventions, conferences, peer discussions, association meetings, getting together with local colleagues for social or business purposes, and other forms of continued learning are part of the investment made in a long-term practice. Whether advanced learning helps the therapist alleviate the boredom of routine work, offers more advanced therapeutic skills that create higher demands and fees, or opens new markets with new skills, it seems to play a role in career longevity. If your commitment is to success, feed and foster your desire to learn.

Gathering Support

The process of moving through the many stages of practice building can be greatly enhanced by gathering support from people who will encourage you through your growth and change. One of the most critical parts of creating a massage career is the time between when the support and structure of the massage school or training ends, and a first job is gained or a financially stable practice is built. Many of my former students dreaded going back into their old environments without the support of their classmates and teachers. In some cases, their old friends were not supportive of their healthier lifestyles or were resentful of their willingness to leave behind the "old gang" for a successful career. Not every parent I encountered at our massage school graduations was thrilled that their child was going into massage. And some spouses, especially husbands, were jealous and felt threatened because their wives were going to be massaging other men. If you are a student, set up a support system while in school to make this transition less lonely and help you keep your dreams alive. Loneliness is a factor that has killed many massage careers, and dreams can die without encouragement, so if your commitment is to success, get support.

Seek support from people you admire, or from friends and family who want to see you succeed, and join a massage organization or group (or start your own). While there are many benefits to belonging to associations, one of the best is that you can talk with people who understand what you are going through. (See Figure 3–3.) A wonderful joy and comfort exists in

Figure 3–3 | **Meet with colleagues on a regular basis for support.**

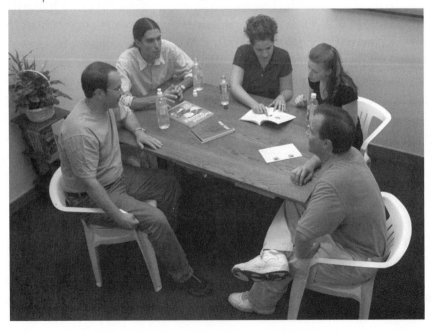

being surrounded by others who really know what it is that you do all day long. One of the best ways to receive support is to give support. Many of the friends that I made from volunteer work to advance the legitimization and acceptance of massage seem to have forged successful careers for themselves over the span of many years, and I believe the factor of support from colleagues was a big part of their success. A note I have taped to my computer simply says, "Whatever you want, give it first." If you want support, start by giving it.

Creating Internal and External Deadlines

Despite all the new discoveries made in physics that challenge our concepts of reality about space and time, to build a successful practice you must deal with the limitations of time. Getting and keeping real clients that pay real money has to occur in real time, and the difference between hopes and wishes in fantasy time and real success is the factor of deadlines. Without deadlines, people tend to procrastinate until opportunity has passed them by. This pushes them to return to options that are less gratifying but are more safe and familiar. To overcome many obstacles or fears, create deadlines for your personal and professional goals. Write out your goals and put them into your calendar so you see them daily. You can keep your plans to yourself, or if you have a support group, tell them your goals and deadlines so you are accountable to them to keep your word. If you procrastinate on a project because you feel uncomfortable or unsure of how to do something new, your accountability to the group will create more discomfort because you know others will know that you never made that call or got your business cards made. In essence, you can motivate yourself by playing the potential pain of other's disappointment off the discomfort or inconvenience of doing what you promised. As a result, you end up pushing yourself over your obstacle.

One of the biggest benefits of deadlines is that they can push you to take action before you feel ready. Successful people know that if they wait until they feel ready, their window of opportunity will have passed. Despite their misgivings, discomfort, or quaking knees, they have trained themselves to jump into things whether ready or not. Certainly, they plan and prepare a great deal, but they do not wait until everything is perfect before they move forward.

Time and again I have heard, read, and experienced that when you make a commitment to something, even if you don't know how you will make it happen, miracles happen, amazing coincidences occur, and you reach your commitment by your deadline in ways you never would have dreamed. Without the focus created by a deadline, creative thoughts and lucky breaks just do not seem to materialize. Make deadlines for yourself, and make commitments to yourself and others. This is how you get results, and results are crucial to attaining success.

Managing Expectations

In addition to managing fear, frustration, anger, growth, and change, successful therapists have the ability to manage their expectations, especially when things do not work out as planned. The ability to manage expectations is a hallmark of maturity, and is often learned only through the proverbial "school of hard knocks." On the opposite end of the maturity scale are those who believe they will get whatever they expect, usually easily and effortlessly, and think they have control over others and their environment.

The danger of this belief to a long-term practice is that people with unrealistic expectations are more likely to quit when the going gets tough. Similarly, a belief that things in life should come quickly and easily can set back a practice when growth takes more work than expected. Building a practice is not like pulling up to the drive-through window of a fast-food restaurant, putting in an order, and then getting a neatly packaged and successful business handed over to you.

A long-term practice requires dealing with adversity, developing patience, and picking yourself up from failure. Miracles, fortunate coincidences, and other good things are a common part of many successful practices, but they are the reward for persevering and not giving up on your dream. There is no room for the concept of entitlement in the massage field. No one owes you anything just because you got a massage certificate or license, and no one is obliged to be your client or give you a job.

On the other hand, don't set expectations too low, either. Your commitment to succeed should balance out somewhere in the reality of this field, which is that we are still a fairly new and growing profession where demand is inconsistent and not at all guaranteed. Create marketing efforts that demonstrate that you have a healthy sense of the value of your work, and combine them with the humility that you must prove your value to your clients or employers on an ongoing basis.

Managing Setbacks

The commitment to succeed demands the ability and willingness to handle setbacks, mistakes, and "failures." Success requires growth, and growth requires mistakes. Therefore, the less fear you have of mistakes, the more quickly you can grow. Handling mistakes and setbacks is not always easy. It is no fun to be embarrassed, or to realize that you were unprepared or ignorant.

This is when your commitment to succeed and your desire to help others become vital. You don't tell a baby that she can have only so many chances to learn to walk before she has to give up. She will fall down and get up again until she can walk, and that is the same spirit you must take into building a practice. Things in a practice "fall down" often. Clients move, clients die, equipment gets stolen, equipment breaks, wrists break, you realize you are out of clean sheets, injuries and illnesses happen, recessions wipe out half your client base, and local laws change, making it impossible to get a business license. It is all part of the package, or at least, it was part of my package. You may have better luck. Whatever your fortune, handle your personal and professional setbacks well and you can succeed in massage.

Managing Success

If success is something you can handle with ease and comfort, then you are a fortunate human being. If you are like most people, though, success can be unfamiliar and scary. Success can make you feel as anxious or out of control as failure does, sometimes even worse. Managing success may take bravery and courage at first, but if you allow success to happen, you will get more comfortable with it. Being at ease with success and radiating the confidence that comes with it sends out a charismatic aura that draws people in and keeps the cycle of success going. Success is not the destination of your career: it is part of the path. Maintaining success over the years usually requires setting new and higher goals, and broadening your personal mission and contribution.

In a paradoxical way, the more "impossible" your mission, the more at ease you can be with your achievements. I, most likely, will not see the end of human suffering in my lifetime, but it is what I strive for every day, and each success I have gets me one step closer to that mission. I'm not afraid that success will go to my head, or that I will reach some point of accomplishment and see a "Dead End" sign. If you want to manage success, put it in the context of your bigger personal mission and life goals. This will keep success in a perspective that is both humbling and motivating. To build a dream practice, welcome and manage success. It may take a little practice, but then, most important skills do.

Creating a Personal Mission

The commitment to succeed can be greatly helped by creating or discovering your own personal mission. A personal mission may seem a bit grandiose for some people, but for me, having grown up with two parents who were and are very mission-driven, it seems natural and valuable to have a bigger reason for life and work besides simply filling time until death inevitably arrives. At times of crisis or during moments where significant decisions must be made, having a bigger picture or mission for your life can be grounding and stabilizing. Having a bigger purpose or mission also has great benefit in sustaining drive and persistence throughout a career. To make mountains into molehills on your road to success, rise high above the basic details of running your life by seeing yourself in the context of your mission and its impact on the world over time. The sobering smallness of our own being and the mere blink of an eye of time we are given here can be both a motivator and a relief. You may want to accomplish much while you are here, but with this mindset, time is neither an enemy nor a burden.

While a larger purpose in life can help sustain one's practice over time, many new therapists don't have a specific personal mission when they begin their practices. Do not wait for a personal mission before you start marketing and building your practice. Just aim for getting your practice started. The experience of working with your clients will help you discover your personal mission, and the sooner you start looking for your purpose within your work, the more satisfying and fulfilling it will be. Therapists who are happy and fulfilled have much greater odds of succeeding, and if having a personal mission can help you succeed over the long haul, then keep it in the back of your mind as we continue with what it takes to build your dream practice.

As you may now recognize, the commitment to succeed has many facets and cannot be waved away with a simple "Oh, of course I want to succeed" statement. This is a marketing book, but the overall purpose of your marketing is to help you reach your version of success. Without a commitment to success, there is no reason to market in order to get and keep clients. Please, if you are going to enter the game, whether it is the game of life or your massage career, enter it to win.

EXERCISE: FIRST DRAFT OF A MISSION STATEMENT

Even if you don't have a clear idea of what your personal mission might be (or even if you do!), take a few moments to write down some of the guiding principles of why you want to help people with massage. Think about what brought you to this profession and what you hope to accomplish over your career. Our career choices are often clear windows into our driving forces. You can simply complete the sentence "I want to be a massage therapist because . . ." as a way to start drafting your mission statement. If you are in a group, talk with others about why they wanted to become massage therapists. Some people might have similar reasons, and some might have very different reasons, but hearing other people's answers may help you learn more about yourself.

_____

_____

_____

_____

_____

_____

MARKETING ATTRIBUTE #3: PROFESSIONALISM

Some of the most important lessons I have learned about marketing have come from talking, not with massage professionals, but with the general public about their experiences with massage. During my cross-country trip, I took every opportunity to ask people about massage, and I got an earful. Whether it was the clerk at the Rite-Aid store in Denham Springs, Louisiana, or fellow Californians sharing a barbecue dinner at an RV park in Orlando, Florida, I got to hear what massage clients thought about their therapists.

While people were generally positive about massage, the conversation sometimes became downright embarrassing when it came to the topic of professionalism. I heard stories of therapists that made me cringe: a male therapist who stripped off his shirt during a session and then dripped sweat on the client; a woman who talked the whole session about who she had slept with the night before; a woman who smelled like she hadn't showered for days; a woman whose blankets were covered with dog hair and whose dogs ran around the treatment room; a man who didn't listen when the client told him not to touch her feet and he did anyway, unleashing very bad memories; and way too many stories about therapists who made unwanted sexual advances on their clients.

The stories told to me by employers at spas weren't much better. Frankly, after what I'd heard, I was beginning to think that if massage therapists could show up at an appointment on time, or show up at all, were willing to wear shoes and decent, appropriate clothing, and could give a full hour of average Swedish massage without talking about their latest sexual escapade or complaining during the entire session about a personal drama or trauma, they would be well on their way to success.

After getting over my initial shock at such widespread stories of unprofessional behavior, my overriding feeling was one of sadness. What a waste and a pity that caring and gifted therapists were losing clients and not getting referrals because they were oblivious to their own lack of basic manners, courtesies, and professionalism. I came to realize that professional common sense isn't all that common!

I doubt the therapists talked about so badly by their former clients would think they had done anything wrong; otherwise, they would not have behaved that way. The trouble was that these therapists had difficulty seeing the world from any perspective or point of view other than their own and could not tell that their behavior was negatively affecting their clients.

Successful therapists maintain their professionalism by seeing themselves through the eyes of their clients, and they adapt themselves to speak, dress, and behave in ways that are appropriate to their clients. Being appropriate does not mean the loss of self-expression, giving up style, or not being yourself. It means having empathy, paying attention to clients, and trying to see, hear, and feel the massage experience from their perspective. As the general public comes to expect higher levels of professionalism from massage, look at yourself from a client's point of view and see if you fit their image of a professional therapist.

Professional Boundaries

Professionalism can take many forms and be expressed in many ways, from how you talk and dress to how you handle a drape. At its core, though, professionalism is a basic attitude of centering your practice around your clients and their needs, desires, attitudes, and goals. There are many ways to demonstrate professionalism, but the most important one is setting appropriate boundaries.

The heart of setting boundaries is simple. You and your client are two different people, and what is desirable, important, or appropriate to you may not be the same for the client. Of all the reasons clients leave their former massage therapists, many come down to a breach of boundaries. Whether a therapist pushes a personal philosophy or religion; gives too much unrequested advice on nutrition, colon cleansing, or meditation; talks about subjects that are too personal for the client's comfort; or just plain talks too much, clients will leave a therapist with good hands-on skills if he or she has poor boundary skills.

The inherent nature of massage makes boundary skills even more important than for other professions. Since most practitioners will be in the position of standing over a client who is lying down, naked under a sheet, and being touched, the normal barriers of clothing, personal space, eye contact, and being on the same physical plane are all removed. Without these common social barriers, the client is vulnerable in countless ways, and what may be tolerable in a normal setting can become frightening or uncomfortable while on the table or floor. (See Figure 3–4).

I recall one story in particular told to me by a client who had been seeing a massage therapist for quite a while. While she liked the therapist's work, at some point, the therapist converted to a particular religion and proceeded to bring it up repeatedly during their sessions. Not sharing her particular faith, this client reluctantly stopped seeing the therapist because she felt uncomfortable and pressured, even though the therapist was "simply telling her own experiences" of her conversion.

Two points are important here. One, the therapist should not have taken the client's massage time to discuss her personal issues, and two, the boundaries of religion and deeply held beliefs are not wise to cross. In a normal setting, these two people could have carried on a dialogue and agreed to disagree, but

Figure 3-4 | **Boundaries are important in massage because the client is more vulnerable.**

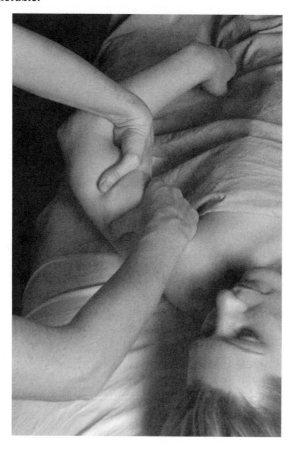

with the client lying down unclothed, she felt defenseless. Sadly, she did not have the heart to tell her therapist why she never rebooked. She just quietly left and never came back. I feel sorry for this obviously skilled and good-hearted therapist who had no concept of the increased significance of boundaries in the massage setting.

Professionalism contains a few basic rules on boundaries, but they really come down to your ability to recognize where you and you clients are different, and then to respect their position. The first step in recognizing where you and your client differ is probably the most difficult, because most people think others think and feel as they do. Neutrality can be very helpful on touchy subjects, especially with new clients who do not know you very well.

Human beings have a very strong sense of "tribe." If you are too different from their tribe and overstep your boundaries on crucial topics such as politics or religion, you can lose them as clients. Remember, marketing is anything that affects your ability to get and keep clients. Stepping over clients' boundaries and threatening their "tribe" can cost you clients and even your massage career.

Some special boundary areas to watch for include:

✳ Religion

✳ Politics

✳ Beliefs about body, nutrition, stress, family, and relationships

✳ Application of bodywork, such as using too much or too little pressure, draping improperly, working areas where client has said not to work, using uncomfortable techniques, and spending too little or too much time working one area

✳ Conversation, including telling personal or intimate stories, asking personal questions, or telling stories about other clients

✳ Improper dress, such as wearing clothing that is revealing, provocative, disrespectful, or greatly different from what the client wears or would expect from his or her stereotypes of massage professionals

✳ Comfort with nudity

✳ Comfort with temperature, lighting, and music preferences

✳ Language such as massage jargon, unfamiliar terms, foul language, or slang

Product Sales

Boundary issues are currently being questioned in the massage industry when product sales are included in a practice. While some people consider product sales unethical because there is a perceived power difference between a therapist and a client, others view product sales as important to customer service. For example, if a therapist working with athletes knows that a cryotherapy product like Biofreeze® can really help relieve pain between sessions, it is smart business and good service to use it during the session so clients get a sense of its effectiveness, and to then make it available to them for purchase if they like it. If a therapist offers spa services with products like Biotone®'s mud wraps or exfoliations, offering take-home scrubs and lotions can be a natural extension of the service. If a therapist does "pamper parties" and brings spa treatments to a person's home for everything from bridal showers to group fundraisers, selling products based on the services offered can be a great revenue generator. Smart marketers then put their contact information on the products sold so people going home from the party or event have a way to contact them later. Stress management therapists can sell lavender eye pillows, aromatherapy candles, or meditation tapes to help their clients better relax. Depending on your clients' needs, you can really help them take better care of themselves in between sessions so that they can progress further on their path to wellness. Some therapists use the products they sell during their services and educate their clients about what they are using and how it will help them. Other therapists just display products and say nothing, only talking about them if the client asks.

That said, even something as seemingly harmless as selling products has the potential to push boundaries and damage a relationship. If you sell products within your practice, don't be pushy. No means no, and if your clients aren't interested, don't keep asking. The biggest problem has come from multilevel marketing companies that have targeted massage therapists as being ideal doorways into various markets. While it may seem like a great idea to enlist clients into becoming your distributors for a product you like, I have heard many horror stories of people who have fled from their therapists, never to return again, because they felt pressured into buying multilevel products or becoming distributors for them. Clients, like most human beings, want to be accepted and loved, and some people may feel pressure to buy something from you for fear that you might otherwise "abandon" them. Combine the fear of losing acceptance with a position of vulnerability, and you may make a sale, but you can also lose a client.

Since this is a marketing book about getting and keeping clients, my emphasis is on keeping the client. Your profit from your massages over the long term is much greater than the percentage of profit you can make from the sale of a few items. Make serving your customer the priority, make product sales a natural extension of your services if selling is comfortable or fun for you, watch your boundaries so that you are appropriate, and you can make product sales something that can help both you and your clients.

Boundaries from Our Perspective

On the other side of this boundary equation are massage therapists, many of whom think it is perfectly acceptable to touch naked strangers for a living. It wasn't until a noticeable number of people asked me how I could stand the thought of "touching all those people," and how "icky" doing massage must be, that I came to realize I have a very different set of boundaries than much of the population. Personally, I have no problem with doing massage, and I enjoy my work very much. However, just because massage is fine with us doesn't mean that everyone likes giving or even getting touch.

Somewhere between the more open boundaries of the typical massage therapist and the more vulnerable boundaries of clients is a flexible line that must be negotiated differently with every client and, sometimes, even from session to session. Pay attention to boundaries and be respectful of them, and your opportunity for long-term success will skyrocket.

Your Professional Self-Definition

Professionalism, especially within the realm of boundaries, calls for an understanding of, recognition of, and respect for the differences between you and your client. Part of your job is to watch, observe, and listen to your clients so you will know what they expect of you as a professional. However, a key factor in meeting their expectations of you is your own understanding or perspective of yourself as a massage professional. (See Figure 3–5.) One of the difficulties our field faces is that because we have such different identities as individual practitioners, it is hard to know what universal "professional behavior" should be.

One story in particular drove home the point of our differences when I heard about a group of elderly men who had been working for years at a hot springs resort in a southern state. Even in the year 2000, they insisted on calling themselves "masseurs," and they were getting paid about $5.00 an hour. Their self-perception was that their massage work was of the same value as the work of the kitchen help and hotel maids. They were deferential, cordial, and "at your service" because that was how a professional at their level behaved.

Figure 3–5 | **How do you see yourself as a professional?**

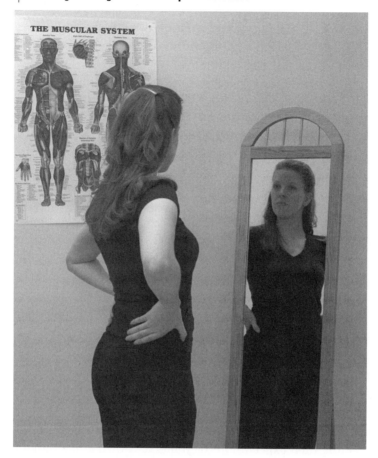

On the other side of professional self-perception are those who believe their work is equal to that of a doctor. Somewhere in the middle are therapists who have professional standards similar to hairstylists, aestheticians, and other service people of that caliber. Others view themselves as artists and live by their own codes and standards. No one way is correct. In each case, the practitioner is directed by his or her own definition of professionalism, and lives by the ethics and behaviors that match it.

As a marketer, your self-definition will affect your marketing message, the kind of client you try to reach, and the behavior you display around your clients. You need to choose it carefully. Each self-definition opens some doors and closes others. If your work is of medical caliber, then your professional presentation will need to be at a similar level to draw clients who want and expect top-quality treatment. However, choosing a medical image will likely turn away people looking for more of a relaxing, spa-type experience. Whatever your choice of self-definition, realize that the consumer wants to trust you and feel safe with you, and your level of professionalism needs to portray to them that you are trustworthy.

Rules and regulations about professionalism can fill pages of text, but I would rather focus on the basics of professionalism that work under any circumstances. Perceive yourself through your clients' eyes, respect your differences, set boundaries, give your clients' needs and wishes priority, and create a self-definition that calls for maturity, stature, and exemplary behavior.

EXERCISE: CREATING YOUR PROFESSIONAL SELF-DEFINITION

Think about what kind of clients you would most enjoy working with. Are they businesspeople, athletes, the elderly, new mothers, people recovering from accidents, or people who are just really stressed? Think about what kind of massage work they would ask you to give them to help with their particular needs. Then think about how they would expect you to look and conduct yourself, given the kind of work you do. Write down your favorite type of client and the type of work you would offer, and write out the details of how you would look and act around those clients. If you are in a group, talk with other people about the kind of clients they want to work with and how they will present themselves as professionals to attract those types of clients.

_____

_____

_____

_____

_____

_____

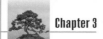

MARKETING ATTRIBUTE #4: EXTRAORDINARY CUSTOMER SERVICE

The difference between professionalism and customer service is that professionalism is about doing what is expected of you, and customer service is about doing what is unexpected. I discovered this distinction during my interviews with massage clients, when I asked them what they liked about their massage experiences. Surprisingly, the happy clients mentioned minor things such as electric foot warmers, flannel sheets, and customized aromatherapy oils. They talked about how much their therapist seemed to care, asked about their lives, and sent birthday cards. Given that many schools and therapists place a primary emphasis on bodywork modalities, I was shocked to discover that most clients I interviewed rarely talked about the technique the therapist used or even mentioned the bodywork itself.

Unless the therapist was hurting the client with too much pressure or was using a painful technique, when an interviewee went back in his or her memory to answer my questions, most talked about what I call the ancillaries: the temperature in the massage room, what kind of music was played during the session, the smell or feel of oils or creams, the softness of pillows, the topics of conversation, the number of minutes in a session's time, the pretty flowers in a waiting room, and other mental bric-a-brac these clients gathered up to form their impression of their massage experience. While good hands-on skills are very important, realize that to your clients, customer service is much more than just efficiently and effectively massaging muscles.

The Center of the Universe

At the soul of customer service is a desire to help your client feel cared for, important, and special. In their heart of hearts, clients believe they are the center of the universe, and, if during a session they feel that you have treated them as such, they will come back to you again and again. (See Figure 3–6.) If you truly aim to help your clients feel cared for and special, it will be natural for you to think of and do the thousands of little things that add up to excellent customer service. Listen to what prospective clients say about what they want, and meet those needs. Imagine what you can do above and beyond those needs, and act on them. Then watch happy clients return and refer their friends.

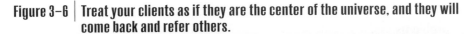

Figure 3-6 | Treat your clients as if they are the center of the universe, and they will come back and refer others.

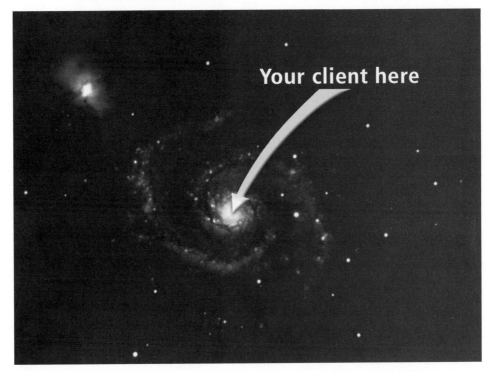

While customer service works primarily for the marketing function of keeping clients you already have, the attitude of genuine caring comes through from you in nearly every situation when you are trying to reach new clients. The word "extraordinary" should be your motto for customer service; it is all the extras on top of the ordinary, or all the unexpecteds on top of the expecteds.

When I asked people what was important to them about their massage therapist, and what they felt shaped their decision to choose or stay with a therapist, these were just some of the many elements of customer service on which they focused:

❋ Personal attention and genuine interest in the client as an individual

❋ Amount of time spent in a session, especially if it felt like a "taximeter" massage

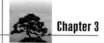
❋ Results of bodywork and whether the therapist could help specific problems

❋ Quality of work and how the therapist's touch felt

❋ Accessibility to book or change appointments, with rapid response to telephone calls

❋ Flexibility of scheduling, including occasional forgiveness for last-minute changes

❋ Preference given for prime-time spots to long-term clients

❋ Caring, remembering details of personal life or stories told, and wanting to help

❋ Compassion for their lives, emotional needs, and physical condition

❋ Friendship and conversation, especially for those who felt lonely or isolated

❋ Education about their bodies and why things were hurting

❋ Information and training on how to care for themselves

❋ Going the extra mile, and researching or learning techniques to help specific problems

❋ Creating an inviting massage environment

As a professional, you will be expected to give a good, quality massage, but add compassion, caring, education, a marvelous place to relax, and real help for physical problems, and you will move into the realm of customer service. Continuously ask yourself how you can make your sessions extraordinary, or even how to make them one of the highlights of your clients' weeks. To do so is to think in a place most businesses do not bother to go. Excellent customer service is quite rare, and if you want to spend more time working and less time marketing, provide great customer care and let your clients market for you.

Many great books have been written about customer service, but of all the books I have read, the one with the most direct application to the personal service of massage is the classic *How to Win Friends and Influence People* by Dale Carnegie. The nature of the client/therapist relationship warrants a deeper understanding of how to relate to and affect others, and if you want to truly serve your clients well, read and reread this book. Human beings have some very core needs that this book can help you understand, and its principles of how to treat other people speak to the heart of customer service.

CHAPTER 3 SUMMARY

Building your dream practice starts with the foundation of the key attributes I found in all of the successful massage therapists I interviewed. These successful therapists were shaped by their desire to serve others and their commitment to succeed, no matter what obstacles lay in their path. They overcame fears, frustrations, and setbacks, and constantly reevaluated themselves and their skills with the intention of always improving. As professionals, they demanded high standards for themselves and their practices, and they put their clients' needs at the top of the list with extraordinary customer service. These people have blazed a trail to success by doing what matters most in building a practice, so use them as role models for your success.

CHAPTER 3 ACTION STEPS

Based on the information in this chapter, do the following to start your dream practice:

- Identify your personal definition of success.
- Write down the elements of your dream practice.
- Review common fears for building a practice, and create a way to succeed in spite of them.
- Review your behavior to keep watch for acts of self-sabotage.
- Create deadlines for reaching your goals, and tell others when those deadlines are due.
- Look at yourself through the eyes of your clients. Do you look and act like what they would want and expect from a professional?
- Review your boundary skills and where your boundaries differ from your clients', and think about how you can best respect those differences.

✳ Review ways you can provide extraordinary customer service by treating clients as if they were the center of the universe.

✳ Create a personal mission that can sustain you throughout the ups and downs of your practice.

CHAPTER 3   KNOWLEDGE CHECK

Check your understanding of the chapter by reviewing these questions and answers.

Q: What is this book's definition of marketing?
A: Marketing is anything you do that affects your ability to get and keep clients.

Q: What are the four attributes of marketing?
A: The desire to serve, the commitment to succeed, professionalism, and extraordinary customer service.

Q: When facing an obstacle to building a practice, what two options are available?
A: Making excuses or getting results.

Q: List three common fears that can affect building a massage practice.
A: The fear of failure, ridicule, rejection, criticism, loss of love, abandonment, making mistakes, not being good enough, not being wanted, and so forth.

Q: What is visualization?
A: Using your imagination for a specific reason.

Q: List two signs of self-sabotage.
A: Being late, procrastination, breaking promises, having accidents, being forgetful, and so forth.

Q: List two ways to continue learning about the massage profession.
A: Seminars, conventions, books, magazines, peer group discussions, and so forth.

Q: What is the biggest benefit of deadlines?
A: They push you to take action before you may feel ready.

Q: List two common social barriers that are removed during a massage.
A: Clothing, personal space, touch, eye contact, an even physical plane, and so forth.

Q: List two conversational boundaries to watch out for with clients.
A: Religion, politics, beliefs, language use, and so forth.

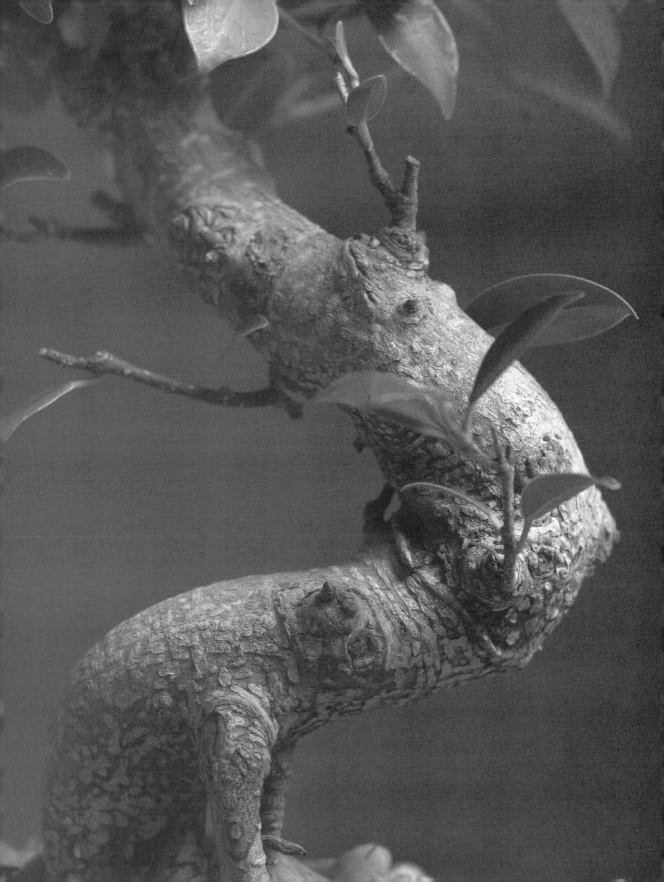

4

Skills at the Soul of Success

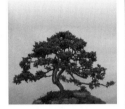

CHAPTER OBJECTIVES

After reading this chapter, you should be able to:

- ❀ Describe the seven levels of the **Perception Continuum** of massage.
- ❀ Educate clients with common misperceptions about massage.
- ❀ Identify elements necessary for creating and maintaining client trust.
- ❀ Describe a professional image you want to convey.
- ❀ Identify six methods of establishing value in your clients' minds.
- ❀ Identify 10 common human needs that massage can meet.
- ❀ Identify factors that affect your prices.
- ❀ Describe three expectations that clients have of their massage experience.
- ❀ Deliver a professional introduction.

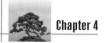

MARKETING SKILLS TO BUILD YOUR DREAM PRACTICE

If attributes are the heart of your marketing, then at the soul of your success are a handful of fundamental skills you must master in order to bring your heart to the people who need it. To build a dream practice requires five necessary skills to reach new clients, rebook those clients, and get personal referrals. Building on the foundation of the four core attributes from the last chapter are the five essential skills of success.

These skills are:

1. Shaping client perception

2. Creating and maintaining trust

3. Establishing value

4. Setting and meeting expectations

5. Reaching out to clients

MARKETING SKILL #1: SHAPING CLIENT PERCEPTION

To build a practice in your community, your marketing strategy needs to take into account what the people in your community think about you and massage. One of the primary goals of marketing is to shape the perception of you and your services in your potential clients' minds. For most businesses, this is a pretty straightforward process. However, massage therapists face some very interesting issues with regard to how the public already sees us, which makes shaping perception a more challenging skill. At this point, massage is going through a period of great transition, and no matter where you work in this country, you must market to a public that fits somewhere along what I call the "Perception Continuum." (See Figure 4–1.)

Figure 4–1 | Understanding how people perceive you will shape your marketing.

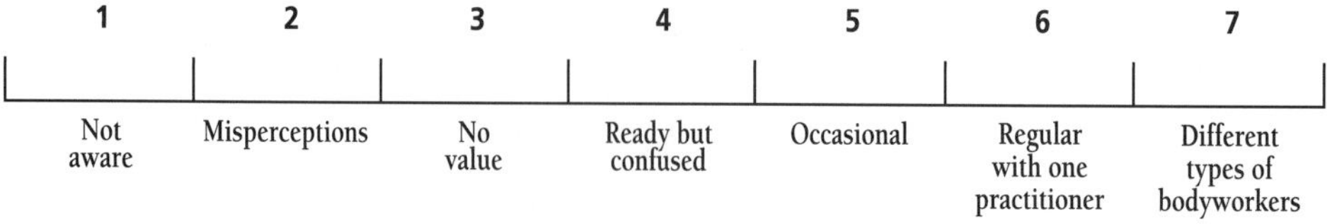

1	2	3	4	5	6	7
Not aware	Misperceptions	No value	Ready but confused	Occasional	Regular with one practitioner	Different types of bodyworkers

The Perception Continuum

The Perception Continuum registers different levels of perception that the public has about massage. It loosely identifies ways you may be perceived by those you encounter, so that you will be better prepared to market accurately and effectively to them. On the Perception Continuum, your potential client is at one of the following levels:

- Level 1: Not aware of massage
- Level 2: Aware of massage, but has misperceptions about it
- Level 3: Aware of massage, but doesn't see its value
- Level 4: Ready and willing to get massage, but confused
- Level 5: Open to massage and gets one occasionally
- Level 6: Regularly gets massage from one practitioner
- Level 7: Gets massage from different types of bodyworkers

Where your potential clients are on this continuum will determine what you need to say or do so they will want to book a massage with you. However, during this time of transition, it is difficult to know what lurks in the minds of those potential clients standing next to you in line at the grocery store. They could think that massage is just for rich people on cruise ships, or they could want a massage and not know how to find a trustworthy therapist. So, how do you create your marketing strategy if you don't know how people see you? In this section on bare-bones marketing, we are simply going to make some educated guesses. In later chapters, we will cover how to create an effective marketing message and develop more specific strategies, but for now, we'll cover the essentials.

Level 1: Not Aware of Massage

Efforts made over many years by thousands of therapists have helped to virtually eliminate this level. Massage is everywhere, advertisements feature massage selling anything from margarine to auto financing, and spas of every size are springing up all over the country. There may be a few people left who haven't heard of massage, but their numbers are dropping daily.

Level 2: Aware of Massage, but Has Misperceptions About It

Level 2 people have heard of massage, but they may have many misconceptions about it, often in the form of negative stereotypes. While these stereotypes are getting replaced, it is important that you know what misgivings or concerns people may have about getting massage because of the history or perception of massage in their minds. The classic unflattering stereotypes usually fit into one of three categories I call the "Three Hs": Helgas, Harlots, or Hippies.

"Helga" is the stereotypical big, beefy Swedish gal in sturdy shoes shown often in advertisements or TV shows (usually about boxing), pummeling the back of some burly man wrapped in a white towel lying down on a table in a steam room. If prospective consumers see this image repeatedly, it can make them think this is what massage is like, and it may not be very appealing to them. Marketing to people who believe this stereotype requires changing their perception. Education is the most effective tool in this case. You can explain to a person that pounding on clients has its place, but by comparison, here's what you do in a typical session. Many people think massage is a painful experience, and since most people don't like pain, you will need to convince them that your touch is wonderful and far from painful.

"Harlots" refers to the unfortunate association that massage therapists are prostitutes, and the confusion between massage parlors and legitimate therapists has hampered efforts to improve regulations that affect therapists, from state licensure and city ordinances to zoning restrictions for offices. While this continues to be an issue in many parts of the country, lobbying by therapists and associations is making it less common for therapists to be harassed by vice squads or to have to get their business licenses at the police department.

However, there are still many potential clients who have believed for years that massage is synonymous with prostitution, and as a marketer, you need to be aware that people you are reaching through your marketing efforts may assume you are offering sex as part of the package. All you have to do is look on the Internet or in the phone book to see that massage is still a cover term for escort services and prostitutes, and if this is a current problem in your area, you need to tailor your marketing accordingly.

If your state or city has outdated, prostitution-based regulations concerning massage, be especially prepared for perceptions about sexual massage. You can take extra caution when reaching out to clients and more clearly define your marketing image so there is no mistaking your legitimacy.

Another persistent stereotype is that of the "hippie," and I have heard people refer to massage therapists as "granola crunchies," "tree huggers," and "woo-woos," complete with the stereotypical imagery of burning incense and "space music." People with this perception can be educated about the benefits and applications of the many methods and modalities of bodywork, but it may take some doing.

A new stereotype is also growing in the public mind, and that is of spas and their many high-priced body treatments I've heard jokingly referred to as "wraps and rubs" or "fluff and buff." Because TV travel shows and glossy magazines show spa treatments of painted-on cocoa paste, avocado rubs, seaweed spreads, mud wraps, Dead Sea salt scrubs, almond exfoliations, and other exotic remedies, many people may think this is all there is to massage. In one of my favorite TV shows, *Great Hotels*, the Travel Channel host, Samantha Brown, goes from one glitzy hotel to another and often gets a treatment at the hotel's spa. If I didn't know better, I would think, after watching many of these shows, that massage was pretty superficial and some of the treatments pretty questionable in their value or effectiveness. Since I teach spa treatment seminars, I know that many spa services are valuable and are wonderfully relaxing, stress reducing, and a viable wellness service, but I suspect a lot of people watching shows like *Great Hotels* will start to confuse massage with spa treatments and will question whether massage is worth the time and money. As a marketer, you need to know that when you talk to people about massage, they may not be interested because they assume you are talking about spa treatments, which are not the same as massage and are valued differently by different markets.

When dealing with any stereotype, your marketing starts with first undoing the false image of massage and then replacing it with an accurate perception of you and your work. Only then can you gain trust and create value in the buyer's mind. Undoing stereotypes and educating people is a large part of marketing massage to Level 2 people, and if you have the desire and patience to aim for this demographic, please read the third section of this book for more tools and skills.

EXERCISE: HANDLING NEGATIVE STEREOTYPES

If you are in a class or group, break up into pairs and designate a Partner A and a Partner B. Partner A acts as a potential new client while Partner B is the massage therapist in an imaginary social conversation at a party. The partners have been introduced briefly by the host, who has also mentioned that Partner B

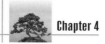

does massage. When the host excuses himself to talk to others, Partner A turns to Partner B.

Scenario 1: Partner A says, "I always thought 'masseuses' worked in massage parlors. What kind of 'masseuse' are you?"

Partner B responds, "Let me tell you about the differences between legitimate massage professionals and massage parlors."

Partner B must find the words to reeducate this potential client so that he or she understands legitimate massage and can value it, and then build up enough trust so this person will book an appointment. Partner B needs to play with words and phrases that educate others without sounding upset, annoyed, or condescending.

Scenario 2: Partner B says, "I see these shows on TV where some lady goes to a spa and they smear chocolate stuff on her and wrap her up in a blanket and then rub her feet. Is that really what massage is?"

Partner A responds, "Well, that's one part of the massage field. Let me tell you about the other kind of work massage therapists do."

Partner A then needs to find a way to reshape a preconceived notion so that the listener is more fully educated about massage.

If you are reading this book by yourself, practice speaking aloud what you would say in response to these two questions. You may never get these two common misperceptions dumped in your lap so unceremoniously, but be prepared. These thoughts may be lurking in the minds of others, and you will do yourself a favor by having a solid, ready answer to versions of these questions.

Level 3: Aware of Massage, but Doesn't See Its Value

Potential clients at Level 3 require different marketing tactics than those at Levels 1 and 2. While Level 1 needs to be informed and Level 2 needs to undo negative stereotypes, Level 3 needs a strong emphasis on the many benefits of massage. Much of the message of massage in our culture doesn't show the many types of massage available. Therapeutic massage, medical massage, energy massage, and many Eastern modalities get very little

publicity, so people who could be helped with work beyond the relaxation and stress reduction modalities don't even know massage can help them. Reaching this market requires a delicate balance between fully informing people about the kind of work you do and how it can help their many different needs, and overwhelming them with too many details about how you work. This is a benefit-driven style of marketing that focuses on telling people how many ways massage can help them, while leaving out all the titles, modalities, and styles of work, so you don't clutter your message. Your message is all about potential clients and their needs, with little emphasis on you and your work.

Level 4: Ready and Willing to Get a Massage, but Confused

Level 4 people are a great market at which to aim. These are people who are interested in getting a massage and either have not had one yet or are not committed to a local practitioner. So what are they confused about? They don't know which massage establishment is legitimate, what modality to get, or where to find a quality therapist. They do not need convincing to try massage, and you are not actively competing with other therapists for their business. Usually, they are simply waiting for the right therapist to come across their path.

As alternative health care has repeatedly proven itself as a viable option for Americans, and as massage continues to gain the credibility and recognition it so richly deserves, the Level 4 group is growing exponentially. More and more people are hearing about or experiencing the value of massage. They are getting results they haven't been able to get elsewhere, and they are increasing their willingness to pay for protecting or improving their health.

People at Level 4 are familiar and comfortable with the images of massage they have seen on television or in magazines. They have come to accept mass media advertisers' promotion of massage as what I call "The Poster Child of the Good Life." In my travels, I have repeatedly had the experience of talking about massage with people who get a wistful look and say, "Oh, I've always wanted a massage!" This remark is usually accompanied by the person's hand instinctively reaching for a sore neck, shoulder, or lower back, and a sort of pitiful moment of rubbing, complete with a sad look in his or her eyes. If ever there were a marketing moment where you could easily begin a working relationship with someone, this is it! Their perception is shaped, their desire is apparent, their need is almost universal, and there you are, ready and eager to help.

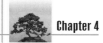

For people who do more than just dream about a good back rub, the typical response is "I've been looking for a good therapist! Are you available, or can you recommend someone?" Many people think marketing is supposed to be harder than this, but the field is ready to be harvested in many places, and for people at Level 4, the best marketing strategy you can use is to show up and start talking.

Level 5: Open to Massage and Gets One Occasionally

Potential clients at Level 5 are often on the hunt for a good massage therapist. They are open to massage, have a little experience, are learning what they like and don't like, and are becoming savvier as consumers. In many ways they are like Level 4 people, in that just meeting you and talking with you may be enough to get them on your table. However, anticipate that they may have had a bad experience, which unfortunately is not uncommon, and be ready to listen to complaints about what a prior therapist has done. Common complaints include being bruised or hurt, especially after so-called "deep tissue" work done by under-trained therapists. Other issues include lack of professionalism and overstepping boundaries, or ineffective work that was little more than someone pushing oil around for an hour. Unpleasant as it can be to listen to complaints about other therapists, as a good marketer you can pay attention to the details and then explain how and why those issues won't come up during your work.

Levels 6 and 7: Regularly Gets Massage from One Practitioner, and Gets Massage from Different Types of Bodyworkers

Gaining clients from the last two levels of the Perception Continuum will take more than just showing up and being seen. With clients at Levels 6 and 7, you now face the marketing issues of competition and differentiation. Most people starting out in massage are neither likely to be actively competing with established practitioners, nor do they know enough about themselves or their markets to know how to differentiate themselves effectively in the minds of their potential clients. If you are at the point in your career where you face great competition or are ready to differentiate yourself so that potential clients will understand and value what you offer, then you need to go beyond the bare-bones marketing of this section and move on to the muscle marketing in the third section of this book, which offers many strategies for dealing with competition.

Most of the successful therapists I have met, though, know their competition is not with other therapists. They know that there are thousands of people in their area who have either never had a massage or are looking for a therapist who suits them. As a marketer in a booming field, if you know your true competition is with ignorance, misperception, and lack of trust and value in the public mind, you will be able to spend your time, energy, and money more effectively to reach the people who are looking for you.

Someday, massage will achieve what many of us have been working toward for years: full public awareness and value of the profession; widespread accurate and positive public perception; demand for bodywork specialties based on needs; and regulatory laws that are clear, consistent, and massage friendly. Until that time arrives, the skill of shaping perception is critical to success. It begins with understanding what public perceptions currently exist, choosing which level of client you are willing and able to work with, and developing a marketing strategy appropriate to that level of perception. That said, for the level of marketing we are dealing with in this section, if you study the four core attributes, go after the many people who are looking for their first good massage, and apply the next four skills, you will have done enough to get and keep clients to start your practice.

MARKETING SKILL #2: GAINING AND MAINTAINING TRUST

As you have seen with the Perception Continuum, many different attitudes, opinions, and beliefs exist about massage. Recognizing and dealing with those perceptions are important elements to your success because they greatly affect your next marketing skill: the ability to gain trust.

Trust is critical in the field of massage for two reasons. First, potential clients must trust the practitioner enough to let themselves be touched. Second, practitioners must trust that the client has no intention to harm or harass them. During this transition time in the massage profession, gaining and maintaining trust is a two-way street between client and practitioner and, therefore, takes more skill and effort than in other professions.

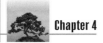

Trusting the Practitioner—How to Help Others Trust You

As humans, our ability to trust is based on our accumulated experiences over time. These experiences teach us how to evaluate and judge other people. For ease of processing the millions of bits of data we encounter every time we meet new people or are in new situations, humans have created a shorthand method of dealing with others and the environment. This shorthand has many facets, but the one we have to deal with most in creating trust is stereotyping. Stereotyping helps us make quick decisions in unfamiliar situations, and it is a skill that has been crucial for survival from time immemorial. The stereotyping in this section is different than what was discussed in the Perception Continuum. There, we looked at common historical stereotypes about massage therapists. Here, we are considering general human stereotypes used especially to evaluate someone's trustworthiness. While stereotyping may not be politically correct, it is deeply imbedded into our psyches.

Handling Stereotypes to Gain Trust

As a massage therapist, you need to know what types of judgments people will be making about you so you can prove you are someone to whom they can entrust their bodies. You will be evaluated and judged, often quite quickly, and will be dealing with what is essentially a form of prejudice, or a prejudgment made about you, before you will be allowed to massage someone. While it may not seem fair that people make instant decisions about your massage work based on how you are dressed, how you talk, or how you stand, that's just the way it is. People have to gather data about whether or not you will be safe and trustworthy, and their strongest first impressions of you will be based on your personal presentation. To let their subconscious minds know you are someone they can trust, people will use as many of their senses as they can to determine their feelings about you.

What Clients See in Your Personal Presentation

The first sense your potential clients most likely will use to evaluate you is sight. People will look at your clothes, your posture, how you move, what your body language says, how you style your hair, and any other visual clues they can gain about you. You don't have to be a beauty queen, dashingly handsome, or dress like a model; you simply have to look like someone who is safe enough to touch them.

If your potential client is a friend or an acquaintance, your personal presentation and appearance may not be as crucial, but it is still important. You need to understand that no matter how well you know people, touching them with massage is a different level of connection and may be scary for them. Regardless of who you are massaging, friends or strangers need to trust you first, so look and act the part of a trustworthy professional, no matter what.

Common sense would suggest that everyone knows to look professional. However, one of the biggest complaints from massage employers is that therapists arrive for work with clothing, hair, and makeup entirely inappropriate for creating trust, safety, and mutual respect between client and practitioner. Some of the following points may seem obvious to you, but personal appearance is such an issue in gaining trust that it must be dealt with directly and spelled out clearly.

Personal Appearance Dos

The rules for a massage professional's personal appearance are pretty basic. Wear clean, comfortable clothes that let you move easily, can be washed frequently, and are acceptable to your clients. Wear hairstyles that keep your hair off your clients and represent the image you want to create. If you wear makeup, keep it professional looking. Wear shoes that are comfortable and can support your feet for hours of standing.

Carry your body with pride. Stand tall, radiate confidence, smile, make good eye contact, hold your head up straight, and look like you are someone who has a good, safe, wonderful touch. Whenever you deal with clients, come across as relaxed, competent, capable, friendly, and ready and willing to be of service. These are attributes clients want before they turn over their time, money, and bodies to someone else. Overall, imagine seeing yourself through your clients' eyes. Ask yourself whether your personal presentation sends the message to your clients that they will be well taken care of.

If you do not feel confident or capable, or are a bit shy, practice carrying your body as if you were confident, capable, and outgoing. Your mind will believe what your face and body are portraying, so when in doubt, smile big, straighten your shoulders, and move with purpose. As one of my very successful colleagues loves to say, "Fake it till you make it!" Most of my best students lacked initial confidence in the quality of their work, but despite their fears, they went out, presented themselves as if they had benefits to offer their clients, and ended up helping people. Their real confidence came later, when they realized they actually did good work. Until that time, they worked at presenting themselves well on the outside despite how they felt on the inside.

Perhaps the best way to decide how you will present yourself can be based on the concept of **congruency**. Basically, congruency means that everything you say, do, wear, and so forth has a feel or an aura to it that is consistent. Congruency is part of what your clients will look for in determining their trust in you, so if you want to be perceived as a professional who offers quality service, you have to look and act the part or they won't believe you. The congruency of your self-presentation is both for you as an individual and you as a stereotype of your clients' perceptions of what a professional massage therapist should look like.

Personal Appearance Don'ts

When creating trust, perhaps more important than the general personal appearance dos are the much more specific personal appearance don'ts. Being taken seriously as a professional is greatly undermined by a poor personal presentation. If you want to command high fees and/or gain new clients, don't do the following.

For women especially, do not wear tight or revealing clothing. This includes leotards, tube tops, halter-tops, tank tops, low-cut blouses, or shirts that show your stomach. Short skirts, short shorts, cutoffs, bicycle shorts, and anything equally revealing or provocative need to be kept out of the professional wardrobe. There are no clothes police out there enforcing these suggestions, but if you want to avoid sexual harassment by clients and be treated as a professional, dress appropriately. As a rule, the less skin you show, the better.

These suggestions have not been made up arbitrarily. They are designed to demonstrate your professional stature, but they also can protect you from sexual harassment or scaring away people who think massage is sexual in nature. Of particular importance are the concerns I have heard from a number of male clients that some men want to try massage, but they don't because they are afraid they would become inadvertently aroused. This fear of arousal and subsequent embarrassment is not talked about very much, but I suspect it keeps many men from getting massage. While this topic is not one to address directly with prospective clients, you can address it indirectly with professional attire and a no-nonsense attitude and energy. If a man is concerned about arousal and sees that the therapist dresses provocatively, he may opt to just say "no" rather than risk the overwhelming training of his body and our culture that touch is primarily for the purpose of sex. For some men, it is difficult at first to be touched and not get aroused. However, as I know from my male clients and students, men can be trained by experience that touch can be pleasurable, nurturing, caring, and therapeutic, and it will no longer always arouse them. Arousal is not harassment, and it is not the practitioner's "fault" if the client gets aroused. That said, your behavior and your clothes make a huge difference between whether arousal becomes harassment or does not occur at all.

The personal presentation of male practitioners needs to be professional as well. In particular, it needs to tell your clients that you will not be coming on to them. Women often express a concern about having male therapists because they are worried about the massage being sexualized, so it is crucial that your appearance and behavior reassure them that you will be trustworthy. On the flip side, professional dress also sends the message that you are not open to them coming on to you, which can certainly happen. I have heard a number of stories in which a woman was moved in the moment by how wonderful a male therapist's touch felt, especially if her own husband or boyfriend didn't touch her well, and she propositioned the male therapist. Needless to say, the therapists who succumbed to the propositions were fired from their jobs or arrested, sometimes on the charge of rape, even though the client started it.

The clothing rules for men are basically the same as for women. The less skin you show, the better. Tank tops, sleeveless shirts, bicycle shorts, tight pants, unbuttoned shirts, or trying to look sexually attractive are all potential signals to female clients that they may need to be on their guard. This keeps them from establishing trust and therefore booking or rebooking appointments. As a general recommendation, stay away from stained, faded, or torn clothes; T-shirts with controversial slogans, images, or pictures of heavy metal bands; "gangsta" or hip-hop wear; ball caps; overalls; and ill-fitting clothing. Droopy pants may look cool on the street, but they look dumb on a professional. If you do choose to wear white clothes, make sure they are nice and white, not dingy and gray. Again, no fashion police will arrest you if you wear such clothes to your sessions, but that type of dress basically marks the wearer as an amateur.

Your goal with your presentation is to gain trust and instill value, so dress sharp. If you work at a spa or business, expect to have a uniform of sorts, often a polo shirt and khaki pants, which isn't a bad idea even if you have your own practice. (See Figure 4–2.)

Figure 4–2 | **What does your personal presentation tell your clients about you?**

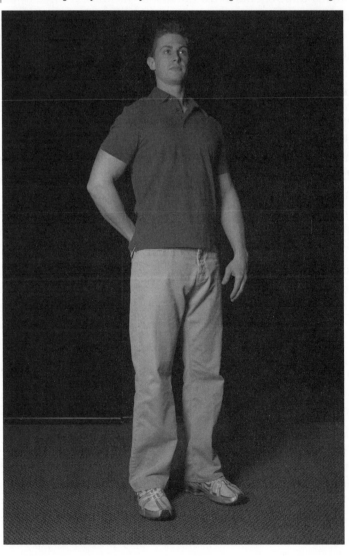

Shoes are another important factor in presentation, and the issue for some people is whether to wear shoes or not. If your practice is going to be barefoot Shiatsu, then this is not an issue, but many therapists face the question of wearing shoes while working. I don't have strong recommendations either way, except for the time you meet new or potential clients, or when your current clients are arriving and leaving. Even with your current clients, wear shoes when you greet them and say good-bye. With first-time clients, shoes are part of shaping their perception and gaining trust, and basically should be worn on introduction.

I feel strongly about this, especially based on a sad but true story one of my clients told me. My client was going to see an acupuncturist, and because I was out of town for an extended period, she decided to try a massage from the therapist who worked in the acupuncturist's office. When it was time for my client's appointment, the massage therapist opened her office door, walked into the lobby in bare feet, and introduced herself. Although a bit surprised, my client figured the therapist fit into the leftover hippie population of massage therapists and let it go, or so she thought. By itself, greeting a new client in bare feet may not seem like a big deal, but it cast an initial doubt in my client's mind as to this person's professional level.

As my client told me later, this first doubt then caused her to notice other trivial things that she might otherwise have overlooked. Once the door of doubt was open about this woman's qualifications or professionalism, things went downhill. By the time the session was over, she had taken her first misgivings, added to them some minor but bothersome observations and feelings, and had come up with the final decision that she would never book another appointment with that therapist.

What intrigued me most about my client's story was that one moment of lost trust virtually undid the rest of the massage therapist's marketing. Amazingly, this therapist had numerous and sophisticated marketing tools, including a great business card, a fancy brochure, a secretary to book her appointments, and inclusion on the office Web site. She even had the great marketing advantage of offering insurance reimbursements through prescriptions written for massage by the acupuncturist she worked for, and, to top it all off, her hourly rates were lower than mine. One would think that, by having all these wonderful elements of marketing in place, success would be guaranteed, but it wasn't. This massage therapist made the mistake of losing her clients' trust through poor self-presentation, and it cost her that client and, I suspect, a few others.

The skill of creating trust has other elements of self-presentation to consider. Personal adornments such as jewelry, makeup, tattoos, and body piercings are also part of how people judge you. Forms of personal self-expression are touchy subjects, and people will have many opinions about them. Therefore, the only way I can rise above opinion is to state what I have experienced. Basically, the older, wealthier, or more conservative your clientele, the more conservatively you will need to present yourself. Of course, there are exceptions to every rule, but for most therapists, multiple body and facial piercings, tattoos, and other counterculture adornments will make it harder to gain trust with clients in mainstream America. Not everyone is bothered by piercings and tattoos, but many people are, and some will worry that if you are willing to hurt or scar your own body, how well are you going to treat theirs?

It is not fair, but in marketing, perception is reality, and much of America still has negative perceptions about piercings and tattoos. I have known a number of successful therapists who are highly decorated, but their bodywork is extraordinary and their marketing consists of almost all word-of-mouth referrals. Their new clients have a high level of trust based on the referrals, which will likely supersede their prior prejudices. However, even though their current clients may be fine with their adornments, I wonder if these same clients hesitate to buy their mothers or fathers massage gift certificates from these therapists.

Jewelry that can scratch clients, long fingernails that can gouge skin or prevent effective hand use, or makeup that looks like it belongs in a nightclub are among many other examples of personal presentation that come down to the basic question: is your need for external self-expression worth risking the loss of a client? Personal presentation isn't about what is right or wrong, or even about what everyone else is doing or wearing. Your choices come down to whether or not it matters to you that your potential clients trust you, even before you touch them. If they do trust you, they are more likely to book, then rebook and refer. If they don't trust you, you will have to keep working to get more new clients.

If no one trusts you, eventually you will have to get out of massage altogether. No trust, no practice. It's that simple. For some people, this is a difficult choice, but now you get to make an educated choice knowing that your personal appearance is a crucial part of building a strong practice.

Reverse Trust

The second element of trust in building a practice revolves around whether or not you, the therapist, can trust your clients. Due to misperceptions about massage and prostitution, and because of unpredictable sexual arousal by clients, this is a topic to be taken seriously. Two primary factors of trusting your clients will greatly affect your ability and willingness to market your services. The first is whether you can trust that your client won't harass or harm you. The second is whether or not you trust that you can reach your clients without harassment by various law enforcement agencies. This isn't much fun to talk about when all you want to do is help others with your massage, but this angle of trust—or rather, mistrust—has shut down the practices of too many quality therapists to not address it with blunt honesty.

Trusting the Client

At this time, a large majority of massage therapists are women, and for women working out of their homes or doing outcall to their clients' homes, being able to trust potential clients is critical for safety as well as success. Obtaining safety and success calls for marketing options that screen out potentially dangerous clients while still making you visible enough to attract legitimate ones.

Unfortunately, many of the traditional marketing strategies of advertising, public relations, and media exposure can attract dangerous callers. I have spoken with colleagues who have phone book ads that clearly state "nonsexual massage" or "therapeutic only," and provide a license number or an association **logo** to add legitimacy, all to no avail. People still call looking for sex. The unwelcome clients are pretty easy to spot. They ask questions such as, "Do you do full body massage?" or "Do you work on all the muscles?" or "Do you do extras?" They use phrases like "happy ending," "prostatic massage," or "full release" to test what kind of therapist you are. These and other transparent code words are a giveaway to what they are really looking for. At the risk of possibly offending a legitimate client, my colleagues who use mass-media marketing have carefully crafted answers and a whole set of questions that don't accuse the caller of anything but do screen out potential trouble.

For anyone who wants to avoid this type of harassment, perhaps the only safe way of marketing is by word-of-mouth referrals, which we will cover in great depth in the following chapters. Whatever type of marketing you use, you will always need to screen your clients (which we will also cover later). For now, just realize that once again we face marketing issues that are unique to our field and require different marketing strategies than anyone else has to use.

Trusting the "Authorities"

The second factor of reverse trust is whether or not you know you can go about your business of getting and keeping clients without being harassed by state or local authorities. This issue is not often talked about, but many therapists work in areas where authorities still conduct what are akin to witch-hunts on legitimate therapists, and it greatly affects their ability to market. In fact, as one of my colleagues who had fought for fair licensure in San Francisco jokingly remarked, at one point just about the only massage people working legally in San Francisco were the prostitutes. Obviously there are legitimate therapists working legally in San Francisco, but it is amazing that even in one of the most liberal cities in the country, massage therapists have a hard time getting a license to practice. How sad that the owners of illegal parlors have the money, connections, and know-how to gather up phony school certificates and pay the right people for licenses for call girls, when qualified therapists have to fight for the right to get a license to practice.

San Francisco is not the only place that makes it difficult to practice legally. A significant number of practitioners I interviewed across the country were working without a business license, either because they could not get one, or because the process was too prohibitive or demeaning. After hearing stories about therapists being forced to put drains in the middle of their office floor so they could hose down the room after each session, or being set up by vice squads with undercover agents harassing therapists for sexual favors so they could bust them, I can see why so many people opt to work without all of their appropriate licenses.

My mother (also a massage therapist), who is a minister's wife and the picture of a quintessential grandmother, had to go through the vice squad ringer to get her city business license. She had to get a doctor's clearance certificate for sexually transmitted diseases, endure a police background check, have mug shots taken, and go through months of foot-dragging before she got a city license to do on-site massage in an office building. Another colleague of mine was told that the city where she lived only gave out four massage permits because "we don't need more than four masseuses in town." Being the 5th or 50th massage therapist in town means practicing illegally.

I look forward to the day that our field is regulated fairly and without the specter of prostitution hanging over it, but that day is not yet here in many parts of the country. Dedicated people have fought for years to be treated fairly by regulating authorities, and their work has paved the way for the profession to grow, but there is still much work to be done. It is only through ongoing efforts that massage will get its due, so it is important that you do what you can to work legally.

If you are fortunate enough to work in an area that treats massage therapy like any other service business, you can have fewer concerns about who you can trust, and you can use more forms of marketing safely. If not, then you will have less room to trust others, and your practice will need to be built almost exclusively from personal referrals. Informal marketing and talking with people you meet can get things started, and the material in a later chapter on **mutual marketing** also can be of great assistance.

Overall, the issue of reverse trust is one of the biggest our profession faces. As our field continues to grow and gain legitimacy, hopefully these concerns will fade off into the distance and just be old war stories that horrified newcomers hear at conventions or read about in old marketing books. Until that day arrives, though, many practitioners who are basically forced to keep a low profile will need to market "under the radar" and trust their intuition about who they can trust in the process of building a practice.

MARKETING SKILL #3: ESTABLISHING VALUE

The third essential marketing skill you need to get people under your hands is the ability to establish the belief in their minds that your work is valuable to them. Fortunately, massage is so valuable to so many people, for so many different reasons, that this skill can be mastered with some good thought and effort.

If gaining trust is the emotional part of a person's decision to get a massage, then believing in its value is the intellectual justification most people need to commit the time and money for your services. Where people are on the

Perception Continuum will affect how much they value massage and how much they are willing to pay for it. If your primary market is the group of people who are already looking for a good massage therapist, creating value will not be too difficult or require a huge marketing campaign. If your primary market needs to be convinced of the value of massage or have their misperceptions changed, then you will have to work harder on this skill.

However, no matter where your potential clients are on the Perception Continuum, they all have basic needs that are core to being human. One way to start a practice is to decide what basic human needs you are able to meet with massage, then market your desire and expertise to meet those needs. The ability to establish value in others' minds will be based on which needs of theirs you can meet and how much they want those needs met.

Following are six questions for establishing value:

1. What **universal needs** do human beings have?

2. How do massage and bodywork meet those needs?

3. What is your ability and desire to meet those needs?

4. Who is your competition that already meets those needs?

5. What are those needs worth to your potential clients?

6. How do you put a price on your ability to meet their needs?

Question 1—What Universal Needs Do Human Beings Have?

Human beings have a vast number of wants. However, we have a much smaller number of true needs that are core to us as a species. Great minds have pondered human needs over hundreds of years and have made lists and pyramid charts trying to synthesize what drives human behavior and motivation. Distilled down, these lists reveal two drives. Simply stated, the two core human needs are to avoid pain and gain pleasure. Basically, we do what we do to feel good, stop hurting, or avoid getting hurt. If this is truly the case, massage therapists are in luck! Of all the other service professions in existence, very few have the ability that we do to offer both pleasure and pain relief. What's even more amazing is that we can do both simultaneously. Even in comparison to other health-care services, we have the advantage because our clients are happy to keep their appointments. Really, how many people truly look forward to seeing their dentist, or say "I've been looking forward to this all week!" when they get their annual medical checkup? Oh, the advantages we have!

As bodyworkers, we address the realms of body, mind, and spirit, and if we mix and match those with the needs to gain pleasure and avoid pain, we can more consciously identify the value we offer to specific markets. (See Figure 4–3.) Clients with mental, emotional, physical, or spiritual/energetic needs want

Figure 4–3 | **The value of massage is flexible, and depends on the wants and need of the client.**

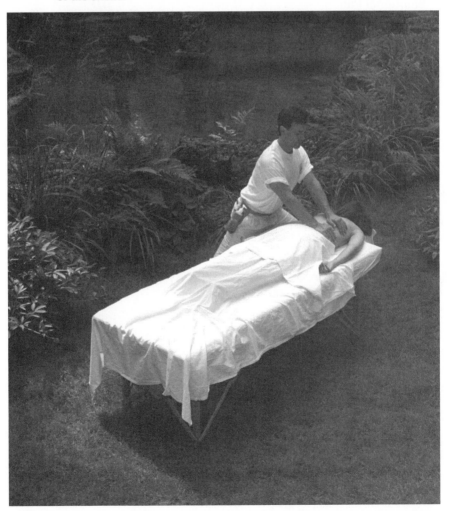

help, and you can offer it. The more you understand these needs, the more valuable you will discover massage to be in meeting so many of them at once. Let's take a closer look at some of the many needs massage therapists can meet.

Pains People Want to Avoid that Massage Can Help

Mental pain

>   Stress

>   Feeling overwhelmed by life or circumstances

>   Boredom

Emotional Pain

>   Loss

>   Insecurity

>   Loneliness

>   Insignificance

>   Isolation

Physical Pain

>   Lack of touch

>   Musculoskeletal soreness or pain

>   Stress-related tension

>   Poor posture

Conditional

>   Tired or fatigued

>   Sleep deprived

Injury

>   Sports related

>   Job related

>   Accident or trauma

Illness

Pleasures People Want to Gain that Massage Can Provide

Mental Pleasure

    Self-awareness

    Self-understanding

    Exploration and learning

    Performance enhancement

    Variety

    Conversation

    Clarity

    Zoning out

Emotional Pleasure

    Feeling loved

    Feeling safe

    Getting attention

    Acceptance

    Feeling popular

    Feeling important

    Feeling successful

    Feeling special

    Feeling better

    Feeling attractive

    Feeling pampered or indulgent

    Feeling deserving

    Happiness

    Having a relationship with you

    Feeling a sense of belonging

    Feeling a sense of significance

Feeling a sense of security

Feeling connected

Feeling needed by you

Making a contribution to you

Physical Pleasure

Touch is healing

Massage feels good

Letting go of stress and tension

Performance enhancement—sports, activities

Looking good—younger, vibrant, posture

Feeling well

Better able to care for self and others, including children

Remaining mobile

Being pain-free

Being healthy

Feeling attractive

The list can go on, but it is clear that massage is valuable to a lot of people for many different reasons. What other reasons can you think of?

EXERCISE: MEETING YOUR CLIENTS' NEEDS

Take another look at the lists of needs and ask yourself these questions.

Which of these needs can I help people with right now? Put an X by those needs.

Which of these needs would I enjoy helping people meet? Underline those needs.

Which of these needs would I want to help people with, but I need more training? Put an O by those.

Which of these needs do I have no real interest in? Draw a line through those.

Now write down how and why massage is valuable. Start with the phrase, "Massage Is Valuable Because I Can Help People . . ."

Below that, review the needs you have underlined or marked with an X, and make a new list that is tailored to you. As you consider each of the basic needs that you are capable of meeting and are interested in as well, make additions to the ones that are meaningful to you. If you can think of needs that you want to meet that are not on these pages, write them in. Your page can look something like this.

Example: Massage Is Valuable Because I Can Help People . . .

Feel less lonely

Figure out why they are hurting and help them make changes

Play tennis without hurting

Let go of their stress

Feel successful, like they've "arrived"

Get touched, especially when no one else touches them

Have a safe place to cry

Just let go and relax

Feel okay about their own bodies

_____

_____

_____

_____

_____

_____

Once you are done, look at your list in amazement. You have so much to give that so many people want and need! And this is just the tip of the iceberg!

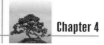

Once you have some idea of what needs massage meets, look at the next five questions for establishing value.

Question 2—How Do Massage and Bodywork Meet Client Needs?

The value of massage can be established with both direct and indirect benefits. Direct benefits are what people often use in traditional marketing. Increased circulation, better range of motion, decreased blood pressure, and other such benefits all sound great, but they aren't usually what people really want to buy. These are results of massage, and they are what we are comfortable talking about. However, they aren't really what motivates people to spend the time and money on your services.

This creates a bit of a dilemma in marketing massage. First, it's not polite or even effective to run ads that say "Are you lonely? Does nobody touch you? Are you embarrassed by your body? Do you want something to brag about to your neighbors? Then come get a massage, and I can help!" The second dilemma is that most people want marketing messages proven to them. How does pressing on muscles help people feel less lonely or learn to accept themselves at a deeper level? There is a lot of anecdotal evidence that it does, but anecdotal evidence on the many indirect benefits of massage is not given much attention in current research. While our field is gathering evidence in research studies proving the value of our work, what people really want to buy is often what we cannot prove.

Not being able to talk about or prove the indirect benefits of massage leaves us with a few options. We can talk about the direct effects, relaxed muscles, lower stress, and other benefits that appeal to the justification side of the brain. We can also get our message across in a more indirect way using the power of intention, one of the most powerful tools utilized during bodywork. If intention can work on the table, it can work in marketing. If you hold in your mind the knowledge of the value of massage, and communicate with silent intention the ways you can really help people, I believe they can hear those silent messages and will know you have so much more to offer that will be meaningful and valuable to them.

Whether you have a formal marketing program or just talk about massage to people you encounter in your everyday life, keep in mind the many needs you can meet, and approach people with the confidence of knowing how much you are able to do for them. Finally, because of all the indirect benefits you offer through your time, attention, and touch, you already provide a valuable service, even if it isn't the latest and greatest bodywork modality to come around. Your power to help address most of the needs on the lists for relieving pain and gaining pleasure can come from good basic massage skills that are applied well, along with compassion, caring, and what most everyone wants: a little attention.

Question 3—What Is Your Ability and Desire to Meet Those Needs?

One of the joys I experienced as a teacher was seeing the marvelous differences among my students. They were all in class to learn the same skills, but I knew each of them would end up with very different types of practices. The beauty of massage is that we can apply our basic skills with very different outcomes depending on the needs of the clients we are drawn to serving.

When you are trying to establish your value in the marketplace, you need to understand and recognize which needs people have that you are able to meet and that you want to meet. To figure out which needs you can best meet, consider the following:

Your inherent personality

Your background, which includes your training and life experience

Your upbringing

Your personal beliefs and values

Your desire to serve

Your ability to serve

For example, if a woman grew up living with a mother who had a lot of pain because of an illness or injury, and the woman gave her mother little massages that helped ease her pain, the woman learned from an early age that she could help people with her touch. She also experienced the value and joy of helping others, and she figured out that giving massages gave her a special connection with people. Or, maybe a man had a bad auto accident and lived with a lot of pain, but it wasn't until a massage therapist helped him that he finally felt better. This person was so grateful that someone could help him, he dedicated his life to being able to do the same for others. Given your background, your experiences, and your personality, what kinds of needs would you most naturally want to help others deal with?

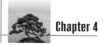

Question 4—Who or What Is Your Competition That Already Meets Those Needs?

Competition is probably one of the most misunderstood facets of marketing massage. Students and practitioners complain about crowded markets, too many other therapists competing in the same neighborhoods, or local schools "pumping out" graduates, all with the firmly held belief that these somehow will take away their access to a tiny pool of clients. Since the pool of clients is comprised of the millions of people who have never even had a massage, we have a huge reservoir of clients from which to draw, and we would be better served exploring our true competition so we can market effectively instead of placing blame and complaining that other people are taking our clients.

If competition is whatever affects people's hearts, minds, and wallets so that they don't book a massage with you, then your biggest competition isn't with other therapists; it is with ignorance. Ignorance about what? About how much massage can help meet people's wants and needs in so many ways. Combine ignorance with mistrust and a lack of value for your services, and you've just identified your main opponent to success. This means that your marketing should be primarily educational, and the purpose of your marketing should be to tell people about the many benefits and values of massage.

Another area of competition we face is from the many other products and services that have nothing to do with massage, but are also able to meet the different needs massage can serve. If you recognize this, you can compete with their draw by addressing your comparative benefits. For example, if you market to clients who need stress reduction, your competition can be psychotherapists, biofeedback experts, or hypnotherapists. The benefit of massage over these services is that you can aid clients in learning stress-management skills while helping undo the physical manifestations of stress in their bodies. None of the other services can use touch as part of their stress-management assistance, leaving us with an incredible and enviable advantage.

Because massage has the great flexibility to serve many markets and needs, we have amazing marketing angles. However, that flexibility can also be a disadvantage. Since our services and fees can be judged and compared with values in other industries, you will have to know more about those industries as you try to establish your value in your buyer's mind.

For example, let's say your market is the group of people in search of relaxation and pampering. Their mental budget for massage can be weighed against other pampering category expenditures such as a nice dinner out, a weekend getaway trip, or a facial. Essentially, you are competing for their pampering dollars, and your value as a pampering experience needs to be the same as or better than other experiences in order to get their business.

Similarly, let's say you are aiming for the market that has a goal of spending money on what makes them look or feel good. Here you are competing with hairstylists, aestheticians, personal trainers, a new pair of shoes, a new makeup kit, or a visit to the plastic surgeon. Discretionary income can be fickle in this market, and if your clients are on a semi-tight budget, their decision may come down to getting a massage from you or buying a new handbag. Your job is to generate enough value in your clients' minds so that if they want that new handbag, they will cut something else from their budget before they cut massage.

If your goal is to build a practice in the medical massage market, you face competition from other medical services. On the marketing front, you will be in competition for medical dollars—an area in which the massage profession has already done quite well—but be careful because you can close doors on other markets if you get too wrapped up in only pushing for clients from the medical model. Overall, massage has proven itself as an effective health-care service for centuries without getting caught in the medical model trap, and individual therapists and the profession as a whole could be risking growth if we try to force massage solely in that direction.

People are fleeing Western medicine in droves and running to alternative therapies for many reasons, so why model ourselves after a sinking ship? Many people go to doctors because they want a professional's time and attention focused on them and their aches and pains, but since insurance companies only allow doctors a few minutes per patient, clients often get a pill but not enough attention. Massage therapists have the ability to give people time, a listening ear, and caring attention, and this is part of why our popularity has soared. Compete in the medical market if that is where your heart is, but realize that the reasons people see doctors are often deeper than the symptoms they claim, and massage can be much more helpful for those silent needs beneath the symptoms.

If you have advanced training and a therapeutic bodywork specialty that gets good results with injuries and soft tissue problems, you can do well in the medical massage field. You may choose to work in a doctor's office or work on your own with referred patients. In this case, your competition can become your ally. As a marketer, when you consider other competitors from other professions, consider the possibility that they also could become allies and great sources of referrals. Those aestheticians, hairstylists, and makeup salespeople all know people who might want massage, so be a smart marketer and befriend your competition.

If you are fortunate enough to live in an area where you experience competition with other massage therapists, consider yourself lucky! This means that other therapists already have been training the general public and moving them further along the Perception Continuum toward accepting and valuing massage. Your job is a lot easier because of those around you simultaneously working to educate the public. Your fellow massage therapists are your allies, not your enemies. Again, your primary battle is with ignorance. Many therapists have sacrificed much of their time, money, and energy to change the hearts and minds of the general public, knowing full well that someone else will reap the rewards of their efforts. Massage therapists have no need for a scarcity mindset. Scarcity makes us miss the opportunities right in front of us, and really, any person who has a body is a potential client. Until every body is being massaged, there is room for us all.

Question 5—What Are Those Needs Worth to Your Potential Clients?

Part of marketing involves evaluating what a product or service is worth to a customer or client, and what factors affect that worth. Why, for example, would people pay $30 for a bottle of wine at a restaurant when they know they can buy it at the grocery store for $15? Has the wine's inherent value suddenly jumped? Of course not. However, the restaurant setting and the experience of being out on the town make the desire stronger at that moment, and the worth becomes negotiable. If a person purchased stock in a new company for $10 and it jumped up to $100 in value, where has the increased value come from? In reality, that stock is just a piece of paper, but its value has changed because the people involved in buying and selling it agree on its new value. As you may notice if you follow the stock market, agreements about a stock's worth change frequently, and often because of factors that are unpredictable or out of the control of the principals involved.

Many factors are involved in trying to establish the worth of massage, but here's the rub: you will find it almost impossible to figure out those factors, and they change constantly. Value and worth are what we agree they are. Is a massage more valuable because it is given at a beachfront resort in Maui instead of in a spare bedroom that now functions as a massage office? Is a massage more valuable to the recipient if it costs $125 instead of $50? Is a massage to help restore range of motion to an injured knee more valuable than a shamanic-style session with burning sage and a crystal layout on the chakras? Is it worth more to a client to be able to brag to neighbors about getting massage at a high-end resort, or to have less lower back pain? Is a massage worth more because the practitioner thinks it is? To all of those questions, the best answer is "It depends." Worth depends on what the practitioner and the client agree it is. Whatever needs you meet will vary in value from client to client, and over time. So, why bring worth up at all? Because worth is flexible, and you have the power to shape it.

The first and most important place worth is shaped is in your own mind. If you truly understand how many needs and wants you fulfill for others, you will have more confidence and belief in the value of your work. With that confidence comes an increased ability to explain how many needs you meet, which in turn persuades others to accept the value you place on massage.

If you set the value, others may agree or disagree, but it is set. I remember seeing this principle in action with a student who had been in his massage training program for about seven weeks. He knew a basic sequence and had rough, unrefined skills, and no prior massage experience. Once he learned his initial sequence, though, he was off and running getting clients, led by his unshakable belief that he offered a great gift to the world. I marveled that he was convincing people that he was skilled, and was amazed that he was charging and getting exorbitant fees. I don't know how many of his initial clients returned or referred others (which are the crucial factors for success), but he sure started off with a bang.

Even more interesting were this man's classmates, many of whom had much stronger innate talent. Despite their better hands-on skills, they lacked confidence to the point that some were even hesitant to work on family and friends for the after-school practice they were encouraged to do. As the teacher, I was concerned and confused. The student with the worst skills and most arrogant attitude was getting clients who were paying higher than average fees, and the students who were truly gifted were having a hard time thinking their talents were worth anything. This experience, and many more like it over my years of teaching, brought me to the realization that the practitioner's confidence is a significant factor in establishing worth at the beginning of a practice.

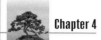

I wish I could say that building a dream practice is fair, but I can't. If you don't understand your own value and how to communicate its worth, success can be elusive, no matter what your skill level. Three primary elements are involved in the process of establishing worth, especially in the beginning stages of building a practice:

1. Self-confidence in skills and abilities

2. Communication skills

3. Hands-on skills

I saw all sorts of combinations of these elements: gifted students with no confidence; arrogant braggarts with no sense of touch; people with caring hearts who were afraid to talk to others; big talkers who were secretly fearful; and students with average skills, save-the-world hearts, and a drive to talk to everybody about massage. In the short run, the advantage seemed to go to those with confidence and the ability to communicate it, regardless of their skills. Over the long run, where repeats and referrals became a factor, the level of hands-on skills became the predominating factor, even for those who lacked confidence.

If you have low self-confidence, work on mastering your hands-on skills, and remember to value the many needs you meet that do not require a high level of skill. Most of my original clients, who were elderly widows, came to me because they were lonely, wanted someone to listen to them, and needed loving touch. Basic Swedish was good enough for them, and it was the level of work I was able to do. Over time, I continued to learn and studied my anatomy when faced with a client problem I didn't understand. With deeper experience and better results, my confidence and understanding of my worth grew. If your confidence isn't the greatest, start somewhere, anywhere, and let your confidence build over time as you practice your skills.

On the other hand, if you think you are the greatest massage student or practitioner to hit the planet, then you have a big advantage in getting your initial clients. If you have the skills to back up your beliefs, then you have what it takes to establish worth over time. That said, I often worried when I had students who thought they were really great right at the start of training. If they were genuinely talented, they could be a real joy; but if they weren't, I feared for their future success. In many ways, the more confident the unskilled students were, the less they seemed able to evaluate their own work and the less coachable they were in improving their skills. Their attitude was,

"If I'm this great, why do I have to pay attention to this teacher or listen to feedback from my classmates? I know what I'm doing!" They were pushy and careless with their classmates, often rough with their work, and were too above-it-all to participate in exercises unless they were in the mood.

Unfortunately, when students like this want to build a practice or get a job, they take their no-room-for-improvement attitude and apply it to their clients. Even if clients tell them the pressure is too hard or say they do not like anyone to touch their feet, these types of practitioners arrogantly ignore them because they maintain the attitude that they know best. The core attribute of the desire to serve becomes lost, and the results are disastrous for the client, the practitioner, and the field.

This type of practitioner manhandles and injures clients all too often, but because of the ability to draw in new clients with their confidence, they may not notice that return and referral clients are few and far between. Clients who have been mauled by therapists with distorted views of their own worth and expertise are rarely likely to try massage again, and certainly do not spread the good word about massage to their friends. By comparison, if a person gets a bad haircut from a new stylist, he or she will look for a new one. However, if that same person gets a bad massage, he or she may never get one again, which is a loss to the whole profession.

If you fit the profile I have just described, please open your mind to the possibility that your skills are not as good as you imagine. If you are in school, look outside of yourself for feedback about your work, ask for help in improving your skills, practice saying "I don't know," and become accustomed to the notion that other's views are as valid as your own. If you think you already know everything and your favorite phrase is "I know," you are in serious trouble for maintaining a long-term practice.

A line I like to use is, "The more you know, the more you know you don't know." If you believe you already know everything about the body or about massage, then you are clueless about the vast amount of knowledge in a wide range of disciplines that would be helpful for your practice. I am not being so blunt to be mean. My goal for this book is to have every therapist become successful, and I have watched too many know-it-alls burn brightly and then flame out to not address this issue.

If you are already practicing, give value to your clients' preferences and be there to serve them instead of dominating them into taking whatever you dish out. Worth is established by agreement between you and your client, and if your view is that your client's wants, needs, and opinions aren't that important, it makes for an unbalanced and often short-lived relationship.

Successful practitioners have an interesting blend of confidence, humility, pride in their work, attentiveness to their clients' needs, and an unquenchable desire to continue learning and growing. They recognize the value of their work, give credence to their clients' feedback, and work together with their clients to set up a trusting and value-driven working relationship with mutually agreed-on worth that improves over time.

Question 6—How Do You Put a Price on Your Ability to Meet Their Needs?

The value of your massage varies from client to client and from day to day, depending on how your clients' needs change or how well you meet those needs. For example, if a carpenter comes to you because of lower back pain, and after a few sessions that pain is gone, his need for massage to help with pain relief will drop. He either will stop getting massage or will find other reasons to continue with you for maintenance or less therapy-oriented purposes. What he valued about massage has changed. Do you change your prices because his needs change? In most cases, no; your prices will remain the same. That is because value is only one of many factors considered when you set the prices for your sessions.

Setting prices is one of the major issues in marketing no matter what field you are in, but it becomes even more of an issue with massage. With so many different needs and markets that we serve, there is no common standard for pricing in the industry. This leaves you to consider other factors for setting your prices besides what other massage therapists are charging.

Your prices may be affected by some or all of the following:

- ✳ What markets you have the desire to serve
- ✳ What needs and expectations you have the ability to meet
- ✳ How big the market is for those needs
- ✳ What your market is willing and able to pay
- ✳ What your "competition" costs

❋ Your personal and business expenses

❋ Your financial goals

❋ Your work location—home, office, outcall, or other settings

❋ Length of session

❋ How you present yourself to your market

❋ What you perceive your work is worth

❋ Your attitude about money

❋ What stage your practice is in—new, growing, or established

Starting out as a new practitioner, your prices will be more affected by these factors. Later on, if you develop an incredible reputation, can help people very quickly, and have established yourself, the rules can definitely change. I've taken seminars from massage experts who charged $100 for a 15-minute session because that's all the time they needed to get the results for which the client came to them. They were world-renowned practitioners and teachers, and believed their method of treatment was superior to what Western medicine and other bodywork modalities had to offer. If you get to that level of expertise, then you have more leeway with prices and how you choose to set them. Until that happens, though, your prices will need to be more in line with what the market will bear.

Value vs. Quality Markets

Two primary groups should be considered when setting prices. One group comprises what is known as the **value market**. These are people who base most of their buying decisions on price; the lower the price, the more likely they are to buy. The second group is the **quality market**. Buyers in this group are willing to pay for the level of quality they want in a product or a service, even if the price is higher.

At this point in our profession's history, most of our clients belong to the quality market. These people are more experimental, willing to be the first to try the latest thing, and will pay for a good experience. The quality market wants a good value, but they are willing to pay well to get what they want. Paradoxically, low prices can turn them off. If you do not put a valid price on your services, this market will perceive your value as beneath their standards.

Their belief is that if the price is too low, something is wrong. This more sophisticated market probably has some dollar amount associated with massage based on what they have seen during their travels to resorts, spas, and hotels. People will usually pay more for most products and services when they travel than they will at home, but they will have a frame of reference, nonetheless, when they start looking for a massage therapist back home.

The value market will become more of a factor as a higher percentage of the population tries massage. However, these "me-too buyers" who follow the trends set by the quality buyers will want a piece of the action, but they will not be as willing or able to pay the price. This group is willing to settle for less, but they want a low price as part of the bargain. There are many more people in the value market, and if you want to appeal to them, offer massage package specials and low-cost, half-hour sessions, and make your prices accessible and appealing. As the value market starts getting interested in massage, pricing may become more competitive, but there will be a larger customer base discovering the joys and benefits of massage. We may soon see the day when "Massage Hut" franchises dot every corner or shopping mall in America, and compete with the "Massage Shack" for clients in search of low-cost rubdowns, but so far, low-cost chains haven't taken over the industry.

To appeal to both markets, use a **massage menu** that can fit almost any budget. Don't have one set price to which people either say "yes" or "no." Maintain multiple options from which to choose. Package deals, couples' discounts, holiday specials, premium add-ons such as aromatherapy, or short, inexpensive sessions all give potential customers the ability to say "yes" to becoming your client. A massage menu lets people select the service level and price they are comfortable with and can afford. The goal of the menu is to move the decision-making process from "yes" or "no" answers to "which option to choose." Your best marketing is the direct demonstration of your hands-on skills, so make it as easy as possible for potential clients to say "yes." Once they are under your hands, you can establish your value so that they choose to return for the same service, or upgrade to a higher service level and price point.

There aren't a lot of hard and fast rules about setting the prices on your menu, but consider having prices containing odd numbers because they are harder for people to mentally divide and assign value. For example, if you charge $60/hour, that amount is easily divisible to a dollar a minute. This may cause some people to pause and wonder if they want to spend a dollar a minute.

If you charge $65 for an hour and 10 minutes, most people can't do the math on the spot and will take the price as a lump sum, which often feels more acceptable.

If you choose to have a massage menu and want a good, high-end option list for the quality market, think for a moment about when people will pay high amounts of money for a product or service. Think about what changes the cost of a particular item so that it becomes more or less expensive.

Within our quirky human nature, there are a number of fairly classic factors for which people will spend more money, and, interestingly, massage touches on quite a few of those factors. Read the following list and ask yourself which of these possibly could affect the prices of your upper-end services.

Factors that Increase Price

People will pay more for things that are:

- Rare
- Exotic
- Unusual
- Status symbols
- Convenient
- Unique
- Highly prized
- Sought after by others
- Extraordinary
- Entertaining
- A break from the routine
- Exclusive
- New and exciting

People also will pay more for: what gains others' approval; what shows superiority or affluence; what others agree is valuable; times of celebration; fast results; and a good reputation.

Whether you work in the world of fine art, fine wine, precious gems, or massage, many of these factors in combination add up to higher demand and, therefore, higher prices. Practitioners who use exotic methods such as working with hot rocks, rain therapy, or soul retrieval have many people come to them who are willing to pay the accompanying exotic prices. The market may be smaller for such specialties, but when the "been there, done that" crowd wants something new and different, the exotic methods are just what they are looking for.

For example, I know a number of practitioners who live and travel between two states every month. Their practices are booming and their prices high. For one thing, they are so hard to book appointments with, people sign up months in advance. These practitioners have a small, exclusive "club" of clients who jealously guard their standing appointments and like to brag about it. Since these massage professionals provide excellent customer service, and have good skills and solid reputations, they have strong appeal and command high prices.

One client I spoke with, who goes to a high-priced, jet-setting massage therapist, thought it was cool that "my masseuse lives in L.A." half the time. Of course, the clients in Los Angeles think it's cool that the massage therapist spends half her month in San Francisco, and 'round it goes.

On a little tangent here, I want to address the ongoing debate about what touch professionals are called, especially with regard to the term "masseuse." Most people in this country do not know the difference between our myriad titles in the many disciplines of massage and bodywork. While it is fine for you to gently train people to call you by your proper title, it is poor marketing to take offense where none was intended if you are called a "masseuse" or "masseur." People use the term "masseuse" with no connection to prostitution or intention of being degrading. This shows that our years of work have changed public opinion, but we're still such a new field that many people don't yet know what to call us. You can educate people about the differences in titles, but getting upset or angry at simple ignorance doesn't help establish trust and value, which is the purpose of your marketing.

THE OTHER SIDE OF PRICING

While the prior material focuses mostly on the market and factors that affect what your potential clients will pay for massage, the other side of pricing covers your financial needs and goals. A dream practice can only last if you are earning enough money. This brings up two issues that have destroyed countless practices. The first issue is how you feel about money; the second is your ability and willingness to make a profit.

Throughout this book, you have learned that the purpose of marketing is to get and keep clients, but now, more specifically, they need to be paying clients. In actuality, the real bottom-line purpose of marketing is to earn money and, more to the point, to make a profit. Now that you have taken a look at the many needs people have and the value you provide for all the needs that you meet, and you have taken into consideration how clients feel about money, it is time to examine how you feel about money.

Practitioners in this field often have mixed feelings about money. Many students I've dealt with felt guilty or shameful about charging money for the "gift" they had been given with massage skills or even an innate healing ability. When I taught classes on marketing and business skills, students would sulk, skip class, or rage against the evil capitalist machine that was devouring the pure sanctity of massage. Money was bad, desire only led to heartache, charging the market rate was discrimination against poor people, selling healing was immoral, having more than enough money to pay the rent and put food on the tables was corrupt, and so on.

Then those same people who said it wasn't fair to charge for massage would gladly go pay $200 for a psychic to tell them what lay ahead in their future. I'll save you the $200 right now. You won't be able to last in a practice if you don't get over negative associations with money. Money is an exchange of energy, and if you are putting out good, helpful energy in the form of massage, you should be paid back in a form of energy of equal value. That energy can return in the form of trading for a service, a product, money, or anything else that balances out what you have given. This is not a subject to be taken lightly, and if receiving money for the value you offer with your massage is difficult for you, treat the issue with serious respect.

Where these negative feelings show up most is in regard to pricing. While it is important to be competitive in your pricing, much damage can be done to long-term success by consistently undervaluing and underpricing services. It's pretty simple, actually. Without adequate income from massage, you can't make a living and pay bills. If that goes on too long, you eventually will have to change professions and make your living another way.

If you are uncomfortable talking about money or telling people your prices, you are actually pretty normal. However, to be successful, you will have to work through that discomfort until you can look potential clients square in the eye and tell them your prices and services without squirming. The value your client perceives starts from you, so you have to exude that value before they will accept your prices. If you feel discomfort, practice standing in front of a mirror and stating your prices. Say them until nothing on you flitters or flutters or flinches, and keep going until your face and body are fully behind those prices.

For further help on this very important topic, I encourage you to read about and explore ways to help you over this hurdle. You need to have clear and healthy distinctions about money because they will help you enjoy your work and your clients, along with the money, compliments, and gifts they give you. One of the hallmarks of being human is that we have the desire and privilege to contribute to other people's lives. If you give a massage and then deny the recipient the ability to contribute back to you in kind, you are, in essence, denying that person his or her humanity. If you give value, be willing and able to receive value. It is a crucial step toward success.

EXERCISE: PRACTICING PRICING

The purpose of this exercise is to get you to a level of comfort with pricing so you can talk to potential clients about money with confidence and ease. If you are in a class or group, get a partner. If you are reading this by yourself, work with a mirror. The partners should sit facing each other, almost knee to knee.

Partner A asks Partner B, "I hear you do massage. What do you charge?" Partner B answers, "I charge $20." Partner A asks Partner B the same question two more times. Each time the answer is $20.

Then Partner A asks the same question, but the new answer is "I charge $50." Repeat that question and answer two more times. Then change the price to $80 and repeat that price two more times.

Then switch and work the other way.

When finished, if you are in a group, take the time to discuss the different feelings that came up at each price point. If it is just you and the mirror, notice how you feel.

For the second half of the exercise, Partner A asks the same question, only this time Partner B answers with the dollar amount he or she plans to charge initially or wants to raise rates to in the future. As Partner B answers, Partner A observes all body language including eye movement, head position, hand movements, breathing changes, color changes, facial expressions, tone of voice, and anything else that can indicate whether or not Partner B is comfortable and confident with that price. Partner A keeps asking the question until Partner B can name the price with no visible signs of discomfort. If there is any form of incongruity, such as dropping the chin, tilting the head, bouncing a knee, or blinking too much, Partner A will tell Partner B what is noticed and keep going with the question-and-answer stage until all symptoms of incongruity stop.

For those working with a mirror, repeat your price to yourself until you come across as sure, confident, and believing that your services are worth the price you are quoting.

WHEN WORTH AND PRICE COLLIDE

Mixing the two issues of worth and setting prices can be a volatile brew. The value of your services is an agreement between you and your clients, and your price becomes a factor of agreement as well. Regardless of which market you are targeting, phrases such as "I deserve . . ." and "I am worth . . ." have to be calculated realistically when competing for your client's dollar. Repeating affirmations about your ideal hourly rate can be great, but if your clients won't pay it, your dream practice may remain a dream. There is a vast difference between what you are worth and what your services cost. Everyone on this planet is a priceless individual and has inherent worth, but that is different than setting a price for a service you offer.

Deserving and earning are two different things. For the sake of your sanity and success, don't mix the critical issue of price into the issue of "deservingness" and personal worth. It is a self-defeating head game that has cost untold numbers of therapists their dream of a successful practice.

To build a practice, accept your inherent worth as a human being, work on your skills so you can have genuine confidence in your ability to serve others, and set prices that work for both you and your clients.

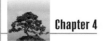

MARKETING SKILL #4: SETTING AND MEETING CLIENT EXPECTATIONS

The fourth marketing skill you must master is the ability to set and meet **client expectations**. However, once again, massage faces some unique issues around expectations. If you were a doctor and a patient came in with a broken leg, the expectations are pretty clear for everyone involved that the leg would be set. Massage, however, has so many modalities and methods of application that it is impossible to know what a client expects without asking. Add to this the variables of the Perception Continuum, and you've got too much potential for misunderstandings and client dissatisfaction.

Clients can have an accurate perception of massage but incorrectly assume that you have certain skills or use a massage method you haven't learned. They may have a misperception and think that all massage has to hurt to be effective; if your work doesn't hurt, they're upset. They might expect you to do Swedish massage and then get upset and think you're lazy if you use a subtle energy technique instead. Whatever clients think, you need to find it out; otherwise, they might leave disappointed and never come back.

Setting and meeting expectations is crucial for building your practice because, without this ability, it is virtually impossible to build trust, establish value, or serve the needs of others. Customer service of any caliber would be difficult to provide if you didn't actually know why someone came to see you. Understanding what clients want allows you to fulfill their hopes and expectations of their time with you. If you are able to ethically and legally give clients what they want and expect, the marketing function of rebooking clients and getting referrals becomes your path to success.

Listening and Educating

Setting expectations requires two major communication skills: the ability to listen and the ability to educate. The listening skill has two parts. There is "listening to," which means you hear and understand the actual words and explicit requests that the client makes, and you respond to them as a professional. Then there is "listening for," which involves reading between the lines or listening to the subtext of the implicit or unspoken requests. Most people won't just come out and say things like they are lonely, want someone to like them, or want someone to listen to them. The basic human needs such as being accepted, valued, respected, and loved are part of the unspoken subtext that is always there, even if it is covered up with official-sounding expectations such as relieving that nagging lower back pain. To be a successful therapist, listen to and for client expectations that are both explicit and implicit, and then meet those expectations.

Each of your clients will have a unique set of expectations, but there are some common ones that most clients have for which you can prepare. Listen for these expectations as you conduct your telephone screening, intake interview, or other pre-massage conversations, and you will be better able to meet your clients' expectations or educate them to change their own expectations.

Some key client expectations to listen for are the:

- ❋ Anticipated results of the session
- ❋ Quality or method of application of massage
- ❋ Modality or technique used
- ❋ Attitude and approach of the therapist
- ❋ Anticipated feelings during and after the session
- ❋ Ambiance of the setting

We will touch briefly on three of these broad expectations so you can better predict what is wanted from you. Understanding these key expectations can help keep clients happy by preventing broken expectations, disappointment, frustration, and misunderstandings. Then we will cover the rest of these expectations thoroughly in the chapter on rebooking, because met expectations are what bring clients back and lead them to refer.

CLIENT EXPECTATION #1: ANTICIPATED RESULTS OF THE SESSION

Clients can expect some interesting results from massage. Depending on their preconceived notions, clients may expect that massage will be a nice rubdown, or they may think they are going to be "fixed" from an old high school football injury in just one session. Your task is to ask questions until both you and your client are clear about what he or she expects. Sometimes, clients do not know what they expect, at least consciously, so get them to talk about their

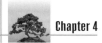

expectations until they can articulate them. This saves them from subconsciously becoming disappointed later when the massage wasn't quite right, but they can't quite say why. In their minds, it wasn't that it was a good or bad massage; it just wasn't right, and they're not coming back. Questions that get people to clarify their expectations can be very simple. Some classic questions are:

"What can I help you with today?"

"What can I do for you today?"

"What are your goals for your session today?"

When they answer, say, "Great! Anything else?" Keep asking them "Anything else?" until they run out of expectations.

If the answers to these more generic questions do not reveal expectations, get more specific and ask about what kind of results they are seeking. Or you can be up front and say, "I want this to be an outstanding massage for you. If you can tell me what your expectations are, I will do my best to get the results you are looking for." Don't be surprised if you see a few jaws drop with a statement like this. Few clients ever experience customer service at this level, but once they have recovered from their shock, they will know they have come to the right place.

If your skill or experience level is not very high yet, stay with the more generic questions. That way, people don't immediately set expectations too high, then become disappointed later. I saw this principle in action at the car dealership where I get my oil changed. An oil change used to be a straightforward process. I booked an appointment, brought in my car, sat in the lobby, drank bad coffee with floating globs of nondairy creamer, watched the news channel, and got my car back in about an hour. I was happy. Then the dealership (I somehow blame the corporate marketing department) got the idea for drop-in service with a 30-minute guaranteed turnaround time. They wouldn't take appointments; they weren't necessary with this new, improved customer service campaign. Unfortunately, reality and marketing departments are often bad combinations. The last two times I "dropped in" for my oil change, the service department was backed up, the wait was longer than 30 minutes, and I left upset because they threw off the schedule I had planned. In reality, I was still sitting in the waiting room drinking bad coffee for about the same amount of time as I was before, but because my expectations were elevated and then not met, I was no longer happy. That is bad marketing, and I've taken my business elsewhere.

If you believe you are able to meet your clients' expectations of the results they are seeking, then, throughout the session, tell your clients what you are doing and how your work is meeting their needs. This form of education is invaluable in creating trust, establishing value, and shaping positive perception. This is "on-the-table marketing," and it is probably the most important form of marketing you can do.

If your clients have expectations of results that you don't believe you can fulfill, you have a number of options.

1. You can bluff your way through the session and hope they can't figure out that what you are doing won't really help them. Not only is this unethical but it's also really bad marketing. People who are upset talk a lot more than people who are happy and satisfied, and bad word-of-mouth is a powerful thing to overcome.

2. You can explain to your clients what you think you can do for them, but be clear that their expectations are too high for your level of skill. This is not uncommon, and I have had many new clients who expected me to have the skill level and diagnostic abilities of orthopedic doctors. There is no shame in saying what you can and can't do. Sometimes, I achieve better results with clients than their doctors do, and sometimes I don't, but I am very up front about my scope of practice and ability level, and I let the client decide if he or she wants to stay. In these cases, I am resetting the expectations to be more realistic, and I have yet to see a client walk out because I won't promise him or her miracles. In cases where expectations are unrealistic, I go to great lengths to educate clients about my strategy, and I discuss my approach or methodology so they know I am making a good-faith effort to meet their needs. Even if I realize that one strategy (such as trigger point therapy) is not working, I tell them so; then I choose a different strategy (such as positional release), explain it, and get back to work.

3. You can refer your clients to other massage therapists or medical practitioners who can meet the level of expectation they have set. Again, there is no shame in this. I have referred a number of clients to a colleague with a whole set of skills I don't come close to having when I think she can meet their needs. Sometimes, good customer service is simply referring the client elsewhere. Be careful with referrals, though. If the client is not satisfied, they can backfire. Only refer clients to someone you know and trust.

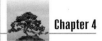

CLIENT EXPECTATION #2: APPLICATION OF MASSAGE, AND MODALITY OR TECHNIQUE USED

Preconceived expectations are not limited to what results clients hope to get from massage. Sometimes, clients think they know how those results are going to occur. For example, if a client says, "Just shove your elbow into that sore point on my shoulder and work it real deep for an hour," the therapist must listen for the real need (the client wants his shoulder to stop hurting) and then educate the client as to how to reach the same goal in a different way. In this kind of scenario, the expectations surround the application of massage and the method used. The client, with his limited knowledge, thinks that direct pressure is the best method, deep work is the best application, and a long period of time on one spot is going to be most effective for releasing pain.

How this exchange is handled makes all the difference in achieving a satisfied client. If you respond by saying, "Well, that's a really bad idea. Pressing in one spot for an hour is pretty stupid," you've just lost a client. I know that most people don't actually use phrases quite as blatant as these, but sometimes this attitude is conveyed by therapists regardless of the words used. One of the major reasons that patients are leaving traditional doctors is because they feel unheard, and they object to having their fears and concerns dismissed. Patients are rarely given credit for their own intelligence and experience of their bodies, and they resent it deeply.

Massage therapists need to avoid the mistakes made in other medical or service professions and be respectful, even if the client has some expectations that are a bit off or unrealistic. A better way to handle the client who believes he knows how you are supposed to work is to reeducate him. You could say something like, "Well, you're the expert on your body, and it sounds like your shoulder is hurting. Tell me more about your shoulder." Once he is done talking, you can say something like, "I hear what you're saying about your shoulder. Now, again, you're the expert on your body, and I'm the expert on massage. I need to tell you that if I just worked on your sore shoulder with deep pressure for an hour, I would probably hurt you more, which I don't think you'd like. Let me give you some options for how we can help your shoulder without hurting it further, and then you can decide."

In this exchange, the client feels heard, learns more about you and your work, retains his power of decision, and has his unspoken needs to be valued and respected met. The odds are high that you will have a grateful client on your hands who now has higher trust and value in you and your work because of how you handled his expectations.

If your massage modality is fairly different from the standard Swedish stereotype, you will need to become good at reeducating clients on how and why your methods work. For example, I use the energy work modalities of Quantum Touch, Polarity, Reiki, and BodyTalk, or Energy Psychology methods such as Emotional Freedom Technique (EFT), which I find to be incredibly powerful tools. Since most people think that they need to feel a lot of pressure to get results, I have to compensate for that expectation. I either mix in heavier work with my lighter energy work, or I take the time before the session to educate my clients about what I am doing and why, and tell them what they can expect to feel. During the work, I ask specific questions that help them focus their attention at a higher level of awareness so that they do feel the work. I frequently retest the area with pressure or range of motion, and ask if it feels better. This further focuses their attention while helping them assign value to the work. They may not feel the work happening, but they feel the changes in their bodies. This lets them maintain their expectation that they feel something, and that, therefore, my method is working.

THE IMPORTANCE OF ANATOMICAL KNOWLEDGE

If you look at the prior examples of how to reeducate a client about results or application, you probably will notice the common denominator of good communication. In these cases, good client communication is grounded in your understanding of your work and of the human body.

The more you understand what you are doing, the better you can set expectations. Underneath this ability to communicate about client expectations is one of the most important marketing skills of all: a thorough and conversant knowledge of anatomy. If you are currently in school, give real focus to your anatomy classes and imagine how you would explain what you are learning to a client. If you are out of school and anatomy wasn't a big part of your training, or it's been so long that some of the details are vague, get some anatomy charts or new books and reenergize your knowledge base.

Understanding anatomy enables you to: explain to clients what is being done during a session; describe why one technique will work when another won't;

demonstrate how the muscles work in relation to one another; and justify strategies, techniques, and amounts of time spent in a given area. Speaking the language of anatomy lets you give words to your clients' vague sensations and show them pain patterns, compensation patterns, and other mysteries that you now seem magical understanding. Clear, anatomy-based communication that validates and illuminates your decisions creates three things unpurchasable in advertising or traditional marketing: a sense of trust, an accurate and positive perception of the therapist, and an understanding of the true value of massage.

Nothing is more fascinating to people than themselves. Educating others about their bodies, how they work, and how they are going to be treated is the ultimate in customer service and marketing. (See Figure 4–4.) Educating a client before, during, and after a session creates the right expectations; delivers what is promised; and reminds the client that what he or she purchased was

Figure 4–4 | **Educating clients about their bodies is some of the best marketing you can do.**

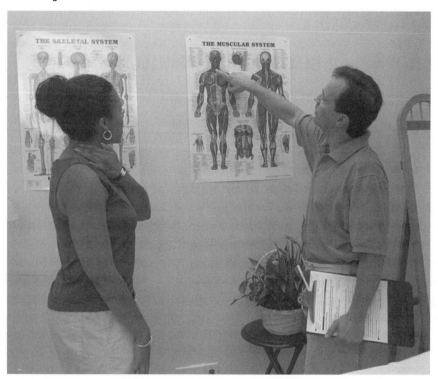

valuable, and worth the time and money spent. When client expectations are met, and they are happy and satisfied, they will market and promote you better than any formal marketing program ever could.

CLIENT EXPECTATION #3: THE ATTITUDE AND APPROACH OF THE THERAPIST

Deep within the hearts of humans is a constant craving for attention. This craving is possibly one of the most important of the silent expectations and human needs that clients have when they come for massage. It is very different from expectations about results or methodologies because it is not based on skills, but on the attitude and personal approach of the therapist. Many people firmly believe they are the center of the universe and want to be given treatment befitting their status.

People aren't just muscles and movable joints. They have hopes and dreams and fears and needs, and your "tableside manner" either lets them feel human and happy or like slabs of meat to be greased up and pushed around until their time slot is over. If you have an excellent attitude, genuinely want to serve people, and treat each client like gold, you probably can have mediocre skills and do quite well for yourself. You also can have excellent skills and a less appealing attitude and get away with it. I know a few therapists who are about as huggable as a cactus, but they do great work, and their clients accept their no-nonsense demeanor and take-care-of-business attitude.

If you are dour, bristly, standoffish, pushy, arrogant, or abrasive, you can make it in a practice, but you'd better be an outstanding clinician. If you will not treat people like they are the center of the universe, be prepared to give them the results for which they came. Since the desire for attention can be met in many ways with the simple mechanical application of touch, you can still meet this need, but the experience will be much better for you and the client if a caring heart is behind the work. Millions of people ache just to have someone look at them and welcome their presence. Have the bigness of heart to do this, and you have already served your client well. The best method for achieving success is to have a positive attitude, make people feel important and special, and provide excellent massage. It is an irresistible combination.

I saw this principle in action, and though the example is not about massage, it speaks to what we need to understand about human nature and our role in healing physical pains and hurting hearts. I went to a fast-food restaurant to get the children's meal so I could get the elaborate toy that my nephew wanted. While I was watching some children to see which toys they got, I saw an interesting drama unfold. A little boy, about two years old, was playing with his brand-new toy when a man entered the restaurant and loudly greeted a little girl who was seated at the table behind the little boy. The girl called back in greeting and immediately raised her toy triumphantly for the man's approval, which he promptly gave. The little boy was sitting with his father, who was obviously tired, distracted, and disinterested in his son's plastic toy. The boy turned to this stranger and raised his toy in hope that the man would give him the same kind of acknowledgment he gave the little girl. The man did not see this boy raise his toy for his approval, but the boy went through a repeated cycle of holding up the toy, not getting acknowledged, and then looking down at his toy with increasing despair.

It was as if the value of his toy was diminishing in his eyes because it didn't get another person's attention and approval. After numerous failed attempts, the boy dejectedly put his toy down and gave out a tremendous shriek, whereupon everyone looked at him and he got all the attention he wanted, even though it was negative. I was fascinated. How core is our desire for attention, for approval, even for a little eye contact? And what damages have so many people suffered from a lifetime of small but painful moments such as I had just witnessed? These wounds are just as painful as torn ligaments or pulled hamstrings, and they are part of what clients bring to us in their silent expectations. There is no job description that says your attitude and approach need to bear these silent hopes in mind, but now you know they are there, and you can do wonders for your business and your clients by meeting them.

MARKETING SKILL #5: REACHING OUT TO CLIENTS

All the work you have done with the first four skills has been preparation for the last bare-bones marketing skill, which is reaching out to clients. So, how do you get clients? According to almost all of the successful massage therapists I have interviewed, they got clients one primary way: they talked to everybody they could about massage. This may not sound very sophisticated or difficult, and actually, it's not. People who built their private practices from scratch started by talking to family, friends, acquaintances, hairstylists, grocery clerks, neighbors, waitresses, people in the park, coworkers, and folks at the gym, in line at the store, or waiting in a restaurant. These casual conversations where massage was discussed often led to a new client being discovered.

The 10 x 10 Rule

I have met very few successful therapists who began with any formal marketing strategy, or who had decided on a **target market** at which to aim when they were new. If someone would come in, lie down, get a massage, and pay, that was good enough.

One strategy, told to me by one of the most successful therapists I know, was to "just get 10 clients." Following her short massage training in a converted back bedroom of her teacher's home, her big marketing strategy was to talk to everyone she could about massage. With no brochures, flyers, public speeches, or a Web site, she talked and talked until somehow she rounded up 10 clients. Now, some 35 years later, her practice has grown and evolved tremendously, but she still feels that the simple goal of "just 10 clients" was a great way to start.

To add another rule of 10, use what one of my colleagues called the "10-foot rule." His policy was this: anyone within 10 feet of him was fair game for a friendly conversation in which he got to mention that he was a massage therapist. He didn't ask for business; he just talked about himself and what he did for a living, which is a pretty standard conversation topic for most Americans. The people who were looking for a therapist were thrilled to meet him, and his informal marketing was more than adequate to get new clients who then rebooked and referred him into a full practice. He now runs a five-room office with multiple therapists working for him, and his marketing has gotten more advanced, but he started off with only this strategy, and it worked.

How do you start a practice? Start with the "10 × 10 Rule." Set a goal for 10 new clients; talk to everyone within 10 feet of you, somehow including the word "massage"; and keep talking until you get those 10 clients. (See Figure 4–5.) It's that easy and that hard. If you have an easy time talking to people, your work will include how to introduce the topic of massage. You can start by asking other people what they do for a living. When they are done and ask you what you do, the door is open for you to step in. One therapist I interviewed gained a significant percentage of her practice by regularly wearing a T-shirt or polo shirt with the word "massage" on it. People who read

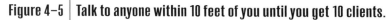

Figure 4–5 | Talk to anyone within 10 feet of you until you get 10 clients.

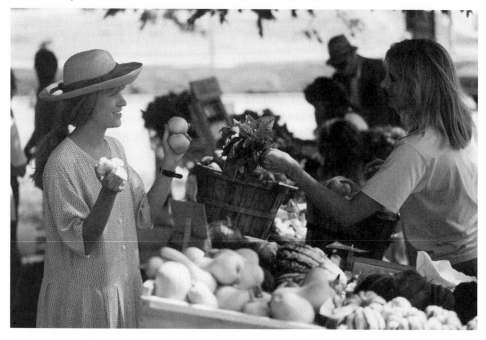

the script on her shirt got into conversations about massage, and that gave her an easy opening to talk about herself and her services.

Ask your family, friends, and neighbors to get the word out that you are starting a practice. If you use e-mail, let your address list know with a simple notice saying you're looking for clients. Ask your e-mail list to spread the word to people on their lists.

Events are a great way to make big announcements, and you can have a party and invite family, friends, coworkers, and others to celebrate the grand opening of your practice. Send written invitations and include business cards for people to give out. Hand out stacks of cards at your party and ask people to distribute them to people they know. You can even have a contest where the first person to get you three new clients gets a free massage. If several people get you three new clients, give them all a thank-you massage, even if they weren't first. It's the least expensive and most effective marketing you could ever do.

To build your business very quickly, hand out gift certificates that your attendees can use for themselves or give as gifts. Massage has a very high dollar perception because of its prominent use in advertising, and certificates are usually quite welcome as gifts.

In your daily life, look at where you spend money and who you pay for their products and services. Do you have a piano teacher, landscaper, coffee shop, craft store, farmers' market, or other business where you go often and know the workers? Tell them you are looking for clients, ask for their help, and give them cards to hand out for you, if they agree to. If you belong to any group or club, announce at a meeting or gathering that you are building a practice. Ask if your fellow members will e-mail or tell their friends about you. Whether you are on a bowling team, are a member of a church, or are in a yoga class or a book club, simply tell people you are looking for new clients and ask for their help. We will cover this in more depth in the later section on getting referrals, but for this bare-bones approach, go to people already in your life and start there.

The next part of this book, muscle marketing, has hundreds of other ideas for building a practice, but the quick and easy steps in this section are plenty to get started. Virtually every massage therapist I have met started with some version of these tactics, and they can work just as well for you.

CHAPTER 4   SUMMARY

In this chapter on bare-bones skills for starting your practice, we covered the fundamentals of how to understand the mindsets of potential clients and what you need to know and do to shape their perceptions about massage and you as a therapist. In today's market, one of the key issues is trust between client and therapist, and we covered numerous ways to both create and maintain trust so that you can touch people for a living. Due to the many kinds of massage and the differing ways they are perceived, you will not only need to create trust in your skills, but also establish the value of your work. Fortunately, massage meets so many needs at the same time, including mental, emotional, physical, and spiritual needs, that massage is given a consistently high market value. Your ability to understand and meet the needs and expectations people have about massage will be one your most important skills in building a long-term practice. Finally, your skills in reaching out to potential clients, even in simple and informal ways, can get you started in your practice, and we covered the skills used by many of the most successful therapists in the country.

CHAPTER 4   ACTION STEPS

Based on the information in this chapter, take the following action steps to start your practice:

- Identify which level of awareness and perception you want your ideal client to have, and tailor your marketing accordingly.

- Evaluate your appearance and behavior, and determine if you can create a sense of safety and trust in potential clients.

- Choose clothing for your work that is appropriate and meets clients' expectations of a professional.

- Evaluate what human needs you are qualified and interested in meeting.

- Establish the value of your benefits to your clients, and set a price for your sessions.

- Determine a set strategy to discover what your clients expect from their massages.

- Continue to study anatomy.

- Get your first 10 clients.

CHAPTER 4   KNOWLEDGE CHECK

Check your understanding of the chapter by reviewing these questions and answers.

Q: What are the Five Skills of Success?
A: Shaping client perception, creating and maintaining trust, establishing value, setting and meeting client expectations, and reaching out to clients.

Q: What are massage therapists' three main forms of competition?
A: Ignorance, misperception, and lack of trust and value.

Q: What are the two basic human needs?
A: To avoid pain and gain pleasure.

Q: What are the primary categories of pain and pleasure that massage can help?
A: Mental, emotional, and physical.

Q: What is the secret of creating value?
A: Understanding what needs you can meet for other people.

Q: What determines the worth of your massage?
A: What the practitioner and client agree upon.

Q: What are the two types of markets with regard to pricing?
A: Value and quality.

Q: What are the two major communication skills for setting client expectations?
A: The ability to listen and the ability to educate.

Q: What is one of the most important marketing skills in handling client expectations?
A: A thorough and conversant knowledge of anatomy.

Q: What is one of the constant human cravings that we can offer our clients?
A: Attention.

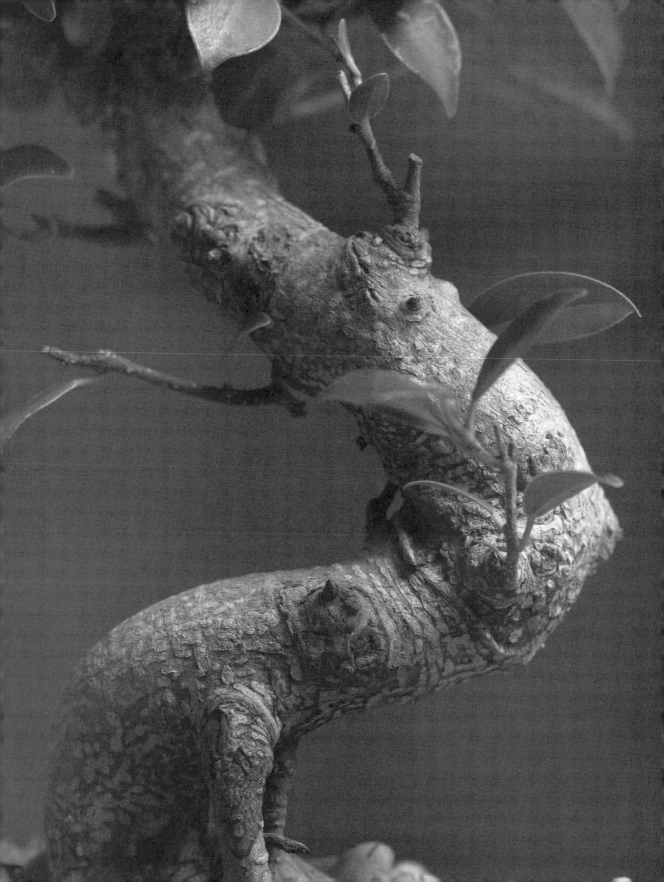

5 The Only Marketing Tools You Really Need

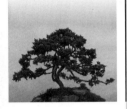

CHAPTER OBJECTIVES

After reading this chapter, you should be able to:

- ❋ Design a basic business card.
- ❋ Select and use an appointment book.
- ❋ Create a professional **contact list** of your clientele.
- ❋ Use the telephone effectively to book and rebook clients.

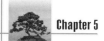
MARKETING TOOLS TO BUILD YOUR DREAM PRACTICE

Your core attributes, marketing skills, and massage abilities will be the primary determining factors in your ability to build your dream practice over the long term. To round out this section on how to start the process of getting and keeping clients, one more key factor needs to be considered: marketing tools, and how to choose and use them.

In this bare-bones section of the book, we are going to review the only marketing tools you really need to start your practice. Yes, you can use e-mail newsletters, four-fold brochures, and Web sites, but when you are beginning a practice, you should start with tools that are inexpensive, simple, easy, and practical. The tools covered in this chapter were chosen because they are the only tools that many successful therapists use. In the upcoming muscle marketing section, we will cover more advanced marketing tools, so if you work in a highly competitive market or want to build a practice very quickly, the advanced tools in the later chapters can help. However, advanced tools take more money, time, and skill to develop. They also take a level of self-knowledge and insight borne only of experience about what kind of work and clients you enjoy most, what level of skill you can promote, and what kind of business identity you want to establish. Too many beginners get excited about developing brochures or Web sites and then have to redo them at more cost later. Many therapists have boxes of leftover brochures featuring a chosen style of work they no longer want to do, or a Web site that gets visitors but doesn't lead to booked appointments because it wasn't right for their target market. In short, if you are a massage professional just starting out, these basic tools are all you need to get your first 10 clients. And they may be all the tools you'll ever need to succeed!

There are only four marketing tools you must have to enable people to gain access to you and book appointments. They are your:

1. Business cards

2. Appointment book

3. Contact list of clientele

4. Telephone and answering machine

BASIC MARKETING TOOL #1: BUSINESS CARDS

Business cards are the most important marketing tool you can use in building a massage practice, and are often the only outreach tool many therapists will ever need. On the surface, the purpose of business cards seems simple. It gives people a way to get in touch with you to book an appointment. However, cards can serve multiple functions, including the ability to act as tiny advocates, spreading the word about you while you are busy elsewhere. The more cards you have out in the world and in other people's hands, the more voices you have speaking on your behalf, multiplying your opportunities to book appointments or reach referrals. A business card gives you leverage, and the more leverage you have, the more you can spend your time doing massage instead of marketing.

A basic business card needs only three things on it: your name, your title, and your phone number. Beyond these three elements, everything else is secondary. You can have a very simple, plain business card that will serve its purpose by letting people remember who you are, what you do, and how to contact you. If most of your clients come to you from personal referrals, which is how most therapists build a practice, your card's appearance is not that critical. For example, if a friend of yours recommends someone to you and that person calls and books an appointment, the first time the person will see your card is after he or she has arrived for the first appointment. At that point your card will be helpful in showing that you are a professional, but it will be the referral, not the card, that brought the person in the door.

When conducting more formal **networking**, such as when you meet with other professionals in order to share business leads, those professionals will be giving out your card to people they know on your behalf, and you may need more than a basic card. Since the recipients of your card from your networking colleague won't see you in person, they will place more importance on how your card looks since it is one of their only ways of judging you. Also, if you are going to post your card in a public place with no other form of personal representation, it must say volumes and give the impressions that people need to make the decision to call. That's when e-mail addresses, Web sites, and graphics matter more, which we'll cover later, but to start with, you will probably be doing most of your own marketing and speaking on your own behalf, so your card primarily will serve as a basic

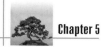

reminder and contact tool. Let's take a closer look at the three elements of a basic card: your name, title, and telephone number.

Basic Business Card Element: Your Name

For most people, a name is a pretty straightforward line on a card. However, if you are planning to change your name for marriage or other reasons after you have started your practice, or will use a nickname on your card, remember that your family and friends may give referrals using your old name, so have a transition card with both names on it, and have your answering machine give both names as well. That way, people with personal referrals or old cards who get your answering machine won't be alarmed by thinking they've reached a wrong number, and then hang up.

Basic Business Card Element: Your Title

The next element on your business card is your title. How you choose to use your title to describe yourself can make a big difference in how you are perceived. The general public still does not have much knowledge about the different titles that massage therapists earn in their schools or specialty seminars, and our field has so many titles, certification levels, and modalities that no one title is the common standard. Since there are no universally agreed-upon titles, consider creating a title that is fitting and appropriate to describe yourself. For example, the title I earned in a 1000-hour massage program was Holistic Health Practitioner and Educator, but no one knew what that title meant and it did not carry much value in the marketplace. A more appealing title to most people at that time and in the area where I lived was the word "massage," so on my card I printed "Professional Massage Therapist." By starting with the word "professional" to set up a positive perception, and by using the word "massage," my title got the right kind of attention from the market in which I was interested.

Marketing is about creating the right impression for your target audience, and your title can be very powerful in telling people that you offer what they want. Ethically and legally, you cannot say you are licensed or certified if you are not, but beyond that, think carefully about how you want to describe yourself. Unless you are required by some local or state regulation to use certain titles, consider using well-crafted words to which the general public will be attracted.

For example, your school certificate may say "Certified Massage Therapist," but if you serve a market of executives, your card can read "Stress Management Expert" or "Stress Management Massage." If you are well trained in sports massage, consider a title such as "Sports Massage Specialist." If you serve multiple markets, you can have two or three different cards with different specialty titles listed.

Basic Business Card Element: Your Telephone Number

Besides your name and title, your card needs to give people some way to contact you. The most common contact method is a telephone, though some people use the Internet more than a phone once the working relationship has been established. If you have an office, list your work number. If you work out of your home or do outcall to your clients' homes or offices, you can list your home phone number. However, for reasons of safety, convenience, privacy, or to control how the phone is answered, you may choose to have a separate telephone line for your business.

Depending on the needs of your practice, you might want numerous ways to be reached. For an outcall practice, a cellular phone is indispensable, letting your clients access you quickly and easily no matter where you are. It helps to be able to call from the road if you get lost or stuck in traffic, and it gives you and your clients a way to connect rapidly for last-minute cancellations or bookings.

Another phone option is to use a separate, remote, voice-mail-only line. If you have a home office and don't want a separate line, but don't like giving out your home or cell phone number to every person you give your card to, remote voice mail offers you a layer of safety, protects your privacy, and is great for stopping telemarketers from bothering you at home. Once someone becomes a client, you can give him or her your private numbers. In addition, a voice mail can be a stable telephone number no matter how often you move, or if your area code changes. This keeps you from having to reprint your cards, and, as an added bonus, stable numbers let clients find you years later.

In conclusion, your name, title, and telephone number are all you need for a bare-bones business card. In a later chapter, we will cover graphics, e-mails, addresses, types of paper, type styles, colors, photos, logos, two-sided cards, folding cards, and layouts. For a basic business card, though, you can walk into any printer or major office supply store, or go to an online printer for your

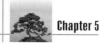

Figure 5–1 | **Don't wait to get your first business cards!**

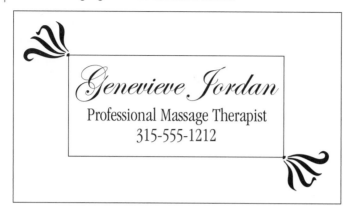

cards. Choose a basic design from their pre-designed layouts, give them your information, and let them do the rest. It really is that easy. (See Figure 5–1.)

Whatever you do, *do not wait* to get your first cards. Do not wait until you design the perfect logo or choose an official business name. Do not wait until you have filed a fictitious business name, or have saved money for a formal photo shoot or graphic artist. This point became clear to me when I was consulting with a therapist who was looking for ways to build her practice. Since a business card is the primary marketing tool for massage therapists, I asked to see her card. Amazingly, she didn't have one, and she had been in business for three years! When I asked her why she had no card, she told me she hadn't had the inspiration yet for what to use as her logo. Please, don't hold your practice up waiting for inspiration to design the perfect card. To get started, just have your first 100 cards made with your name, title, and telephone number, and get them into people's hands. Do not make any excuses; just make cards and give them all away. Later, when your practice is under way, you can put more time, money, and understanding into creating a graphic representation of you and your work. And, whatever you do, don't leave home without your business cards. Potential clients are everywhere!

EXERCISE: DRAFT A BASIC BUSINESS CARD

Sketch out the information you want to include on a basic business card. Include your name, phone number(s), and title you plan to use. If you want to include other information or have an idea for how you want it to look, draw it freehand. Then take it down to the printer and get it printed! It really is that simple.

_____

_____

_____

_____

_____

_____

_____

_____

_____

_____

_____

BASIC MARKETING TOOL #2: THE APPOINTMENT BOOK

Owning your own business requires some tools and disciplines you may have never had to fully use before. For a massage therapist, an appointment book is a crucial tool for managing a practice or building a new one because you basically sell two things: your reputation and your time. (See Figure 5–2.) Most marketing is about creating your reputation, but how you manage your time, and how you book and keep your appointments, are all important to your ultimate success.

If you are building your own practice and have never used an appointment book or **time management system**, it may take some getting used to, but it is vital for your business. Even if you have used a calendar or appointment book before, scheduling your life and practice together takes forethought and planning. In addition, your appointment book is a marketing tool. How you

Figure 5–2 | A month-at-a-glace calendar can let you book appointments quickly and easily.

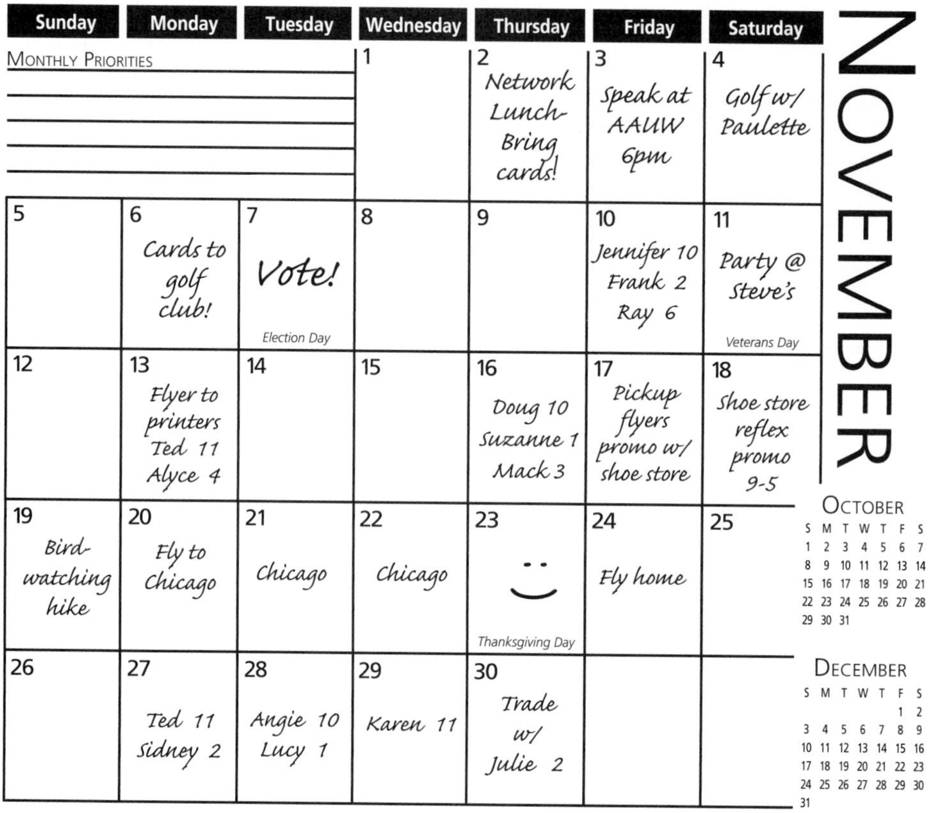

Sunday	Monday	Tuesday	Wednesday	Thursday	Friday	Saturday	
Monthly Priorities _____ _____ _____ _____			1	2 Network Lunch- Bring cards!	3 Speak at AAUW 6pm	4 Golf w/ Paulette	**N**
5	6 Cards to golf club!	7 *Vote!* Election Day	8	9	10 Jennifer 10 Frank 2 Ray 6	11 Party @ Steve's Veterans Day	**O**
12	13 Flyer to printers Ted 11 Alyce 4	14	15	16 Doug 10 Suzanne 1 Mack 3	17 Pickup flyers promo w/ shoe store	18 Shoe store reflex promo 9-5	**V**
19 Bird- watching hike	20 Fly to Chicago	21 Chicago	22 Chicago	23 :-) Thanksgiving Day	24 Fly home	25	**E**
26	27 Ted 11 Sidney 2	28 Angie 10 Lucy 1	29 Karen 11	30 Trade w/ Julie 2			**M B E R**

OCTOBER

S	M	T	W	T	F	S
1	2	3	4	5	6	7
8	9	10	11	12	13	14
15	16	17	18	19	20	21
22	23	24	25	26	27	28
29	30	31				

DECEMBER

S	M	T	W	T	F	S
					1	2
3	4	5	6	7	8	9
10	11	12	13	14	15	16
17	18	19	20	21	22	23
24	25	26	27	28	29	30
31						

use it while booking appointments can create trust with your client, instill value in your services, and shape the perception of you as a professional.

An appointment book not only schedules your time, it also can serve to hold your business cards and give you a place to put all those checks that clients give you. While personal digital assistants (PDAs) like Palm Pilots, BlackBerries, or other electronic devices can certainly schedule your time, we're going to start with the simple and inexpensive approach for this bare-bones section. Besides, paper never crashes or has to be left at home to recharge.

Calendars

Time management systems such as Day Runner® or Day-Timer® are available at office supply or stationery stores, and are ideal for scheduling your time, setting boundaries, setting goals, and booking appointments. These are portable ringed binders with multiple sections you can purchase individually. The sections can include: month-at-a-glance pages where you can schedule the times of your appointments; daily pages where you write your to-do lists; contact pages where you write in telephone numbers, addresses, and e-mail addresses; project pages where you record reminders of things to do for your personal and professional goals; expense pages for business purchases and mileage; and more.

The key benefit is that this system is portable, so you have only one calendar system. This lets you take it with you to your office, your clients, or anywhere you will need to know your schedule and when you are available for appointments. Do not try to cross-reference two calendars, and don't try to keep appointments in your head or on scraps of paper. As a professional, you need to book clients confidently without worrying about accidentally double-booking with some faintly remembered dentist appointment written on your home calendar. Organizing a practice is very different from going to a job or school. You will be booking your time, sometimes to the minute, and you need the right tool to keep you relaxed and confident that you will be in the right place at the right time.

When building your practice, there are four primary uses for an appointment book:

1. Scheduling your time

2. Setting boundaries

3. Setting goals

4. Booking appointments

Scheduling Your Time

Massage therapy is a service typically sold by time. Clients can book an hour session or a 15-minute session, and they pay for your time, often by the minute. Therefore, how you handle your time greatly affects your ability to make a living with massage. The first principle to consider is that time, like money, is a commodity, and there are ways to perceive and handle time that can lead to business success or failure.

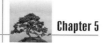

One of the key principles of time is that it is fluid and malleable. For the therapist, time can often seem to stand still when doing massage, though at other times it can seem to fly. Your clients also experience odd distortions of time during their sessions, usually concluding that a good session is too short and a bad session feels interminable. Even though your clients are paying for a set amount of time, their personal experience of that time is malleable, and that can alter how they perceive the value of their session and affect their decision to rebook.

There is a subtle but important difference between when the clock says a client is done and when the client "feels" done. One of the complaints I have heard repeatedly from people who go to large massage establishments is the feeling they get that the therapist is doing a "taximeter massage." Throughout the session, the clients feel that the therapist is looking at the clock the whole time, like their taximeter is running, and the moment their time is up, the therapist just stops and walks out of the room. As one client described it to me, "The therapist suddenly stopped what she was doing, lifted her hands off of me like she'd been burned, and walked off." After hearing people describe this experience so many times, I have come to the conclusion that the therapist's attitude about time greatly affects the clients' perceptions of how much they trust them and value their work. If the therapist feels rushed or focused on the clock, the client feels that the session seemed too short or was even a rip-off. However, if the therapist is relaxed and focuses his or her attention and energy on clients, even for short sessions, the clients will feel that they got their money's worth. In my experience, giving a few extra minutes of free work past client expectation points makes their experience of time expand, and their trust and gratitude rises exponentially. Somehow, just as with money, if you have a spirit of generosity with time and give from a place of abundance, you are blessed back tenfold. Those few free minutes you give away are precious to many clients. That extra time happily given can instill what I have experienced as fierce loyalty, where clients don't want to get massage from anyone else and gladly give referrals.

If you, or your client, are on a tight schedule and don't have the luxury of adding on a few minutes, you can still create the expansive sense of time. Focus your energy on the person, not the clock, and have a concluding ritual that is unhurried, deliberate, and makes the body feel whole and integrated. This gives the impression that the session is full and complete, not stopped at an arbitrary place because the clock ran out.

Where the practicality of time crosses the marketing need to maintain trust, demonstrate value, and shape perception is a middle ground of scheduling, which brings us back to the appointment book. As you schedule your work time, it can be valuable for you to pad your session time with a few extra minutes. Even if you have a very busy practice and can sell every minute you have available, a little leeway can go a long way toward keeping you and your clients happy.

For your clients' benefit, these spare moments give you the option to work longer, let a client lie on the table and snore, or not feel rushed getting changed. For you, those extra minutes scheduled can make the difference between an enjoyable, productive day and one where you are stressed because clients are backed up and kept waiting. More important, though, massage is a physically and often emotionally demanding profession, and the risks of burnout and injury are increased with booking clients too close together. The stress of rushing, working too fast, or becoming anxious because a client is slow getting up and is cutting into the next appointment is very detrimental to your health and your practice. It will do your blood pressure a lot of good to be prepared for unanticipated delays and to plan accordingly. Padding your schedule with a little extra time can compensate for all those unpredictable delays that throw off tight schedules. Besides, you can take that time to do a little stretching, get in a short meditation, drink water, get a quick snack, and otherwise take care of yourself.

If you have an office, anticipate people being late, taking a long time changing, fumbling for their checkbooks, talking while they get out their appointment books, and so on. If you do outcalls, give yourself time for traffic, getting lost, and stopping for gas or food. Sessions booked without building in time for these little delays can result in having to hurry, which does not create the atmosphere of calm that your clients highly value. Rushing around also might give the impression that your client is just another hassle or inconvenience in your day. Clients who sense that they are just another booking in your overcrowded schedule resent getting what I have heard called a "conveyor belt massage" because they feel treated like just another product coming down an assembly line. When people don't feel like they are unique and special to you, they will find another massage therapist, so block out the time to be able to give your full focus and attention to whomever you are with at each moment. (See Figure 5–3.)

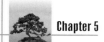

Figure 5–3 | **To be in the right place at the right time, use daily calendar pages.**

the week of the 4th-10th • January 20XX

Monday, January 4	Tuesday, January 5
8:00 AM	8:00 AM Breakfast Presentation - Rotary Club
8:30 Dr. Hofstra (45 min)	8:30
9:00	9:00
9:30 Suzanne (1 1/2 hrs)	9:30 Community Center 1 hr sessions
10:00	10:00
10:30	10:30 c. c.
11:00 Frank	11:00
11:30	11:30 c. c.
12:00 12:15 - 12:55 Lunch w/Sally	12:00
12:30	12:30 Lunch at Community Center
1:00 Work for Dr. H, 1/2 hr sessions	1:00
1:30 - session	1:30 Mr & Mrs Foxworth (1 1/2 hr each)
2:00 - session	2:00
2:30 - session	2:30
3:00 - session	3:00
3:30 - session	3:30
4:00 Drive to gym	4:00
4:30 Work out	4:30 Drive home
5:00	5:00 Snack, WATER PLANTS
5:30	5:30 Joel (REMEMBER TO
6:00 Dinner w/Steve	6:00 SAY HAPPY ANNIVERSARY)
6:30	6:30
7:00 Donald (first time client)	7:00
7:30 DO SOAP CHART	7:30 Do laundry
8:00	8:00
8:30 Tape golf game	8:30
9:00	9:00

Setting Boundaries

In the start-up stage of a practice, it is common to take any client who calls and to book sessions whenever possible. If you can, be flexible in the beginning in order to get new clients, but once you are more established, it is appropriate for you to set more boundaries or limitations on how you schedule your clients. Therapists who try to accommodate early, late, and weekend bookings and set no boundaries around their schedules are likely candidates for burnout. Your job is to create a balance between serving your customers when they are available and taking care of your own physical and emotional well-being.

It is easy to become unbalanced with regard to scheduling. If you are a people-pleaser, have weak boundary skills, or struggle with codependency and have a tendency to take care of others to your own detriment, plan accordingly. Use your calendar to help you preplan, and write in your personal appointments, socializing time, and recreation so you don't give clients time slots that are reserved just for you. In this way you can avoid the temptation to cancel things in your personal life just because a client happens to want that time slot. The more inclined you are to overbook, the more important it is that you schedule your personal life into your calendar.

Once your personal time is set aside, set up your work schedule and only book clients into those preset time blocks. In this way you take care of yourself and your clients, which gives you a great foundation for having a long, happy massage career.

Setting Goals

When you start out building your practice, set a goal for how many clients you want each week, then use your calendar to visually remind you of that goal. Block in the hours you want to work, and, as you plan your week, look for empty spots to alert you to focus on getting a client for those specific times. By knowing when to make a more concerted marketing effort to fill those specific time slots, you can more effectively meet your goals. For example, it is more powerful to have a goal of getting a client for a 4:00 p.m. time slot on Thursday than it is to tell yourself "I need to get new clients." With a specific goal set, your subconscious mind will keep alert during chance meetings and conversations, looking for that one person who meets your needs.

In addition, creating a time frame for the hours you will work helps you appear more established when people call for appointments. After all, it sounds much better to say "I have appointments available on Monday at 2:00 p.m. or at 3:30 p.m." than to say "My schedule is totally open and I can book you any time." People believe that busy therapists are that way because they're good at massage, so don't sound like you're sitting around waiting for your first client to call.

Finally, using a calendar to set your goals can help to make them real. Once you have figured out what you can realistically charge your clients per session, you can then look at what time you have available to book those sessions and

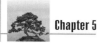

calculate an initial ceiling on your financial goals. The key word here is "realistic." Too many new therapists hear about the high costs of hourly sessions at spas and think that they can charge the same. Similarly, they hear about what a top therapist with years of experience charges, and believe they can command those rates as well. So many times I have heard of new therapists "doing the math" by multiplying high hourly rates by 40-hour workweeks, and envisioning themselves making tons of money. It is crucial for your long-term success that you not make this common mistake. Too many therapists believe they will make much more money than is possible, either due to the physical demands of massage, the time it takes to build a practice, and what the market will actually pay, either with private clients or as an employee. When the money isn't what they expect, they drop out, which is a loss both to them and to their potential clients. The goal of this book is to help you have a successful career in massage, and using your calendar to make and monitor realistic financial goals can make the difference between giving up on pipe dreams and building your dream practice.

Booking Appointments

Booking appointments enables your calendar to become a valuable marketing tool beyond managing your time. In short, your marketing efforts culminate in the moment when you book a paying appointment. There are two distinct types of booking moments, and they each require two distinct skills:

* Booking a new client for a first appointment
* Rebooking a current client

In both cases, your appointment book is part of the marketing process, and how you physically handle your book sends volumes of information to your client. First of all, just having an appointment book in your hand indicates you are serious about doing business. Second, how you hold your book, or gesture with it or around it while you talk, gives signals that you are ready to move the conversation to a moment of decision.

First-Time Appointments

First-time appointments may be made on the telephone or in person, but opening your appointment book tells you and your client it is time to get serious. Somehow, when a piece of paper becomes part of the process, it means an expectation is now present that a commitment is requested. If you can see your potential client while you open your calendar to book an appointment, watch for signs about levels of readiness to get a massage. An appointment book out with a pen or pencil poised over it is a signal to decide, and if you see hesitation or resistance, your marketing is not yet done. Your prospective client may need more information about you and your work, want more reassurance that you can help his or her specific needs, or just want to talk with you further before making a decision. If your potential client is ready to book, look for one of those empty spots you highlighted for client sessions and fill it in. Then write down that date and time on a card, and give it to your new client. You are on your way!

Rebooking Appointments

When rebooking clients, your calendar can also be a useful tool to move the post-massage conversation forward. With clients who book on a session-by-session basis, the time after the massage is when some of them can get clingy and want a few more moments of special attention. There is a delicate balance between cutting to the chase of setting up your next appointment and having your time wasted. With some of my elderly clients who are rarely in a hurry, this is when I especially notice that I am judged on being genuinely caring. What I've learned is that if I talk a few minutes and then start opening my appointment book, they subconsciously know that their time is up and I will be leaving soon. Perhaps I am overly protective of my clients in their hazy, happy moments after the massage, but I have scheduled in time for those moments, and I use my appointment book as the signal for them to conclude this session and plan for the next one.

After your session is over and your client is dressed, sit down for a debriefing and talk about how you worked toward the goals and results discussed in the pre-massage intake session. If the client agrees that you delivered the massage expected, simply ask for a rebooking. Even if you are nervous or feel you could have done a better session, don't make excuses for your work. If you are constantly trying to improve and learn to be a better practitioner, then you can be confident that you did your best at the time, and you can exude that confidence in your rebooking conversation. Touch your appointment book, indicating that you are ready to talk business, and say something like, "I enjoyed working with you today, and I'm glad I could help with your (whatever the goal was). Would you like to book another massage?" Then be still and listen. If your client says yes, open your appointment book, pick up your pen or pencil, set a time, fill in an appointment card, hand it over, and close your book. Rebooking can be that simple. However, if your client does not want to rebook, then read the chapter coming up on rebooking. Clients who rebook are going to be your best source of returns and referrals, so take the time and have the right tools to make the rebooking process simple, smooth, and professional.

Keeping Your Appointments

Using an appointment book is a discipline, and it may take practice to get used to looking at it regularly and not making promises without it. When you write down an appointment, you have given your word, and you need to do everything in your power to keep your word. The marketing function of gaining trust is dependent upon you **keeping your word** and your appointments. To be head and shoulders above your massage competition, make sure you show up for your appointments, and make sure you are on time.

I interviewed a woman in the Hollywood area who made upward of $200 a session in 1999 doing **outcall massage** to high-end hotels. She had a 200-hour education and used only basic Swedish skills, but when I asked her why she got so many exclusive, high-paying assignments from the hotels, she had a simple answer: she was one of the only therapists the hotels trusted to show up when she promised, and she was always on time. From her story, and many others like it across the country, I realized that responsible and punctual therapists can be, unfortunately, a rarity, and this one factor put her well above her competition.

Having an appointment book can help you with the details of keeping your word, scheduling your time realistically, and managing your responsibilities. However, it is up to you only to make promises you can keep, and then keep them. If you don't want to book a person as a client or work on a Saturday, say no. The word "no" is one of the best words you can learn to say, because when you say "yes," you can trust that you mean it.

If you often find yourself running late, needing to cancel at the last minute, or forgetting things that are important to your work, you will need to make some adjustments beyond using an appointment book. Your reasons can be as deep as sabotaging your business due to a subconscious fear of success, or just plain inexperience in the discipline of managing your time and commitments. Whatever your reasons are for not keeping your word, remember, you either get good excuses or good results, and you can't have both. Your friends and family may tolerate you being late or not showing up when you said you would, but when you run a business, your clients will not. You are selling your reputation, and the better it is, the more money you can command, and the more people will rebook and refer.

If you do break a lot of promises, big or small, or often show up late, take serious steps to change those habits. One of my favorite ways to break the habit of making excuses for being late is to ask the question, "If I got a million dollars for making it there on time, could I do it?" If I recognize that I can, I realize I am justifying my excuses, and I look at what I'm doing that is getting me off to a late start. If you are just plain forgetful, make your appointment book your constant companion. Write down everything you have agreed to, refer to your book often, and use it to help you learn the discipline of keeping your word.

Use It, and Don't Lose It

The last factor of using an appointment book is being able to find it when you need it. Whatever style of calendar you choose, what matters most is having one you can easily find when a client calls to book an appointment. You don't want to be running around the house or office shouting "Hold on, hold on!" into the phone while a client waits for you to unearth your appointment book.

If you are prone to misplacing things, or always seem to be looking for your missing keys or wallet, you will need to develop a better set of habits for yourself. One of my mentors, Ted Frey, gave me a great tool to change a bad habit into a good one. The tool is comprised of two simple phrases, but the words can shape your self-perception, personal beliefs about yourself, and, ultimately, your behavior. The phrases are: "That's like me" and "That's not like me." First, to help you not misplace your appointment book, pick a designated place to put it when you are at home, at work, or wherever you use it. Make a commitment to yourself to always put your book in that one spot. Then, when you go into your home or office, head right to that spot and put your book there. When you put it down, acknowledge yourself with a simple "That's like me." This trains your mind to keep repeating your new habit. If you race into the house and start to put your book down somewhere else, simply say, "That's not like me." Habits often are based on self-perception, and when your self-perception expects you to do one thing but you do another, it jars your awareness. This momentary jarring is your signal to pick up your appointment book and move it to its designated spot. When you put it down in the right place, say, "That's like me," and get on with whatever you were doing.

Simple things such as being able to immediately find your appointment book when a client calls may seem trivial, but they are not. The little details are what end up shaping your clients' perceptions, and, added together, they determine your overall image as a professional.

Finally, make photocopies of your appointment book pages on a regular basis or input your data into your computer and burn backup disks. That way, if you should lose your book, you will still have that invaluable information. This is crucial for running your business as well as maintaining your **paper trail** records for taxes.

BASIC MARKETING TOOL #3: A CONTACT LIST OF YOUR CLIENTELE

In a service business such as massage, your primary asset is your client contact list. Keeping track of your clients in an organized manner gives you the ability to access them for scheduling, marketing, sending birthday and holiday cards, or any other reason you want to get in touch with them. (See Figure 5–4.) Your client list also can be used to demonstrate the value of your practice. If you want to get a business loan, enroll investors, sell your practice, rent an office, or otherwise prove your creditworthiness and earning potential, your client list may be required as one of the tools you use to back your income claims. Your client list is also part of your tax records, and may be needed to prove to an auditor that you are a legitimate business and have rights to the **tax deductions** you claim. In addition, it is critical that, like doctors or psychologists, you take every precaution to ensure the privacy of your client list. In short, make sure you keep your list maintained and well guarded.

Dozens of ways to document your client list are available, ranging from customizable software programs with business-card scanners, to PDAs with wireless interface, to basic paper address books. The best paper option is a time management system with the insertable contact or address pages where you can write in all your client contact information. Using this system, when a client calls and leaves a message on your machine to change an appointment

Figure 5–4 | A contact list helps you keep in touch with your clientele.

ADDRESSES

Name **Angie Frost**
Address **4 Golf Club Ave, Pleasant Hill 94523**
☎ **925-555-1212**
Ⓞ ✆

Name **Suzanne Garcia**
Address **1920 Bonita Road, Concord 94518**
☎ **800-555-1212**
Ⓞ ✆

Name **Karen Smith**
Address **22 Elm St, Alamo 94507**
☎ **707-555-1212**
Ⓞ ✆

Name **Doug Wong**
Address **123 Buena Vista, Berkeley 94618**
☎ **510-555-1212**
Ⓞ ✆

Name **Ted Johnson**
Address **789 Moraga Circle, Lafayette 94509**
☎ **888-555-1212**
Ⓞ ✆

Name **Lucy Outlaw**
Address **456 Pleasant Drive, Walnut Creek 94597**
☎ **866-555-1212**
Ⓞ ✆

Name **Frank Jump**
Address **123 Main St. Pittsburg 94565**
☎ **877-555-1212**
Ⓞ ✆

☎ Telephone ✆ Fax Ⓞ Mobile Telephone/E-Mail/Web Address

but doesn't leave a telephone number, you can find the number and your schedule in one book. To make your life easier, consider having one section in your address pages for clients (perhaps under the letter "C" for clients), and do not list your clients separately by last name throughout the alphabetical pages. In this way, you can quickly find their names all in one place, and for clients you see infrequently or whose last names have slipped your mind, you won't lose them in the alphabetical pages.

Even if you have in-office files and forms with all of your clients' information in them, a centralized and portable list makes it easier to reach your clients, especially if you do outcalls. You can write down addresses and telephone numbers only, but for each client, you can also include his or her:

❋ Name

❋ Address

❋ Home telephone number

- ✳ Work telephone number
- ✳ Cell phone number
- ✳ E-mail address
- ✳ Birthday
- ✳ Date of first massage
- ✳ Directions to home or office, if you do outcall

For bare-bones basics, this simple time management system is enough to get your practice off the ground without too much expense, hassle, and delay. When starting out, go to a business supply store, get an appointment book or time management system with an address section, and start using it. Later, when you want an electronic organizer, programmable cell phone, or computer program to hold all your information in one place, you will know better what you want and need to keep track of your clients and business.

As with your appointment pages, maintain a regular backup of your client information. Whether on your computer with backup disks, or by photocopying your pages, keep your client list in a few places so if you lose one source, you will still have this most valuable information.

BASIC MARKETING TOOL #4: A TELEPHONE AND ANSWERING MACHINE

One of the primary ways you will conduct your marketing is over the telephone. How you handle the telephone can tell your callers a lot about your level of professionalism, and your phone manner can greatly affect their level of trust in you.

I remember one vivid instance of this principle in action when I was returning a call to a massage therapist I had never met before. She had called me and left a message, and when I called her back, I did not have any major impressions of her. However, when her teenage son picked up the telephone and greeted me with a surly "Yeah?" that was bad impression number one. Not knowing if I had called the wrong number, I asked for the massage therapist, whereupon the boy dropped the phone on the counter with a loud bang and yelled, "Mom! Phone!" Somehow, no matter what this woman had to say after that, I already had created my initial impression of her, and it wasn't good. It may seem unfair that we are judged as professionals by our non-massage skills or by others around us, but if I were an apprehensive new client alert to every detail to see if I was going to feel safe in this therapist's home office, such a telephone reception would have sent me running.

Marketing on the telephone works in two ways: incoming calls, when potential or current clients call you; and outgoing calls, when you call them. Each situation requires different communication skills, so let's take a closer look at what it takes to market on the telephone.

Incoming Calls

Incoming calls have two possible outcomes: your callers either reach you in person, or they don't. Both scenarios create a lasting impression on your caller. For that reason, the telephone etiquette used by you, a family member, colleague, receptionist, or your outgoing message on your answering machine or voice mail is important. It can very well make a difference in the success of your practice. There are a few elements in your telephone manner that indicate to your caller whether you are a trustworthy professional or an amateur. These are very basic rules, and may seem simplistic, but in calling massage professionals across the country, I have so often experienced these rules broken that I am including them here.

To represent yourself as a professional, when your telephone rings:

- ❋ Assume every call is a business call and answer it like a new client is on the line.

- ❋ Smile before you pick up the telephone; it brightens your voice.

- ❋ Always say who you are; immediately answer with your name and/or your business name.

- ❋ Remember to be of service and sound happy to hear from the caller.

- ❋ Greet the caller by name, and ask "What can I do for you today?"

- ❋ Be quiet and listen when he or she talks.

- ❋ Have a pen and paper handy, and know where to locate your appointment book.

If a potential client or **prospect** calls, he or she is in one of two possible states. One is a state of readiness and desire to book an appointment with minimal conversation. In my experience, when prospects called me because one of my clients referred them to me for massage, they already had made up their minds. All they wanted to do was go over a few details and book the appointment.

The first time this happened to me, I assumed the man calling would need to know all sorts of things about me and my work before he would book a session. I was wrong. This man was a high-powered executive who had very little time, knew what he wanted, had made up his mind, and, quite frankly, wasn't interested in what I had to say. He had heard from a friend of his that I was a good massage therapist, and that was all he needed to know. With clients like this, give a simple greeting such as, "I'm glad you called. What can I do for you today?" and then be quiet while they lead the conversation the way they want it to go.

The second state of caller readiness is when the prospect has heard about you from a referral or some other source, but wants to know more before making a decision to book an appointment. In the beginning of the conversation, ask as many questions as you can to find out what the caller wants or needs.

Ask questions to get them talking, such as:

> "How can I help you?"

> "How did you hear about me?" (Create common ground if from a personal referral)

> "Have you had massage before?"

> "What are you looking for from a massage?" (This is a good screening question)

Then:

✳ Listen as long as you can before you answer their questions.

✳ Take notes as they talk, especially on which words they use so you can use them later.

✳ Rephrase their questions or answers if you are not clear what they mean.

✳ Think as if you will have a long-term relationship, not just book one session.

✳ Ask for some form of decision to move the caller to booking.

✳ Trust your gut reaction if you don't feel okay about scheduling a session.

Early on in my practice, I learned to trust my gut instinct, and I turned down new clients a number of times because of an intuitive feeling. In a number of cases, I never really knew why my internal warnings went off, but in a few instances, I later learned that the person had a severe medical condition that I could have aggravated. When I worked for a large company while I was going to massage school, one of my coworkers asked me to give her a massage, but I refused because something felt very wrong to me. Even though she got angry, I stayed with my intuition, which I'm glad about because a week or so later, she left work in an ambulance because she had a bleeding ulcer. My guess is that, based on her personality, she would have blamed me for aggravating her medical condition and probably would have sued me. When booking unfamiliar people, listen to your intuition, and pay attention to hunches, inclinations, uneasy feelings, or hesitations. Whatever you decide, pay attention to what happens as a result so that you can learn to trust your intuition on ever more subtle levels.

Common Questions During Incoming Calls

There are three questions you need to anticipate and be ready for when dealing with incoming calls. These questions will be about your work and your fees, and occasional questions may test your legitimacy. If your caller asks a question that doesn't make sense to you, respond with your own question and get clarification before you answer. The more your prospects talk before you say much, the better you will understand their needs so that when you do finally talk, you can tailor what you say to show that you are the right massage therapist for them.

Following are three versions of these common questions, including suggested answers and the rationale for those answers. Every question you are asked is an opportunity to market yourself, so formulate answers that you can smoothly and professionally give to shape your caller's perception, establish value, and create trust.

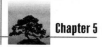

Common Questions

Q: What kind of work do you do?
A: That depends. I have a wide range of skills, and depending on what my client needs from me, I pick and choose what will help him or her most. What can I help you with?

Rationale: Massage therapists, like most professionals, can become so used to their own industry terminology that they no longer notice when they are using it. For instance, if a woman calls and asks you what you do, and you say you do Quantum Touch, Neuromuscular Therapy, or some other very specific style of massage she hasn't heard of, her immediate perception may be that what you offer is not what she wants. It does not matter that the modality you named can meet her needs; she may have already made up her mind and won't listen well to whatever else you say. To avoid this mistake, ask her what she wants first, then tell her how you can help her and meet her needs, especially using the same words and phrases she used when she was talking.

Q: How much do you charge?
A: That depends. I offer a wide variety of services in my practice. What kind of work are you looking for?

Rationale: When people ask your rates, avoid giving out a price until you have a good idea of what the client wants. It is ideal to have a massage menu that includes a variety of services of different lengths and modalities that cost different amounts. Having only one service and one fee means potential clients' only choices in response to you are "yes" or "no," or to negotiate, which puts them in charge of the conversation. With a range of services and prices, your options greatly increase the odds of a "yes." Just like a menu at a good restaurant, a variety of offerings can tantalize more buyers than if you just have one item on the menu.

If your caller is looking for a special anniversary massage for his wife, you could offer a 90-minute session with an exotic aromatherapy add-on. If the caller is having a wedding party and wants a therapist to do chair massage for the bridesmaids, be glad that you didn't just answer his or her initial question by saying you charge $80 an hour for deep tissue massage. By answering the question about what work you do or what you charge before you know what they want, you might miss a sale. As you listen to your caller talk, think about how you can best be of service and make offers that will get him or her under your hands. Also, listen for elements that will affect your prices, such as how long a session they want or need, what time of day they want a session, or even how long you may work together. If it sounds like the caller just wants one massage, you can give an hourly rate, but if he or she wants and needs ongoing treatment and is looking for a regular weekly massage, offer package deals or discounts for loyal clients based on frequency of sessions. If you do outcall, your price will also be affected by how far you have to drive and how long that drive will take. However, instead of charging extra by the mile, wait until you learn where the caller lives, then give a flat rate that will absorb the cost of driving time and expenses.

Q: Do you do full-body massage/give extras/do release massage?

(These are some common euphemisms or code phrases that really ask if sexual favors are part of the session. Other phrases may be used, so if a question of this nature sounds odd, you may be dealing with someone you need to screen out.)

A: Let me clarify what you mean. I work holistically and feel it is important to massage the body as a whole, but unfortunately for my profession, sometimes the term "full body" means that the customer is expecting a sexual massage, which is not what I do. If that is not what you meant, my apologies, and please understand that this, unfortunately, is an issue with which my profession still has to deal.

Rationale: The link between massage and prostitution has not been eliminated yet, and massage advertisements in phone books, newspapers, magazines, and on the Internet continue to lead men soliciting prostitutes to inadvertently call legitimate massage therapists. Therefore, there is a possibility that the caller may be a real threat to you. Questions of this nature need to be dealt with firmly and directly. If the client is looking for sexual massage, or is a vice squad officer checking on your legitimacy, this is your safest opportunity to protect yourself. It may be uncomfortable in the moment to accuse someone essentially of soliciting you, but once you hang up, it's over. Not dealing with it directly, but instead booking an appointment, endangers you greatly, so you must have the courage to confront the caller on the telephone if you suspect anything. If you still are not sure about the caller after your initial conversation, you can simply ask, "So, what is it that you are looking for?" Then be quiet and listen until you feel confident in the response. It is better to risk annoying a real client than getting trapped in a dangerous situation.

Finally, callers may ask you many questions before they decide to invest their time and money in your services, so be patient. Some questions may seem dumb or obvious, but remember that ignorance is your biggest competition. Take time to answer questions, assume nothing about what your client knows about massage, and listen well so that you can best educate your caller about massage in general, and your work specifically. Education is still one of our field's best forms of marketing, and incoming calls are your golden opportunity to get people excited about getting massage from you.

Incoming Calls You Don't Answer in Person

The prior material was based on the premise that you actually answered your telephone. If you are busy with your life and practice, however, you will have fewer opportunities to answer your telephone in person. If you do not answer your telephone, then someone or something else should, because most people will probably not bother calling back if your telephone just rings and rings. This results in your caller's first impressions being created for you by another person and/or a machine.

When Other People Answer Your Phone

If you have a home-based or **outcall practice**, it is likely that your home is your office. If you live alone, one telephone is fine, but as discussed earlier in the section on developing a business card, if you have family, children, roommates, or anyone else living with you, you would be wise to get a separate business line. You need tight control over the impressions created for your callers, and unless those living with you are well trained in business phone manners, do not let them speak on your behalf. By getting a separate line and a machine, you control your message, and you have sole access to creating your business image. (See Figure 5–5.) Equally important, you don't lose any calls, and information is recorded accurately so you can call people back. Plus, a separate line makes it easier to deduct your business telephone and calls as a clearly definable tax expense.

If you have an office, you can answer the telephone yourself, have a machine or receptionist, or use a booking agency. Since we are in the bare-bones section of the book, a receptionist or agency is not usually part of a beginner's scenario, but if one is, be very choosy in your hiring. Receptionists can make or break a business, so if you are hiring one, screen well, do good training,

Figure 5–5 | Professional telephone skills are crucial to building a successful practice.

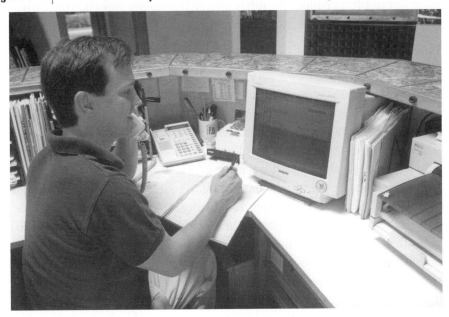

practice with scripts, pay well, give acknowledgment, and treat this person as a full-fledged marketing representative who establishes and maintains your professional image.

Answering Machines and Voice Mail

For the price of one or two massages, you can buy an answering machine. If you don't have one, get one. Even if you don't like technology very much, an answering machine is a necessity for starting and running a massage practice. For a prospect or client to call you and not be able to reach you or leave a message is confusing and annoying. If the caller is new to you and has some hesitancy about getting massage or is evaluating your level of professionalism, a ringing telephone with no answer can be interpreted as being suspiciously unprofessional. After all, what other business or service profession does not have some immediate response to a caller? Plumbers, dentists, carpet cleaners, and other businesses answer their calls, and people expect massage therapists to do the same.

Clients who want to set or change appointments need to be able to call once and leave a message, not call back until they happen to get lucky enough to

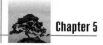

reach you in person. If having an answering system sounds like common sense, it is, but I have called enough massage therapists over the years who simply let the telephone ring to consider this topic worth emphasizing.

Choosing Your Message Machine

If you exclusively use your cell phone, you won't need a machine, but make sure you have enough memory for long messages. If your calls go to a home or office line, make sure you have a machine there. If you don't already have a message machine, or you have an old one that doesn't have a good-sounding outgoing message, get a new one, especially one with a capacity for long incoming messages. Clients will be leaving long messages to book or change appointments, tell you about a friend they are referring, leave directions, or give other data-rich messages that need more than 30 seconds to provide the details you need. Machines that cut off the caller after 30 seconds create an abrupt, jarring feeling. You want callers to feel special and important, but if your machine or "telephone representative" cuts them off without warning, that feeling is lost. Because the need for trust is so high in such a personal service as massage, therapists are judged more intensely on seemingly little things like message machines, so you need to give a lot of thought to those little things that make up your marketing package and professional image.

If you are buying a new machine, it is preferable to get one with electronic chips instead of cassette tapes for incoming and outgoing messages. Cassette tapes are harder and slower to rewind to hear a message again, or to retrieve remotely, and they can sound worn or wobbly after a while. Saving and deleting messages can be done more easily and accurately with chips, though if you need to save messages for long-term purposes, such as court cases where you are working with workers' compensation or injury cases, you may prefer tapes.

Message machines come with a wide variety of features, and while you may not use them all, you should still get a high-end model for your business. Cheap machines are never a bargain. One lost message can mean one lost client or appointment, which could more than make up the difference in cost between a junky machine and a great machine you can rely on for years.

How to Leave a Professional Outgoing Message

We covered outgoing messages in an earlier chapter about making a good impression on an employer calling you for an interview, but now we need to look at an outgoing message as an important marketing tool. As a marketing tool, your outgoing message has the task of greeting your callers, informing them that they have reached you, and otherwise enhancing or maintaining your professional image. In setting the tone of your message, imagine who may be calling you and what they will want from you. A professional message can include the following elements:

- A greeting
- Your name and/or business name
- Request for further information, such as their number or the best time to call back
- Information on other ways to reach you
- Information about when you will return the call

You may choose to add more elements, but these are the bare minimum components to include. Their primary purpose is to help your callers trust that they have left a message with you, not with a wrong number, and that they know what to expect as a next step. Before you record your message, write it down and practice it until it comes out smoothly and easily. Make your sentences short so that you can breathe naturally, and do a few takes on the machine until your message is perfect.

Your Telephone Voice

When you create your message, your voice is just as important in shaping your professional image as the words you choose. Use a friendly voice, speak clearly, and sound as if you are genuinely happy to hear from the caller. Imagine your favorite client or the kind of person you want as a client getting your message, and speak as if you were talking directly to that person. You don't have to fake being perky or sound chirpy; just smile, be confident, and talk.

Sample Messages

Here are a few sample messages that put all these elements together under a variety of circumstances. These messages cover the bases and can help you write your own message for your own situations.

- "Hello! You have reached the voice mail of Monica Roseberry. I'm sorry I missed your call, but if you leave your name and number, I'll be happy to call you back as soon as possible. Thank you for calling, and remember to wait for the beep."

✳ "You have reached the massage therapy office of Katy Woods. I am either out of the office or with a client at the moment, but your call is important to me. If you leave your name and number at the tone, I will be happy to call you back as soon as possible."

✳ "Thank you for calling the office of Maria Hernandez, massage therapist. My office hours are 11 a.m. to 7 p.m., Monday through Friday, or by special appointment. If you would like to schedule an appointment or book with me for a free consultation, please leave your name and number, and the best times available for you, and I will call you back within 24 hours."

✳ "Hello! You have reached the message center for Floyd Gambalie. I will be out of the office until October 6, but I will be checking my messages every evening and will call you back as soon as possible."

✳ "Hello! You have reached the message machine for Doug Wong. I am out of the office today, but I will call you back when I return on Friday the 12th. If you need to speak with me before then, please call my cell phone at . . ."

✳ Hi! This is Lucy O'Connor. I can't come to the phone right now, but if you want to book an appointment or learn more about my massage services, please go to my Web site at . . . Otherwise, leave a message and I'll get back to you within 90 minutes."

You can add other words to these few elements, but don't make the message too long or use it as a miniature advertisement. It is better that you create your first impressions yourself, and you want to know more about your caller before you start crafting those impressions. Live conversations let you speak more rapidly and get to the point with executive-type callers, or talk slower and more personably with elderly clients. You can be more familiar in tone with long-term clients and more formal with new ones, and you want to choose your tone in person, not let your machine do it. Therefore, keep your message short and simple enough to get your information across while still being professional.

Anything beyond a simple message risks alienating a client who is very different from you. Cutesy sayings can be annoying to no-nonsense businesspeople, and background music of any type can put off callers who don't like your musical selections. I have gotten massage therapists' outgoing messages ranging from seemingly endless New Age music, followed by a dreamy-voiced "Leave a message!" to heavy-metal riffs with "You know what to do!" shouted as the only message. Then the therapists wonder why no one leaves a message and why they don't have enough clients. To make the best impression, use professional wording and keep the music off your outgoing message.

Establishing your preference in music as the first impression a prospect gets of you sets a number of precedents. First, it subconsciously suggests that your practice is about you, not about your clients. This distinction is really subtle, but it is important to understand. It may sound harsh, but in essence you are forcing other people to listen to your music whether they like it or not. This one factor has the potential of warning the caller that other elements of your practice may be based on your preferences as well. Clients who have been forced to endure a prior therapist's conversation topics, music selections, pressure preferences, and temperature settings are wary of getting another therapist who is self-centered, not client-centered, so don't set off their alarm systems with your choice of music. You may like wooden flutes or Led Zeppelin, but leave it off your outgoing message and just enjoy it yourself.

The second precedent that music sets is the possibility that the caller may leap to a narrow and incorrect stereotype of you that may be difficult to overcome. If the caller is hoping for a therapeutic, no-nonsense practitioner and is treated to a minute of what I have heard labeled as "ding-dong" music, she may conclude that the therapist is one of those hippie types and will not be what she was looking for. The odds of her leaving a message have decreased, and, even if she does, the therapist will have to spend precious marketing minutes later undoing the caller's negative stereotype and creating a new impression.

Finally, if you do choose to have a long message, get a machine that will give people an opt-out such as, "To skip this message, press #," so regular callers don't have to listen to the whole message every time.

EXERCISE: CREATING YOUR OUTGOING MESSAGE

Write down two outgoing messages that will represent you and your business well. If you are in a group, practice your outgoing messages with five other people and get their feedback. If suggestions are made that can improve your messages, rework them until you find one that works well for you.

_____

_____

_____

_____

_____

_____

Taking Messages

How you document all the information that comes through your phone line can greatly affect your success. Telephone numbers, addresses, driving directions, appointment times, referral names, and the like should be written down in a place where they can be retrieved quickly and easily. Taking messages on scraps of paper, backs of envelopes, or sticky notes may be convenient in the moment, but this can lead to lost or misplaced information, which can cost you business.

For a basic, bare-bones message system, go to an office supply store and get a spiral-bound telephone message book with carbonless copy pages and tear-out message sheets. (See Figure 5–6.) Then attach a pen to it with unbreakable dental floss! These books have many advantages. First, the big message books are hard to lose in a pile, and if you have a home office, no one is likely to walk off with your book to make a grocery list. When the telephone rings, you know you always have something to write on, which isn't a big deal until you have a client on hold while you rummage around for a piece of paper. Second, the tear-out sheets let you take a message with you, but the carbonless copy page stays as a permanent record you can refer to months later, which can be invaluable. In addition, if you need to prove that your telephone is a tax-deductible business expense, these message books can serve as a record of your business use. Using a message book may take a little discipline at first if you aren't used to it, but in the long run, it will save you time, frustration, and valuable information. The process of getting and keeping clients requires

Figure 5-6 | Keep track of your incoming messages with carbonless message pads.

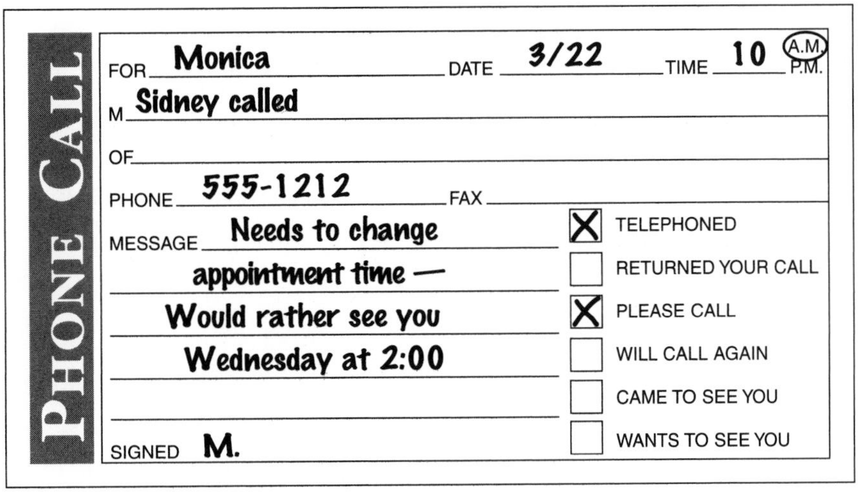

PHONE CALL

FOR **Monica**   DATE **3/22**   TIME **10** A.M. / P.M.

M **Sidney called**

OF

PHONE **555-1212**   FAX

MESSAGE **Needs to change**
appointment time —
Would rather see you
Wednesday at 2:00

☒	TELEPHONED
☐	RETURNED YOUR CALL
☒	PLEASE CALL
☐	WILL CALL AGAIN
☐	CAME TO SEE YOU
☐	WANTS TO SEE YOU

SIGNED **M.**

calling people back, so get good at, and be consistent with, how you store the information that lets you reach your callers.

Outgoing Calls

Marketing on the telephone also occurs during your outgoing calls. Since making cold calls to strangers is not recommended for building a practice, you don't have to work up a sales pitch, but you still need to be prepared for calling prospective clients. Outgoing calls can be first-contact calls, such as when clients or networking partners hand you a telephone number and say they have a referral interested in massage. Other outgoing marketing calls occur when you return calls from current or potential clients, confirm appointments, or make follow-up calls after a massage session.

These topics will be covered thoroughly in later chapters, but for now, what matters most is what to do with messages left on your answering system, because how you handle the return call can mean the difference between a paying client and a lost lead. Here are some basic, professional rules for returning calls. First and foremost, you must call back the people who left you a message. Return calls within 24 hours at the latest, and within 90 minutes if you can. When incoming calls are about scheduling appointments, it is a professional courtesy and smart business sense to return the call promptly so that your clients can solidify their schedules. For clientele who book massage as an impulse buy, your turnaround time for callbacks is even more important; otherwise, you may miss opportunities in the short and long term.

When you call back a client (a familiar person) or a prospect (an unfamiliar person), a few simple courtesies can help create trust and demonstrate your professionalism. Your call can go one of three ways:

- ❋ You can reach your caller in person at home, at work, or elsewhere.
- ❋ You can get someone else on the telephone.
- ❋ You can get an answering system.

The Unfamiliar Caller

When you return a call to someone who is unfamiliar to you, start the conversation by giving your name and asking for the caller by name. For example, you can say, "Yes, hello, this is Jeannine Rossol. I am returning a call from Tom Armstrong." If you have reached the person directly, remind him who you are. "I'm the massage therapist you called this morning. Is this a good time to talk?" If he says yes, then simply say something like, "Great, how can I help you?" Then be quiet and listen closely. Ask as many questions as you can to figure out his needs before you talk, so that you can craft your responses well. Notice that the call starts with the word "yes." This is a powerful word, and opening your introduction with it starts you off with a positive feel and leads the person answering toward a more open position. Experiment with saying "yes" early and often, and notice if people lighten up a bit.

If you do not reach your unfamiliar caller directly and someone else answers the telephone, be careful. If you have reached your caller's place of work, state that you are returning a call, which makes it more likely that you will be forwarded through the answering system with less delay. Since this is not a current client, staff will not be familiar with you, so do not tell anyone else about the purpose of your call or say, "I'm calling Tom Armstrong about getting a massage." This can cause a serious breach of privacy and can be embarrassing to a potential client who might not want his staff or coworkers to know details of his private life.

Even if you have reached a home telephone, be judicious if your caller isn't in. Tom may have called you to book a surprise session for his wife, and if she answers the phone, you could spoil the surprise. If you get a different person than you are trying to reach, leave a message, but keep it vague. "Yes, this is Jeannine Rossol. Please let Tom know I returned his call from this morning. He can reach me at this number until 5:00 p.m. today, or after 10:00 a.m. tomorrow morning. Thank you!" If you have to wait while the person searches for a pen and paper to take down your message, smile to yourself and remember why you got that big message pad.

Reaching a machine or voice mail is a good possibility, so be prepared with a brief but also vague message. "Yes, hello, this is Andrew Botter. I got your message this morning, and I'm sorry I missed you. I will try back this evening, or if you get this message before I get a chance to call back, you can reach me at this number between 3:00 and 5:00 p.m. today." This tells the person what next step to take, but also gives you the opening to call back in case you don't hear from the caller again, which can happen. Finally, and perhaps most importantly, when you leave your phone number in a message, be sure to speak clearly and slowly and say the number twice so the person can write it down and check its accuracy when you say it again.

The Familiar Caller

When current clients or people you know leave a message, you can be a little less formal in the return call, but still keep it professional. When calling familiar people, you can reach them in person, another person can answer, or you can get an answering system. If you reach your client, still start with your name, and use your full name. Whatever you do, don't say, "Hey, it's me!" This gives your clients only three words to figure out who you are, and it can be embarrassing for both of you if they don't.

After you give your name, get to the point, especially if your client is at work. You can say something like, "Hi, Jennifer. It's Alyce Maria. I got your call from this morning. What can I do for you?" Notice that the customary greeting, "How are you?" is missing. This is because you want to be sure you are not interrupting their work, or yours, and with lonely or talkative clients, it can sometimes take a bit of time to steer the conversation back to the point of your call.

Current clients are usually more specific with needs such as changing times or booking appointments. However, if they are not, ask them to tell you exactly what they want if they leave you a message. That way, when you call back, you have a ready answer, whether you reach them directly or leave a message.

Oftentimes you can book a session without talking to anyone in person, as long as you are clear. For example: "Hi, Crystal. It's Marla McKibbin. I got your call about needing to cancel on Wednesday at 3:00. I can either rebook you on Thursday at 3:30 or 5:00, or on Friday at 5:00, so let me know which works best and I'll book you in. If none of those times work, let me know and we'll try some other options. Bye!" When you hang up, make a note in your appointment book, such as in the daily pages, that you called and left those options. In that way, you keep a call log and know to call back if you don't hear from the client soon.

In conclusion, your telephone will most likely be the main marketing medium through which you build your practice. Professional telephone skills can be your ticket to your dream practice, so pay attention to all the little details on the phone, and the big details of success become possible.

CHAPTER 5 SUMMARY

Marketing is a process of blending your attributes, skills, and tools together to help you get and keep massage clients. In this chapter, we focused on the only tools you really need to reach, book, and rebook your clients to get your practice started. We covered the bare-bones tools, including business cards, calendars, contact lists, and telephones and answering machines. For the business card, what matters most at this point is your name, title, and phone number, and not procrastinating in getting them printed. The appointment book section included topics about how to schedule your time, set boundaries, set goals, and book new or returning clients. The contact list section discussed key information points to include in your list, and emphasized that client lists need to be maintained, backed up, and kept private. Finally, we covered the telephone and answering machine, which included how to professionally handle incoming and outgoing calls, whether in person or by machine.

The goal of this chapter is to help you use your tools to build trust between you and your clients, establish the value of working with you, and shape your clients' perceptions so that they view you as a professional. This chapter has a lot of "dos and don'ts" with the intention of keeping you from making mistakes that have cost many therapists their careers and using what successful therapists have proven to be effective. Finally, the real goal of this chapter is to give you the realization that you don't need a lot of fancy marketing to be very successful in massage.

CHAPTER 5   ACTION STEPS

Based on the information in this chapter, do the following to start your private practice:

- ✳ Design and order at least 100 basic business cards.
- ✳ Select and purchase an appointment book or time management system.
- ✳ Create a professional contact list.
- ✳ Get an answering machine or voice mail, if you don't have one.
- ✳ Create a professional outgoing message.
- ✳ Practice being on time for everything so that punctuality becomes your standard.

CHAPTER 5   KNOWLEDGE CHECK

Check your understanding of the chapter by reviewing these questions and answers.

Q: What is one of your most important marketing tools?
A: A business card.

Q: What are the three elements of a basic business card?
A: Your name, title, and telephone number.

Q: What are the four primary uses for an appointment book?
A: Scheduling your time, setting boundaries, setting goals, and booking appointments.

Q: What are two possible risks of overbooking your schedule?
A: Burnout and injury.

Q: What are the two types of bookings you will face?
A: Booking new clients for a first appointment, and rebooking current clients.

Q: What are the two phrases you can use to change bad habits into good ones?
A: "That's like me"; "that's not like me."

Q: What is your primary asset in a service business?
A: Your client list.

Q: What are the two possible results of an incoming call?
A: Your caller reaches you in person, or doesn't.

Q: What are the five elements of a professional outgoing message?
A: A greeting; your name and/or business name; request for further information (name, number, when to call back); information on other ways to call you; and information about when you will return the call.

Q: True or False? Music on your outgoing message is fine, as long as it's instrumental.
A: False.

Muscle Marketing: Reaching, Rebooking, and Referrals

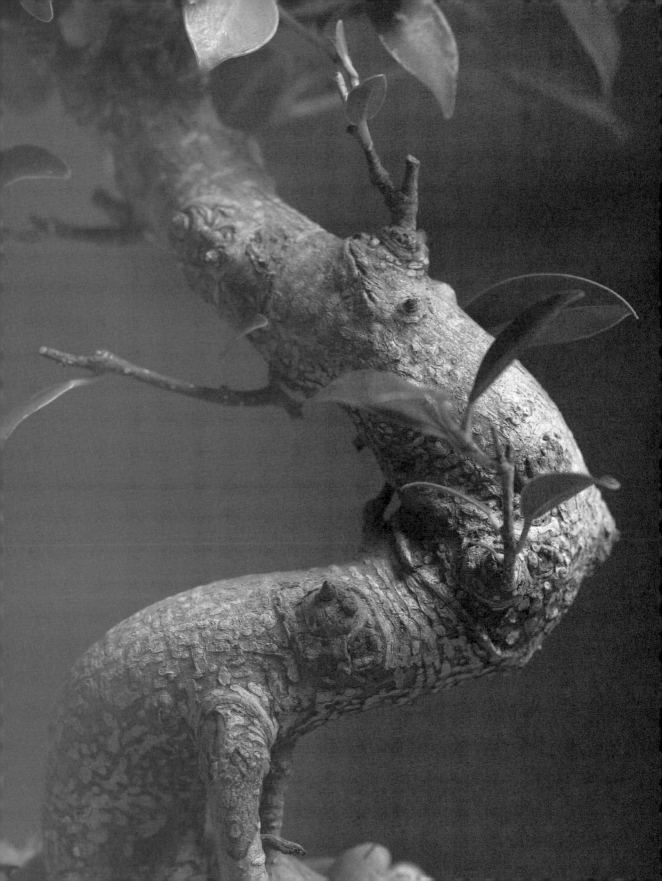

6 | Reaching Skills

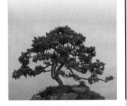

CHAPTER OBJECTIVES

After reading this chapter, you should be able to:

- Identify factors of your ideal life and work.
- Identify elements of an ideal practice.
- Explain how to choose a niche market.
- Select the best places to market in order to reach your ideal clients.
- Describe the elements of prequalifying clients.
- Explain the five levels of mutual marketing.

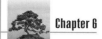

MUSCLE MARKETING

In the prior section of this book, we focused on the bare-bones marketing attributes, skills, and tools that successful therapists have used for decades to build their practices. These basics are the foundation of success for countless therapists and are necessary for sustaining a long-term practice.

Most massage professionals have not needed to do a lot of advanced marketing because they have followed the fundamental principles covered in the prior section, and have built their practices on direct marketing and word-of-mouth referral. However, as the massage field grows and moves into broader acceptance by the general public, more and more avenues of marketing are becoming available to us. This third section of the book aims to take advantage of marketing skills and tools that can propel your practice from dreams to reality. These skills and tools will take more thought, more time, more money, more skill, and more maturity than bare-bones marketing, but if you are ready to move from being an employee to starting a practice, or you want take your current practice to the next level, start a new practice in a different location, or open your own day spa or clinic, and you are willing to commit yourself to do what it takes to succeed, then buckle up for this section on muscle marketing.

Muscle marketing gives you two things that are hard to come by with bare-bones marketing: speed and control. If you want to build your practice quickly, and if you want to reach a bigger target market that you directly aim for, keep reading. We will cover many ways to market your practice, and while not every option suggested here may be right for your current circumstances or your personality, consider them for use later in your career.

Muscle marketing covers the "Three Rs" of marketing, and within them we will examine more advanced skills and tools to help you quickly and effectively:

- ❋ **R**each your prospective clients
- ❋ **R**ebook your current clients
- ❋ Get personal **R**eferrals from multiple and ongoing sources

Reaching Skills to Build Your Dream Practice

The primary skills for reaching prospective clients in the bare-bones section were: informal networking, social events, and talking to people yourself, including using what we called the "10 × 10 Rule." The goal of getting

10 new clients by talking to anyone within 10 feet of you can be very fast and effective, and getting client referrals from family and friends can be very helpful, but these can bring in a random clientele, leading to a practice that may not be totally satisfying. As you build your practice, you will discover your preferences for types of people you enjoy working with, massage modalities you find more effective, or other facets of a practice you will want to adapt or adopt toward making your dream practice a reality. The more you know what you want, the more quickly and effectively you can build your practice. Therefore, the next level of reaching clients requires these three skills:

1. Knowing yourself

2. Choosing your **ideal clients/niche market**

3. Selecting the best places to market in order to find your clients

Two primary philosophies of marketing exist for massage. One says you should see what needs there are in the marketplace, then prepare and shape yourself to meet those specific needs. It's the "find a need and fill it" approach. An example might be that you notice the growing percentage of the elderly population as the Baby Boomers age, and you decide you would be smart to train yourself to be better skilled at working with them.

The other way is to take the time to think about who you are and what you enjoy, then attract clients who want what you offer. You may love dance, art, or music, and decide you want to build your practice serving professionals in those fields. Neither way of choosing is right or wrong, but they are very different approaches.

I saw the first principle in action with a friend of mine. Her father, wanting his daughter to succeed, urged her to get a degree in computer science because he knew she could always find a well-paying job by doing so. She followed his advice and, sure enough, she got a good job and was secure in the knowledge that she could always find work. Unfortunately, lurking under the surface of this widely accepted thinking is the fact that she's bored out of her mind, and is doing daily work that doesn't inspire or move her. She is going through the motions of life, but she is not living it. Security is virtually guaranteed for her because she chose to shape herself to meet the needs of the marketplace, but in many ways, she has traded her soul in the process. She has no idea what is important to her or where her real passions lie. But she is now trapped by her bills and her lifestyle, and I doubt she will ever get out of the rat race into which her well-meaning father steered her.

When you are developing your practice or shifting it in some way, I would advise the second principle, which is to first know who you are and what you want, and to then use your marketing to find the right clients for you. With more daily satisfaction, happiness, and passion, your odds of succeeding soar.

Reaching Skill #1: Knowing Yourself

Getting to know and accept yourself is not always an easy or obvious path. However, it is interesting that the second commandment of the Bible is pretty emphatic about this point: "You shall love your neighbor as you love yourself." Whether you read the Bible or not, American culture has placed much emphasis on the loving-your-neighbor part. However, what is most intriguing is the command to love yourself. After all, if you don't love yourself much, you can't love your neighbor much either. If you want to serve and care for, or love, others, your first step is to care for and love yourself. Part of loving yourself is getting to know who you are and what is most important to you. Once you know that, it will be easier to figure out how to serve your clients.

EXERCISE: CREATING YOUR IDEAL LIFE

There are many avenues to discovering your beliefs, values, passions, goals, dreams, and lifestyle desires, and although this discovery is a lifelong process, we'll start here with a mental stretch to open your mind to new or additional levels of awareness of what's really important to you. Now is the time to let your imagination fly. We're going to do an exercise to create a no-holds-barred ideal day, week, month, year, and life by writing down how you want to spend your most valuable asset, your time. Since no one else will see what you write unless you want them to, you don't have to sound like a Miss America contestant, with everything being about saving the world. For most of us, making the world a better place is an underlying foundation of our goals, but it helps to be more specific.

Oh, and have some fun with this. After all, it's your life you're planning. I recommend that you do the following "Ideal Life" exercises at the rate of three to five minutes per exercise. Our brains create miracles when we are on a deadline, and given too much time, our "mental editors" wake up and tell us to write down elements of the ideal life that will impress other people, make parents happy, or otherwise have nothing to do with what we really want our lives to be like. Be prepared! Your answers may surprise you.

Here's what to do. First, take a minute to look at the list below of possible elements to consider in your ideal day, week, month, year, and life. On the following blank pages, set yourself a time limit of three minutes per time frame, and write as quickly and freely as you can about your ideal day, ideal week, ideal month, ideal year, and ideal life. In between each time frame, look at the elements again to spark new ideas.

Ideal Life Elements

- Relationships
- Friends
- Family
- Personal growth
- Finances
- Health
- Hobbies
- Work
- Leisure/travel/entertainment
- Sleep
- Contributions

Ideal Day

_____

_____

_____

_____

_____

_____

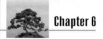

Ideal Week

_____

_____

_____

_____

_____

_____

Ideal Month

_____

_____

_____

_____

_____

_____

Ideal Year

_____

_____

_____

_____

_____

_____

Ideal Life

_____

_____

_____

_____

_____

_____

_____

If this is the first time you have been given the opportunity, or perhaps even the permission, to think so freely, so boldly about how to live your life, notice how you feel. The first time I did this kind of thinking and writing, I was exhilarated, frightened, hopeful, doubtful, surprised, and suspicious. I experienced mixed and contradictory feelings rattling my self-perception and identity. If your "Ideal Life" exercises came up with a surprise for you like "I want to draw greeting cards" instead of "I want to do sports massage for the U.S. Olympic Team," like you thought it should, don't worry. What bubbles up from your subconscious mind is a set of thoughts to consider, evaluate, accept, or let go of. These are not commandments written in stone. However, if a revelation comes to you in the process that needs serious thought, even if it has nothing to do with massage, go ahead and consider it.

Knowing Your Ideal Practice

If your ideal life didn't include any work or clients, then we may be in a bit of trouble here, since this is supposed to be a marketing book for how to get and keep clients. However, if you see that much of your passion revolves around one of your hobbies, say, surfing, cooking, gardening, bicycling, and so forth, then consider a practice that caters to like-minded people. Whatever passions and interests came up in the prior exercise, keep them in mind as we now turn to focus more specifically on your practice.

The skill of knowing yourself enough to reach new clients includes knowing:

✽ What kind of hands-on work you want to do

✽ What benefits you want to offer your clients

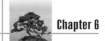

✳ What services you can offer in addition to massage

✳ What setting you would work best in

✳ What work time frame is most suitable for you

✳ What kinds of clients you want to have

Choose Your Work

Given your ideal life, and your passions and interests, here are some questions to consider as you choose your ideal work.

✳ What kind of hands-on work do you want to do?

✳ What convictions do you have about the body and about health?

✳ What kind of touch do you want to give?

✳ What is the intention of your work?

✳ What are you trained and qualified to do?

✳ Where do you have depth and experience, both in massage and outside of the field?

✳ Where do you foresee areas of growth for your work?

✳ What areas do you want to specialize in?

For example, do you want to do massage more for stress reduction or as an indulgent, marvelous luxury? Do you want to work with tricky injuries and holding patterns, and use in-depth anatomy knowledge and complex strategies? Do you have a gift for releasing chronic tension or compensation patterns? Do you prefer the emotional aspect of massage and know that touch can help in ways that words never could? Do you like digging deep into tissue, or do you prefer laying-on-of-hands styles like Therapeutic Touch or Polarity?

Choosing your work is part of the process of creating a niche for yourself, which is a big step toward developing your marketing plan. In essence, you are choosing your own persona and are identifying yourself in the marketplace based on the work you choose. Since public perception about massage is still vague, you can create your own titles and massage categories to fit your work, becoming the expert and establishing a marketing angle for defining yourself in your prospective clients' minds.

Having clearly defined work lets you differentiate yourself in your marketing, especially if you face competition. You can develop a unique specialty and become the first in your community to offer services in specialty categories such as massage for entrepreneurs, carpenters, patients following hip replacements or plastic surgery, or anything else that can distinguish you from your competition.

In this time of transition in our profession, we have ample room to explore and invent ourselves, and to create niches that never previously existed. Start with what you know and like, and don't worry about others with advanced certificates, more experience, or better brochures. There is always room if you know how to make it. Please don't wait until you are "good enough" to choose a niche. Start with a niche doing work you think you will enjoy, and make a conscious effort over the years to continuously improve. That is how you become good enough.

In the section on "Establishing Value" in Chapter 4, we looked at what needs humans have that massage can help. Addressing those many needs to relieve or avoid pain, and to gain pleasure, can be one of the factors of choosing your work. Wherever you can cross-match your passions and interests with other people's needs can become the point where you develop your work. If you have a passion for acting, market your practice to a movie studio or theater group. If you love archaeology, dig up a group you can accompany to an excavation site. Do they need massage after days of lifting stones and carefully brushing dust off ancient pottery shards? Of course they do!

Do you love river rafting, snow skiing, mountain climbing, or race car driving? Can you imagine your table set up where the rafts come ashore, in the ski lodge, or at the bottom of the mountain where all those aching bodies are desperate for you? (See Figure 6–1.) Since massage is portable and useful in endless settings, let your mind open to the possibilities of where and how you can work. Given this vast variety of markets, if one segment of the market seems overcrowded with other massage therapists, you can adapt your work, create a new marketing message, and appeal to a whole new segment that other therapists haven't reached yet. With the broad appeal and flexibility of massage, this won't be hard to do, and it's how you can create work you love for many years.

Know What Benefits You Want to Offer

One way to further identify the kind of work you want to do is to consider what kind of benefits you want to offer your clients. We are fortunate in our profession because massage offers a vast array of benefits to countless

Figure 6–1 | Massage can go just about anywhere! (Image courtesy of Getty Images)

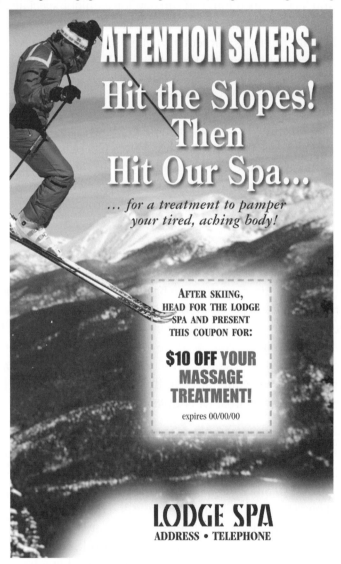

markets. Massage can offer pain relief to football players, dentists, post-surgery patients, assembly line workers, secretaries, and artists. Massage can offer pleasure, touch, and companionship to elderly shut-ins, infants, single mothers, ministers, gardeners, and traveling salespeople. Human touch, applied with caring and skill, can meet a host of needs from heartaches to muscle aches.

Marketing Motherliness

My favorite example of understanding and marketing your unique benefits comes from my mother. She saw how much I enjoyed my work and decided to go to the massage school where I taught so she could become a massage therapist. Since I was her teacher, she got the notion that her work and practice should be similar to mine. Long story short, her natural affinity for massage was different than mine, so after trying unsuccessfully to fit into my mold of work, she broke out and devised her own style and benefits.

In the case of benefits, mine were primarily about relieving stress in uptight business professionals, whereas hers were much more about nurturing. It was hard for her to give much value to such an etheric benefit as nurturing, but that was her true healing gift. Eventually she built a practice being, among other things, a "mommy" to motherless adults. Here she could shine, touching and stroking and caring for her clients in a way many of them had never experienced from their own mothers, or for clients whose mothers had died and were sorely missed. Most marketing books would not consider motherliness an asset or a salable benefit, but it was the perfect niche for my mother's practice. When she retired from massage, I inherited some of her clients, and while a few stuck with me, most just disappeared. Does this mean my work isn't good or effective? No, it doesn't, but being motherly is not my strong suit. It's not my main benefit, and I could not provide her clients with what they wanted most from their massage, which was a gentle mother's touch.

Special Additions

Beyond the modalities or types of work you want in your practice, there are a few nuances to consider as you create your niche and design your ideal practice. These elements may be where you become a "specialist," and they could be the factor that will be most attractive to your target market. Being unique and different can make you memorable in a competitive marketplace, and when you know yourself, value yourself, and want to break into a certain market segment, having special additions can make all the difference in the world.

Do you have skills or training in such additions as guided visualization, hypnotherapy, biofeedback, meditation, hydrotherapy, stretching, fitness training, nutrition, healthy cooking, yoga, tai chi, crystal work, breathwork, spa treatments, or hot stones? Imagine building a practice around a uniquely desirable combination of services for which clients are out there looking.

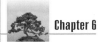

To amplify this concept, let's look at another industry for some ideas on the power and profitability of additions.

The Diet Expert

While thumbing through an issue of a fashion magazine, I came across an article on diet experts, people who work under the broad umbrella of the nutrition field. The spotlight was aimed on said experts who cater to those who want to be healthy (especially movie and music stars), and as I read, I was surprised that many of these experts had no formal training. Their "weight-loss wizard" titles were earned with gems such as recommending fruits, vegetables, lean proteins, and cutting down on fat. What made these people stand out from the crowd was not their sage advice, but the additions they tacked on to otherwise humdrum, everybody-knows-that information. What made these experts special were the amount and kinds of attention they paid to their clients. Whether the diet expert had weekly sessions to discuss increasing metabolism rates, did hair sample analysis for mineral levels, designed a tailored eating program, or reviewed blood samples, the clients felt like they got more than they would from a standard nutritionist. After all, who would you rather go to? Someone who "ooh"ed and "ahh"ed over your food journal, nodded sympathetically while you explained your turmoil over ice cream, and then gave you a customized protein shake, or someone who simply weighed you and then handed you a load of frozen dinners and a calorie counter?

I marvel at the thought that a man with no nutrition training but with a strong background in "motivational psychology" can be elevated to diet guru status enough to be written up in a magazine; but he gave consumers the attention and additions they wanted, and he has a waiting list of eight months for those who want his help.

While massage is a more tightly monitored industry than nutrition, at least in some states, we would do ourselves a disservice to scoff at the marketing methods and "additions" used by the people just mentioned. Your future clients want to feel special, be fussed over, be listened to, have customized strategies designed for them, be motivated and supported through life changes, and learn more about their bodies. Offer additions like an aroma-therapy concoction mixed exclusively for each client, a specially selected chakra-balancing music sampling, or a computer-generated astrology chart that points out which area of the body needs more work at a certain phase of the moon. This may cause a few snickers or eye rolls, but if it fits your target market, it will help you build your practice.

Your additions to your ideal practice can run the gamut from having a bowl of fresh fruit and a bottle of sparkling water ready when your client leaves the massage room, to having a team of specialists working with you, offering cholesterol and blood pressure screenings, back-strengthening exercises, herbal remedies, or biofeedback training. As you ponder what additions, if any, you want to incorporate into your massage practice, consider the following categories of what you can include in your work or setting that can make you memorable and appreciated. In my experience of interviewing clients, the additions are what they seem to remember and talk about, even more than the massage itself, so think about what you can add that will enhance your clients' overall massage experience. This is just a short list of additions to consider. If you come up with something else that can build your perfect practice, by all means include it.

What Additions Do Your Clients:

- ✺ See—art work, equipment, wall color, certificates, reading material
- ✺ Touch—oils and crèmes, sheets, table, face rest, temperature, your hands
- ✺ Hear—music, chanting, toning, silence, conversation, drums, ambient sound
- ✺ Taste—refreshments, drinks
- ✺ Smell—aromatherapy, body and breath, sheets, oils and lotions, candles
- ✺ Feel—showers, hot tubs, pools, saunas, steam baths, mineral soaks
- ✺ Learn—new skills, self-awareness, understanding of the body
- ✺ Act on—exercise, stretching, posture, movement

Remember, what makes you different makes you memorable. If you want to expand on your additions to draw a clientele that wants more than basic massage, create an aura or atmosphere that is interesting or unusual. In today's market, where people frequently see advertisements or TV shows featuring high-end luxury spas, your additions and environment are being compared to higher and higher standards, and you need to know how to meet your clients' increasingly demanding expectations.

EXERCISE: SPECIAL ADDITIONS

Write down five services or additions you can include in your practice that will appeal to your market and help differentiate you from your competition. Look at the list of additions and think about what more you can add that your ideal clients would enjoy.

_____

_____

_____

_____

_____

Your Ideal Setting

Another important facet in creating your ideal practice is deciding on your ideal work setting. Do you want to do fast-paced, on-site work, moving quickly from person to person within an office or business setting? Do you want to work at one place, and if so, by yourself or in conjunction with other therapists, colleagues, or doctors? What would that space look like, what kind of sounds or music would you hear, how would it smell, and how would it feel? In short, what can you do to your setting to create the energy and atmosphere that matches your work? Do you want to work at home, turning a spare room or space into your massage room? Do you like the variety of outcalls, going to offices or homes? If so, in what areas or neighborhoods? Do you want more of a spa setting, and can you set up your own day spa?

Do you want more of an alternative setting, especially more on-site oriented, such as wildlife safaris, truck stops, motor home campsites, airports, convention centers, coffee shops, health food stores, malls, seminars, psychic fairs, movie shoots, street fairs, festivals, and so on? (See Figure 6–2.) While you're imagining, think about places you've always wanted to go, or careers you dreamed of having but never got around to, and ask if you can bring your massage into those worlds.

Figure 6-2 | **Chair massage can let you take massage to many settings.**

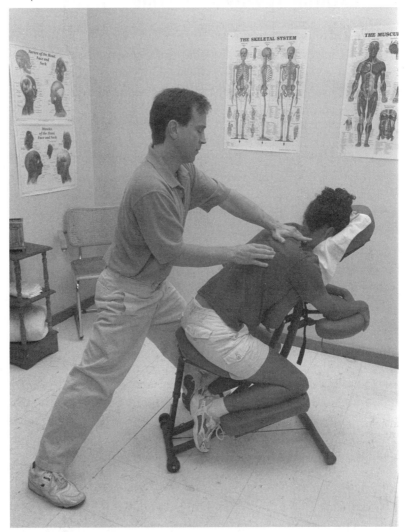

If you are more into sports massage, can you see yourself in sports-oriented settings like bird-watching hikes, dance companies, college or professional teams' training rooms, gyms, at an endless variety of competitions, boat races, fund-raising sports events, the Iditarod, and the like? Now that sports massage has become an accepted part of the Olympics, the Ironman Triathlon, and other such events, more doors are open than ever for massage therapists to find their place among world-class athletes.

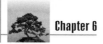

EXERCISE: CREATING YOUR IDEAL SETTING

What settings will make you happiest? Unshackle your mind from any limited options you may have and really think about who you are, what you want, and where you want to spend most of your waking hours. Then write down those ideas, uncensored and unedited, and notice what shows up. Create as many settings as you would like.

_____

_____

_____

_____

_____

_____

Your Ideal Time

In a perfect world, what would be your ideal number of days to work per week, and ideal number of hours in those days? How many days a month do you want to work, and will that vary depending on the month? Some therapists I know are skiing buffs, so they work hard during the warm months, then take off for a month or more during ski season.

Time for each session also needs to be considered in your ideal practice. Do you like working for 15 minutes, 30 minutes, an hour, or more than an hour? This is a preference you will learn from experience, but given your inherent nature, you can probably make some good guesses here and now. If you are naturally slower, laid back, and methodical, anticipate that you may be more physically and energetically comfortable with sessions that go over an hour. If you are more brisk and efficient, you can probably be happy working 50 minutes to an hour. If you are downright speedy, like action and change, and enjoy the stimulation of a variety of clients, you may be more suited for the shorter sessions appropriate for on-site or chair massage, pre- and post-event sports massage, or working with chiropractors doing patient prep massage.

No one way is better or more admirable than another. The trick is to know who you are, accept yourself, and build your ideal timing around that. Forcing yourself to work against your inherent nature may be okay while you experiment with what works best for you, but over the long haul, being true to yourself is the best choice.

EXERCISE: CHOOSING YOUR IDEAL TIME

Write down the ideal time structure for your work. Include the days per week, hours per day, times of day, special time off, and length of sessions you would like to be working.

_____

_____

_____

_____

_____

Reaching Skill #2: Choosing Your Ideal Client

After all the work you have done in the prior sections toward creating your ideal practice, you probably have noticed some patterns emerging about yourself. Knowing the factors of your dream practice, you now can formulate the ideal client who would fit into that scenario. While these perfect creatures may not be roaming the face of the earth by the thousands, having a firm grasp on what kind of practice you want will produce enough of a generic client profile that you can start to develop your marketing program around how to reach them and educate them on the value of your work.

One former student of mine needed only one client to make up her dream practice, and she finally found him: a world-famous singer who wanted a massage therapist to go on the road with him while he toured in concert. Not only was the pay marvelous, but she traveled all over the world, stayed in some pretty plush places, and saw sights she probably never would have seen. So,

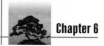

before you dismiss the idea of dreaming big, miracles have happened in the lives of many therapists who weren't willing to give up on getting what they really wanted.

In your ideal practice, do you want to work mostly with men, women, or both? Do you want to work with people in certain professions, people who are rich, middle class, blue collar, struggling artists, or entrepreneurs? Do you want to work with pregnant women, new parents, newborns, kids, or teens? Do you enjoy the elderly? Do you want people who are just learning how to take care of themselves, and massage is their first step into raised consciousness, or do you want people who are very evolved, spiritually developed, compassionate, vegetarian, and so on?

One therapist I know required that anyone who wanted to be his client had to be an athlete or exercise regularly, and even though he was charging $80 to $100 an hour in 1985, when most people thought $40 was high, he had to turn many clients away. His work was good, but he had that added twist that made him different, and his exercise requirement created such a buzz and reputation that people flocked to him. He knew what he wanted, and the clearer he got about his ideal clients, the more he was able to find them, and they were able to find him.

Do you want to work with people who share your religion or belief system, or who share a common hobby, sport, recreational activity, or art? A common ground is a wonderful opportunity for getting some of your first clients, especially if you are new to an area. On the other hand, do you want to work with people you want to be more like, such as world travelers, adventurers, inventors, computer whizzes, business leaders, athletes, writers, musicians, activists, or speakers?

As with charting any course, knowing your destination is critical. The clearer your destination, the less time, money, and energy you'll waste along the way, and the more you'll get to enjoy the fruits of your labor. When you talk to others about building your practice, and you know what you want and maybe even know what's in the way of your getting what you want, people can be much more helpful if they have a specific idea in mind of how to give you a hand. For some wonderful reason, many Americans see themselves as problem solvers. If you tell them your problem is that you need one or two new clients who fit your target market, they instinctively take the problem on as their own and try to solve it for you. And, the more clearly they know what you want, the faster they can help you with it.

If you want clients from a number of categories, that's fine. It is good protection for your practice to have at least two primary target markets. That way, if the economy takes a dive in one of your target markets, you will have a backup market. When I began my practice in 1984, my two main markets were wealthy, entrepreneurial couples and retired, elderly women. The entrepreneurial couples were charged more, but mostly because they were difficult to schedule, prone to last-minute cancellations, and I was never quite sure I could count on them. More than a few times, I was met at the door by the maid of one client who handed me a check and apologized that the couple had to leave unexpectedly in their private plane. My "little old ladies," as they liked to call themselves, were charged a much lower rate, but I could count on them being there every week for their massages. And besides, they were fun to talk to. When the economy took a tumble that affected a number of my wealthy couples, the little old ladies floated my monetary boat while I rebuilt my practice.

Preselecting a target market may feel a bit funny, but the reason we're doing this is because many business owners don't take the time or have the guts to either choose a market or limit markets in any way, especially if they are feeling desperate. One of the biggest marketing fallacies is that if you cast a bigger net, you'll catch more fish. Again and again, research in marketing and advertising campaigns has found that by casting a narrow net, businesses reach their most profitable market sooner. When you have the courage to select a niche market and appeal to it, amazing things can happen.

For example, let's say you just moved to a new community and you want to start a practice. You could try to send a flyer to every address, but that would be expensive and wasteful. You want clients from your community, but that group is too big to market to. So, to narrow things down, you could select a niche market you would enjoy, and market to them. Let's say you like horseback riding and antiques collecting, and you think clients with similar interests would be fun to work with. By narrowing down your market to people who ride horses and collect antiques, suddenly your market is easy to reach. You could go to local horse shows, attend competitions, and just talk to people; do a presentation on massage at a local horse-training center; send out a letter to the members of local riding clubs; and more. For your antiques collectors, you could set up a massage booth at a flea market or antiques fair; post a flyer at a local antiques shop; make friends with a local antiques dealer and ask that he or she help you get clients; and more. Don't worry if you don't quite know how to do all these things; that's what the rest of this book is for!

To summarize this point on choosing and understanding your ideal clients, remember that this is your life, and if you value your time, you should think hard about what kind of people you want to spend it with. What kind of clients will contribute conversations that will fascinate you, offer words of wisdom, give gifts, and show appreciation for your hard work? If each moment of your life is precious, how do you want to spend it with the people you work with? You will be spending cumulative years with your clients, sharing your lives on a regular basis. Your client relationships will motivate you to learn and continue to improve your ability and competency. Do not take that lightly. If you wake up on workdays looking forward to the clients you get to see, you virtually can guarantee yourself long-term success.

EXERCISE: CHOOSING YOUR IDEAL CLIENT

Write down a brief description of your ideal client using the demographic factors below. You can start the sentence with "My ideal client is . . ." You don't have to use every element, and you can add other elements that matter to you. You also can list additional ideal client profiles if you want to work with multiple markets. I'll give a few examples from my own practice to get you started. A little hint: if you have a hard time imagining your ideal client, think of who you don't want to work on, and why; then write the opposite.

Example: my ideal client is a woman between 30 and 70 years old who is an entrepreneur earning $70,000 or more annually, and is involved in a sport or physical activity. My ideal client has previous experience with massage, wants sessions every other week for stress management "maintenance massage," and sports performance enhancement or injury recovery work. She lives within 15 miles of my home office.

Example: my second ideal client is a married man between 45 and 70 years old who is an executive earning $100,000 or more annually, and travels extensively. This ideal client has previous experience with massage, wants sessions monthly for stress management and relaxation, and lives within 15 miles of my home office.

Example: my third ideal client is an elderly widow who is retired. She wants weekly sessions for a variety of small aches and pains, as well as for conversation, companionship, and touch.

Now you try it, using the list below.

Client Demographics List

- ✺ Male and/or female
- ✺ Primary massage need
- ✺ Profession
- ✺ Hobby or recreation specialty
- ✺ Income level
- ✺ Perception Continuum level
- ✺ Age
- ✺ Massage experience
- ✺ Education
- ✺ Frequency of sessions
- ✺ Marital status

_____

_____

_____

_____

_____

_____

Congratulations! You have just finished one of the hardest parts of this book. You now are unlike most people in this world who aren't sure what they want, aren't even sure what they don't want, and have never nailed down a dream on paper. Virtually every success book ever written emphasizes the power of knowing what you want and writing it down. That way, when the door of opportunity is opened to you, sometimes for just a fraction of a second, you can say to yourself, "Yes, that's exactly what I want!" and step into a life that makes people marvel about how lucky you are. This book isn't about hope or luck; it's about knowing what you want, and doing what it takes to have the practice and life that you love.

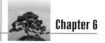
Reaching Skill #3: Finding Your Ideal Clients

During this time of transition for our profession, we still face issues of lack of trust and value, and misperceptions about massage. Many people genuinely want to receive massage due to its growing popularity, but because of the very personal nature of massage, they want some form of referral to reduce the risks of literally placing themselves in a stranger's hands. Most traditional marketing is anonymous; advertising, direct mail marketing, posted flyers, and the like do not reduce the worries of the buyer that the massage being advertised is going to be a good experience. In addition, therapists face risks as well by blindly marketing to an unscreened populace. What both clients and therapists want are personal referrals that are prescreened and safe. With this factor in mind, one of our best ways to find clients is through a process I call "mutual marketing."

MUTUAL MARKETING

The foundation of mutual marketing is built on three fundamental questions you can ask yourself to build your successful practice. We will go through each of these questions thoroughly.

Three Key Questions

1. Who is my target market?

2. What small businesses already serve my target market?

3. What do I have to offer that business to get my hands on its customers?

We just covered the first question when we identified your ideal client. Now we will look at the second question, and I ask that you keep an open mind because literally hundreds of possibilities exist for working with small businesses. Embrace the thought process here and you will start opening your eyes to all the ways you and your clients can safely and easily find each other.

What Small Businesses Already Serve My Target Market?

This is where the fun and creativity of marketing start. Somewhere out there, one or two small business owners have been working, perhaps for years, and they already have a client list that matches your target market. If you can find that one business, or even two or three of them, you can, in essence, knock on one door and have your whole practice waiting for you behind it.

Why should you consider partnering with a small business for your source of personal referrals? Because it is one of the fastest, easiest, safest, and most controllable ways to access new clients through a source that vouches for your trustworthiness and value. If you are new in town; if your friends and family don't know anyone who can afford massage; or if your handful of clients aren't willing, able, or keep forgetting to refer you, who else would be willing to help you build your practice? Someone who can mutually benefit from marketing your service of massage.

The act of cross-referring customers has been used by everything from huge corporations to sole-proprietor businesses, and because of where massage is now, it is time our profession starts making better use of this wonderful resource of clients.

I remember one of the first times I saw this cross-referring principle in action with a small business. I had just arrived at a friend's house, and she was finishing up some paperwork with a dusty looking man who turned out to be a chimney sweep. My friend had been thinking about getting her chimney cleaned but she had been putting it off. Then she got a coupon in the mail that offered a free, one-month membership at a local gym if she used this particular chimney sweep's services. The cross-offer did two things. One, it motivated her to finally get her chimney cleaned since there was a deadline on the gym offer; and two, of all the choices she had available, she made a decision to choose this particular chimney sweep just so she could get the gym membership. Also, she figured if the gym was willing to risk its reputation by being associated with a chimney sweep, he must be pretty reputable. As she paid him for his work, he gave her a pass card that got her into the gym. I was intrigued. There was no obvious link between chimneys and gyms that I could see, but the cross-reference got her to take action and choose this chimney sweep over all the others, and, when she went to the gym later, they had a chance to sell her a regular membership. The chimney sweep probably paid nothing to the gym, it didn't cost the gym anything but a pass card, and both businesses helped each other out with a very low-cost marketing campaign.

The beauty of massage over almost any other service business is that it is in the enviable position of being able to be easily associated with almost any kind of business for this type of cross-referral. Since massage is viewed as a luxury service, a medically beneficial service, an avenue for sports enhancement, and part of the good life, among many things, we can partner with any small or big business.

With its broad and valuable appeal, massage can be linked with a wide number of seemingly unrelated businesses to the benefit of that business and you. Small businesses are always in competition for customers, and they are in need of an edge over other similar businesses. They advertise and market, and spend a lot of money keeping their doors open, so if you can help bring in new customers or keep their current customers coming back, they will help you build your practice by giving you direct access and trustworthy referrals to their customer base. Small businesses are the ideal mutual marketing partners because you can give them a strong incentive to help you, they help screen potentially dangerous clients, they vouch for your value and trustworthiness, and as you grow your practice over time, you can refer business in their direction as well.

Choosing Your Ideal Mutual Marketing Partner

You can approach almost any type of business to be a mutual marketing partner, but some businesses will be able to help you more than others. When considering businesses to approach, consider the following questions.

- Do they already serve your ideal clients or target market?
- Do they have a good, linkable association to the needs you want to meet?
- Are they located in close proximity to your home or office?
- Are they amenable to partnership projects?
- Do they have a wide sphere of influence or contact in the community?
- Can they benefit from partnering with you?

Example: in using the reaching skills we have covered so far, I start with the skills of knowing myself, and mix my passions and interests with the needs of my target market. By doing so, I can see that it is a natural fit for me to want to work with golfers. I love golf, most people who golf can afford massage, golfers seem to keep hurting themselves, and I keep needing to fix them. If I wanted a clientele of golfers, I would consider partnering with a golf instructor.

To select a potential partner, think about who you are, what kind of clients you want, what needs you want to serve, and what businesses already serve your target market. To help you think, look at the different categories below and imagine what businesses would be best for you to approach in order to work together.

Factors to Consider for a Mutual Marketing Partner

Type of Business

Service

Product/manufacturing

Nonprofit

Government

Business Image

Conservative/traditional—eldercare lawyer, accountant, banker, architect

Professional—real estate agent, sports agent, wedding planner (see Figure 6–3)

Informal—dance school, florist, pet sitter

Manual—carpenter, maid service, pool cleaner, building contractor

Extreme—bungee jump, sky dive school, white-water rafting, rodeo

Customer Base

Large—serves your main target market and your secondary ideal client profiles

Narrow—serves only your main market

Contact Frequency

Regular repeat—piano teacher, gardener, hairstylist, tai chi instructor

Occasional repeat—travel agent, restaurant, nutritionist, herbalist, yoga teacher

Seasonal repeat—tax preparer, landscaper, sailing club, spring cleaner

Figure 6–3 | You can partner with many types of businesses to reach new clients. (Image courtesy of Getty Images)

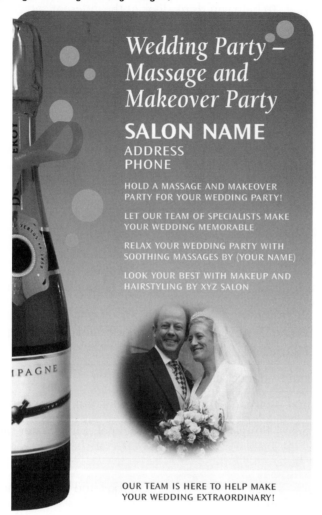

One time only—spa builder, real estate agent, moving company, photographer

Impulse buyer—novelty store, jeweler, boutique, antiques dealer

Emergency buyer—electrician, plumber, roofer, contractor, computer repair

Customer Needs

Basic needs—grocer, baker, water delivery, pet store

Essential service—barber, mechanic, printer

Preferred service—personal trainer, aesthetician, interior decorator, athletic trainer

Nonessential—dog psychologist, tanning salon, riding stable, diaper service

Novelty/impulse—psychic, rock-climbing gym

Contact Value (how much the customer spends per contact)

$1 to $100—winery, restaurant, bookstore, kayak rental, parasailing

$100 to $500—camera shop, shoe store, building supply store, exercise equipment

$500 to $2,000—bicycle shop, computer store, home furnishings store

$2,000 and up—car dealer, RV sales, boat sales, hot tub sales, motorcycle dealer

Contact Quality with Business Owner

Low personal contact—telephone, e-mail, employees handle customers

Medium personal contact—acquaintance, small background knowledge

Intensive personal contact; occasional—tuxedo rental, retreat center, broker

Intensive personal contact; regular—manicurist, tutor, speech therapist

Here are some other places to look for mutual marketing partners:

✳ Associations

✳ Philanthropic organizations, such as Lions Club, Rotary Club, Kiwanis

✳ Walk around your town and look at businesses

✳ Go through your phone book business pages

✳ Visit your Chamber of Commerce

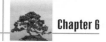

EXERCISE: CHOOSING A MUTUAL MARKETING PARTNER

Now that you have even just a few ideas for mutual marketing partners, write down 10 businesses with whom you can work. Be creative and think about what businesses would be good partners to work with in reaching your ideal clients. Ten is a lot to come up with, but stretch your mind! You may be surprised by the answers that come up after you've thought through the obvious ones.

_____

_____

_____

_____

_____

What Do I Have to Offer a Business to "Get My Hands" on Its Customers?

The third key question of mutual marketing basically asks, "What do I have to offer small business owners so they would be thrilled to refer me to their customers?" You have a number of options and they can vary, depending on the business owners' needs. You can trade massage with the owner or staff for referrals, ask for referrals as a personal favor, or offer some form of massage promotion they can use to increase business.

You can concoct all sorts of promotions, gift premiums, and rewards of massage to customers, all of which can help that business gain and keep customers. As we go through the upcoming examples of this process, be creative and see if you can come up with other offers, deals, or ideas that will make small businesses thrilled to help you as you help them.

Please note that, in contrast to many other businesses, giving your mutual marketing partner access to your clients is not included as one of the options here. Due to confidentiality issues, you should not give anyone access to your client list. You can tell your clients about the great landscaper or nice restaurant you are doing a promotion for, but don't give out your client information.

How to Create a Mutual Marketing Partnership

The first thing to know about any business, including yours, is that there are some universal requirements for success. The more you understand the specific requirements your mutual marketing partner has, the more you can tailor your offers to meet their needs. Businesses need to:

- Attract attention to bring new customers in the door
- Find a way to stand out from their competition
- Make a sale once a customer is in the door
- Bring the customer back again
- Upsell current customers to spend more on higher volume or quality
- Have current customers refer other qualified buyers

When you are considering potential partners, look for businesses that are motivated to work with you. They could be facing new competition, losing market share, wanting to get in touch with missing customers, trying to attract attention to get people in the door, or needing an incentive to close a sale.

The Shoe Store

One of my massage clients is a business consultant, and he told me a story that illustrates the importance of understanding what needs a business really has. He was consulting with the owner of an upscale men's shoe store who ran the store with her daughter. Their sales were slipping from previous levels and they weren't sure what to do about it. When he asked the mother and daughter what they perceived was needed to turn the store around, they gave different answers. The daughter's primary goal was to "get customers in the chair." Her mother's goal was to "sell shoes." They realized that the daughter had spent a lot of time and energy getting people into the store, and even sitting in the chair to try on shoes, but that was when she stopped the selling process. She had met her goal, but it was the wrong goal. When she was in charge of the store, people came in as she'd planned, but they didn't buy.

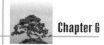

Figure 6–4 | By helping other businesses, you can also reach your ideal clients quickly and easily.

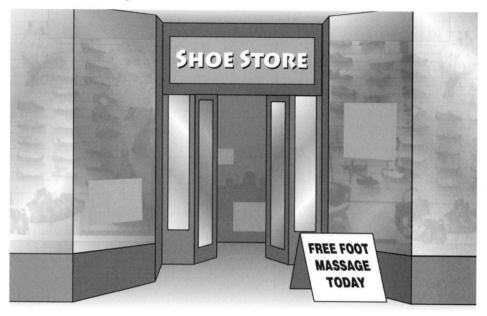

If you knew the goal of the owner was to get people in the door, into the chair, and then make a sale, what could you offer her to gain access to her upscale customers? To get people in the door, she could run an advertisement or send out a coupon saying that anyone who bought a pair of shoes could get a free foot reflexology, either on-site on a particular sale day, or by booking a later appointment with you. (See Figure 6–4.) She could hand out discount coupons for your massage as a thank-you gift for visiting the store, in order to create good will and "buzz." If she wanted repeat sales over time or more shoes sold in one visit, she could give out a **frequent buyer card**. If the buyer buys three pairs of shoes, he gets a certificate for a free half-hour massage or half-off the price for a full hour. If the owner wanted her current customers to refer their friends, she could offer a frequent buyer card to the buyer and any friend who purchased enough shoes for a free massage.

In all of these cases, your name and contact number would be given to these upscale buyers. In this way, you have been introduced to a desirable market, been associated with an upscale store, gained trust by association, shaped perception, and created a one-stop-shopping avenue for a strong source of direct referrals. You have helped a small business handle a serious problem, and you get prequalified referrals for minimal cost, if any. Now that is smart marketing!

If promotions such as these don't work for your circumstances, ask to leave your cards or brochures in the store for a trade of massage, or just as a favor. It is amazing how much others are willing to help, if only you ask. If you think that mutual marketing requires giving away a lot of massage for free, it doesn't. Some promotional setups can work better if you give away a few massages to gain access to your target market, and many successful therapists have benefited greatly from a few well-placed and well-timed donated massages.

The Five Levels of Mutual Marketing

Working with a business partner can be a very involved relationship, or it can be fairly removed. We will cover five levels of interrelationship so that you can consider what type of connection would work best for you. Each level of relationship has variations on a number of different elements. These elements are the:

* Actions you take

* Actions your partner takes

* Marketing tools you use

* Benefits of your joint projects to your partner

* Benefits of your joint projects to yourself

* Drawbacks of each level of project

Level 1: You Get a Mailing List of Your Partner's Customers and Do the Work Yourself

You can mail out a marketing postcard, card, letter, flyer, or coupon.

You may or may not mention your partner in your marketing piece.

> Benefits to Business
>> Payment for the list
>> Trade massage for list
>> Goodwill or favor to you

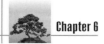

Benefits to You

> Your message reaches a large number of prospects quickly

> Minimal expenditure of time and money to reach your target market

Drawback to You

> Prospects unscreened, and it's harder to prove your value or create trust

Level 2: You Get a Mailing List Plus a Personal Endorsement from Your Partner

You can mail a marketing piece, such as a letter on their stationery, or use quotes or endorsement from the owner; the ad copy reflects their business.

Benefits to Business

> Pay/trade/goodwill

> You pay to market for them when you mention them in your letter

> Your letter gives them attention, association to image of massage, and free advertising

Benefit to You

> You reach a large audience quickly and cheaply. With the endorsement, you gain more trust and value by association and personal referral

Drawback to You

> If you are working without full licensure, you create a risk for yourself and your partner and therefore shouldn't use endorsements

Level 3: You Create a Marketing Piece with Their Endorsement, but They Distribute It

They can send your marketing piece as a special mailer, include it with billing or invoices, send it as a regular mailer or in a newsletter, or promote you on their Web site.

Benefit to Business

> Get to have image of massage and "good life" associated with their business

Benefits to You

> Direct access to qualified customers in your target market
>
> Less expense to you since they do the distribution
>
> More interaction with partner, with more possibility of personal referral

Drawbacks to You

> Some elements of the marketing process may be out of your control
>
> The process may be slow
>
> Your prospect still has to make the decision to buy a massage
>
> Your partner's incentive to refer you is low
>
> Their business needs won't be helped much
>
> Words on paper are no match for hands-on experience of your work

Level 4: You Sell Massage Packages and Promote Your Partner's Business by Offering the Bonus of Their Service Free or at a Discount

Examples:

> The customer buys five massages and gets a free, half-hour golf lesson.
>
> You get your partner's client list and write and mail a marketing piece offering your joint package deal, call the client list offering the package deal, or e-mail the client list offering the package deal.

And/Or

> Your partner distributes your marketing piece at the business site, as an enclosure with an invoice, or through their own mailer or other means.

Benefits to Business

> They stay in contact with current customers without "selling"
>
> If you pay, they market cost-free

Their offer can reinitiate a business relationship with former customers

Their offer can be converted to a better sale with upselling

They gain goodwill with their customers for making a valuable offer

Benefits to You

You get money up front for package deals, a good short-term strategy

It gets people under your hands to demonstrate cumulative value of massage

People who experience your work are more willing to rebook and refer

Your partner is closely involved, which means more personal referrals

Drawbacks to You

Purchasing a package of massage without testing your work may be a leap for some

It requires a decision to buy

The agreement of your partner's bonus can cost you money

If your partner can't resell or upsell, or gets no benefit from the deal, it may be difficult

There is a lower return percentage, but each lead is more valuable and committed

Level 5: Your Partner Uses Massage Certificates or Events to Promote Their Business

"Buy five golf lessons and get a free massage or discount coupon for massage."

Massage has wide appeal to many markets and can help generate sales.

The image of massage draws many types of people, and can be used in:

- Broadcast advertisements with an image of you working
- Ads to promote a sale or event with on-site massage at business location

❋ Direct mail promotion to customer list

❋ Direct mail promotion to purchased list

❋ Ads offering gift certificates or discount coupons in exchange for:

- X number of repeat sales (within X amount of time)

- X number of dollars spent

- X amount of service time booked

- X number of referrals to new customers

Benefits to Business

New marketing angle for advantage over competition

Massage appeals to a huge range of markets and attracts everyone

Massage is easy to associate to their product or service for good ads

Massage creates strong association to the "good life"

Promotions can attract new clients and missing clients, or create loyalty

Massage angle gets attention; is novel, different, and unique; and creates a buzz

Promotion gets people in, gets people to buy, and gets people to become regular buyers

Your partner gets money up front for package deals

Promotion gets people to upgrade the value of their purchase

Benefits to You

You reach your narrow target market and ideal client quickly

Your association with the business improves your market's perception of massage

You reach prospects you are more able to trust, with one level of screening

The association with your partner decreases odds of harassment

The client's decision to buy is removed; they don't have to have value proven beforehand

The promotion gets people under your hands quickly

The benefits of massage are more evident from your work than other forms of marketing

Getting a chance to prove your work leads to opportunity to rebook

If you are new, a big promotion gives you a lot of experience trying out techniques and learning what you like and don't like; it gives you a fast learning curve. If no one rebooks, you can find out quickly what's wrong

Drawbacks to You

You may have a lot of work up front with little short-term return. This is a long-term strategy

You can become resentful of doing free or discounted work if you're not careful. Promotional work won't pay off if you don't have good rebooking skills

EXERCISE: MAKING AN OFFER TO A MUTUAL PARTNER

Look at your list of potential mutual marketing partners. Pick one partner from your list that you think would give you the best access to your ideal client or target market. Then review the five levels of mutual marketing and create three offers to make to your partner for a mutual marketing project.

Partner:

_____

_____

_____

Project 1:

_____

_____

_____

Project 2:

_____

_____

_____

_____

Project 3:

_____

_____

_____

_____

Gaining Trust First

As a concept, mutual marketing is actually very simple. Many other businesses have been using partnership or joint venture marketing for years. Companies around the world have realized that if they share each other's customers, their profits will increase because they do not need to spend as much money finding and advertising to their target markets. Some massage therapists have taken the first step toward mutual marketing by putting up cards or signs in other businesses, such as gyms or health food stores. However, posted cards are passive, easily ignored pieces of paper, and we are now ready for proactive marketing with direct recommendations from small businesses. Since massage is enjoying a growing, widespread, positive public perception, your job of finding a mutual marketing partner will be much easier than it would have been even a few years ago. Finding a mutual marketing partner may take time, or you may build a successful partnership with the first business you approach.

One important element of creating a mutual marketing partnership is trust. Before any of these ideas can be implemented, you must create a professional relationship with your potential partners. You can offer your mutual marketing partners free massages, do on-site work in their offices, or do whatever you must so they know your work is of the highest quality. Don't expect them to trust you on your word that you're good. You'll have to prove it. Then, once you have established their trust, you can work on numerous projects together to build both of your businesses. Trust, depending on the past experience of the other person, may be easy to build or could take a while. Trust cannot be forced, and don't take it personally if the other person seems distrustful of you or your offer.

Being an Equal and Professional Partner

Since this is an official business agreement, it is important that you discuss your arrangements and agreements clearly and get them down in writing. I strongly suggest that you draw up a contract: one, so that you can be clear about what it is you've agreed upon; and two, so that you are treated in a professional manner. You are a professional in your field and you can be a great asset to another business, so approach a potential partner as an equal and handle your relationship as a peer.

To make the most out of your partnership, talk with your partner about what needs the business has and strategize together about various cross-promotional projects. Before you even meet, create some interesting options for how to promote their business first, and they will be much more open to any kind of working relationship. If you are fortunate, you will be able to partner with a business owner with good marketing skills. However, many small business owners may be good at what they do, but they may not be good at marketing. To maximize the value of your time, energy, and investment, you may need to help your partner realize how to make the best use of your joint projects.

For example, if I were to partner with a Pilates instructor, I would go the extra step to make sure she was following up with the leads she got when we did the "buy five massages, get a half-hour Pilates lesson free" project. Instructors, like most professionals, would rather be teaching than marketing, so if I want to make it a win-win project, I would consider helping her with encouragement or reminders to follow up on the leads we generated. This may not be necessary, but if you get many valuable clients from your partner, do what you can to maintain and move forward the relationship. One good partner, as I have learned, can provide you with the majority of your clients without you ever having to market again, so invest well in the relationship.

Client Net Worth

If you are going to do any form of marketing beyond the 10×10 method, you will be making a more serious investment of time and money. When you consider marketing methods such as mutual marketing or more traditional forms of reaching prospective buyers, understand that eventually you must gain or profit more than you spend; otherwise, you can put yourself out of business. The reason I like mutual marketing so much is that you can reach large numbers of your target market inexpensively with a very high potential for a good return on your investment. If you are a new therapist starting out, you will probably have more time than money, and many of these projects can be set up to take time, with little money spent.

As you evaluate your use of mutual marketing, I'd like to introduce a term that I call **client net worth** (CNW). Client net worth is the sum of what one massage client is potentially worth to you financially over the lifetime of your working relationship. This net worth is critical to know because it will determine how much you are willing and able to spend, or give away, to get a client.

While the income you anticipate earning from each client will start off as an estimate, if you plan to do numerous marketing campaigns, you will need to sit down and figure out what it really costs you to land a new client. However, if you follow the principles in the bare-bones marketing section, all you need are a few good clients to build a practice. You may only have to conduct a few marketing campaigns, then let the rebookings and referrals do the rest. For now, though, let's work with some general numbers so you can see the value of one client and why it is worth getting him or her.

Client Net Worth Examples

Let's consider some of my first clients, a couple I began massaging in 1985. I started by massaging the husband, a former boss of mine, every Friday. Then I moved to working with him and his wife every Friday, and then every other Friday, until I broke my wrist and had to give up my practice. Over the span of time I have known them, I have earned around $46,000 from them. Adding the income from some of the people they have referred to me brings their CNW closer to $50,000. Do I make them a priority, hold my Friday nights open, and treat them well? Do I go the extra mile, play with their dog, and wait a few extra minutes while he takes a shower after his massage before starting her massage, since he doesn't like getting dressed when he's oily? Do I bring in special aromatherapy oil for her, since that makes her feel special? Of course I do. Do I listen to her discussion of the topics of the television talk shows that day without giving my opinion? No, I have to draw the line of customer service somewhere.

My point is, I serve, pamper, and care for my clients in every way that I can, and in this case, the CNW of those extra miles I walked have resulted in more than $50,000 in sales with no advertising expenses. Advertising is a huge expense for many businesses and takes much of their budget, but if you can retain a client of this caliber, you can save your marketing and advertising expenses, and have each return visit be that much more profitable.

Doing Client Net Worth Math

Depending on your target market, you may do mostly weekly, biweekly, or monthly massage, and since the average American moves every five years, let's keep that in the equation. Let's say you get a new client who comes in once a week for a $60 session. He is out of town for summer vacations, Christmas, and assorted other trips, so he comes in for 45 of the 52 weeks in the year. This brings his total to $2,700 a year. If you only work with him for three years, his CNW is $8,100 ($60 a session × 45 sessions a year = $2,700 a year × 3 years = $8,100 CNW).

Let's say you get a client who comes in every other week at $60 a session, and she comes in 26 times a year. Her yearly worth to you is $1,560, and if she stayed three years, she'd gross you close to $5,000. If she stayed with you for 10 years, her CNW would be $15,000 not including price raises. That's a lot of money, and if it only costs you one free gift certificate to get that caliber of client, do you think it's a worthwhile investment ($60 a session × 26 sessions a year = $1,560 a year × 3 years = $4,680)?

If you do top-quality work, provide excellent customer service, and really take care of your clients in the way they like, they should become regulars, if that is the kind of practice you have. More clinic-oriented practices won't have multiyear client rebookings, but many practices have a foundation of long-standing repeat clients. We'll talk about how to build a repeat client practice in the chapter on rebooking, but for now I simply want to emphasize the value of rebookings and referrals for CNW so when I present unusual ideas later, you'll understand my rationale.

MUTUAL MARKETING EXAMPLES

Mutual marketing can happen in any type of business, and if you know who you are, what needs you want to meet, what kind of work you want to do, and the potential profitability of your mutual marketing projects, you can get to work. If you still want more ideas, I will go through a few examples to show mutual marketing in action.

Partnering with a Travel Agent

Let's say your target market consists of upper-management executives or older, wealthy women. If your specialty is more geared toward pain reduction, then ask yourself, when are these people sore, tired, and otherwise in need of your services? One possible answer is when they have been traveling. The next question is, what small businesses serve them when they travel? An answer to that would be a travel agency, and a potential mutual marketing partner could be a travel agent. So let's look at some of the ways you can work with this one well-connected mutual marketing partner.

The first thing to do is establish what needs a travel agent has. At this point, travel agents are in serious trouble. Airlines are cutting the percentages that agents get for bookings, and airlines are giving travelers incentives to book online or directly through the carrier, leaving out the agent altogether. As a partner, a travel agent needs to get new customers, but the primary need is retaining current customers. Therefore, your offer would need to include some promotion that rewarded the agent's customers for using her services instead of booking their flights, cruises, or vacations themselves.

Using Gift Certificates

To meet the travel agent's needs while getting rapid access to her customers, you can use the Level 5 strategy and give away free massage as part of a promotion. One way to do that is to print a stack of numbered gift certificates and give them to the travel agent, along with some brochures or educational materials. Let her know who your target market is and ask that she give the certificates to them. Give her some of the following ideas on how to increase her business by using your certificates, but also let her be creative.

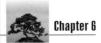

Travel Agent Promotions

There are a number of ways the agent can use your certificates to promote both of your businesses simultaneously. One way is for the agent to use the certificates as a promotion: buy a cruise from me and you get two massage certificates; book 10,000 miles in three months and get a free massage after your long flight; or buy a vacation package to Hawaii and get two massages for the price of one, or one massage free. If you do outcalls and the recipient of your gift certificate is a couple, try to massage both of them. Your odds of returning for two paid sessions are higher.

Another way is to piggyback on ads. If your travel agent uses advertising to promote travel specials, ask the agent to include your name or offer in her ad or promotional literature. This gives you valuable exposure, offers piggyback marketing for you, and, even if people don't buy from the travel agent, you still get exposure. If massage is offered as a free gift for purchasing travel specials, it creates a valuable premium for her customers. This differentiates her from other agents and may bring her new or repeat business. (See Figure 6–5.)

If she is a great resource for repeat clients and you want to continue the relationship after your initial project, keep giving her free massage gift certificates that she can use to build her business. This increases her incentive to send you quality prospects and refer you often, since she will benefit when you massage her clients. If you are trading massage for her referrals, figure out a formula for how many massages you will give her in exchange for a set number of referrals. Keep accurate books and keep up your end of the agreement without reminder, and she will think she really got lucky. The lucky one is you, however, because if her clients expect to pay $100 or more for a massage because they are used to massage prices at hotels or resorts, your profit from this venture can be substantial. You have not had to pay for expensive advertising, you created trust by word of mouth, and you helped someone else. I believe this makes it a win-win experience. If you think you can convert the certificate receiver into an ongoing client, this strategy gives you the opportunity to build a practice fairly quickly.

Remember, doing a lot of free massage will increase your new client workload initially, but it raises your odds of gaining repeat customers. And, you don't have to do it forever. If you need cash right away, this arrangement won't

Figure 6–5 | Travel agents can connect you to numerous target markets. (Image courtesy of Getty Images)

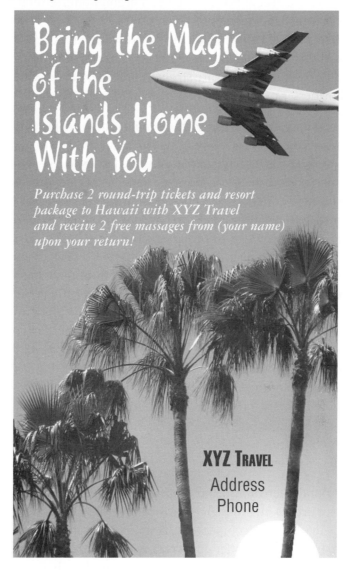

work, because this is a long-term, profit-building process. If you want money right away, you might presell the certificates at a volume discount to the agent. That way, you receive some money up-front, and the agent will be more selective about whom she gives your gift certificates to, since she has to pay for them. Be creative, meet her needs, and meet your needs, and you may never have to market again.

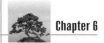

Real Estate Agents

Let's consider another scenario of the Level 5 promotional strategy. Let's say you want to do stress management massage with employees of a large company that is growing quickly and hiring people in your area. Using the same key questions, ask yourself what small businesses already serve your ideal client or market when they are stressed, and think about what you can offer those businesses to gain access to their customers.

In this case, you have multiple windows of opportunity. People who sit in offices or work at computers all day often have sore necks and backs, risk carpal tunnel syndrome, and otherwise perpetually need massage. However, if they don't value massage much, don't consider massage as an option, or are so wrapped up in their work they don't notice they hurt, they can be difficult to market to. In this case, your marketing focus needs to narrow to a smaller window of opportunity where you can identify a small business that serves this market in a shorter time frame. One time frame to consider is when there is a break in their normal routine, such as when they are moving. Their physical and emotional stress will be greater at that time, their need for massage will be higher than during their normal routine of life, and they will be dealing with a small business through which you can easily access them— namely, a real estate agent. If a large company is bringing in many new employees, it may be using a specific agent to help relocate its people. Getting access to that real estate agent gives you incredible access to all the new employees moving into your area. In this scenario, the agent already has the relocation business and needs no promotion, so what you have to offer him is massage in exchange for his referrals, or he may promote you as a favor to you and his clients.

On the other hand, there may be an agent you would like to work with who is trying to entice prospective homebuyers to choose her over other agents, and she needs an edge over the competition. To gain her as a mutual marketing partner, go to her office and offer gift certificates that she can give to people who buy a home from her. The agent can use this angle in her advertising or promotions to slant to upscale customers, using the gift of massage to create the image that by using her, the prospective buyer will have an easy, relaxing experience during the highly emotional and volatile time of home buying. Her marketing can use images of massage, which will give the new homeowners something to look forward to. They can imagine the massage therapist arriving (compliments of the real estate agent) after the deal closes, the boxes are moved in, and the moving truck has gone.

Another, less complicated or involved way to work with a real estate agent as a partner is to have him give to his current or prospective customers (courtesy of you) a plastic map of the local area with a star marked over your office, and a gold foil label at the bottom of the map that includes your name, address, and telephone number. New people in the area will need to learn their way around, and will probably use the map all the time. They will see your name, and be more inclined to call you to schedule an appointment. The main benefit of a map is that, unlike business cards, it is difficult to lose and is usually kept in one place, such as the glove box.

Preemptive Strikes

One of the biggest benefits of working with a real estate agent is that you get first access to many new people moving into your area. This is a preemptive strike in a highly competitive market, giving you an edge over other therapists or massage businesses in the area because it gives you first contact and creates a loyalty similar to imprinting on newborns. You may be their first friendly contact in a new area, creating a unique attachment and commitment. One of the major tenets of marketing is that being first in the customer's mind is crucial for success. Those who come second either need to have a better product or service, a better price, or some other unique advantage to take the customer away. And even then, people often will not switch.

Finding a Real Estate Agent

If you want to work with a real estate agent but don't know which one caters to your target market, pick up a home sales or rental magazine, look in the real estate section in your newspaper, or look at the homes or neighborhoods in which you think your target market is likely to be interested. Then notice who is selling or renting the homes or apartments, and approach the agent to suggest ways of working together as mutual marketing partners.

Finding New People in Town

If you want to find new people in town but not work through a real estate agent, pick up the business section of the paper and watch for the days when new executives in the area are welcomed. Send them a "2-for-1" coupon or some other promotion, and introduce yourself. (See Figure 6–6.) One way of finding new people in the area is to go to your local Chamber of Commerce for lists of new residents. This method does not give you the screening that a

Figure 6–6 | Real estate agents or the Chamber of Commerce can refer you to new people in the community. (Image courtesy of iStock)

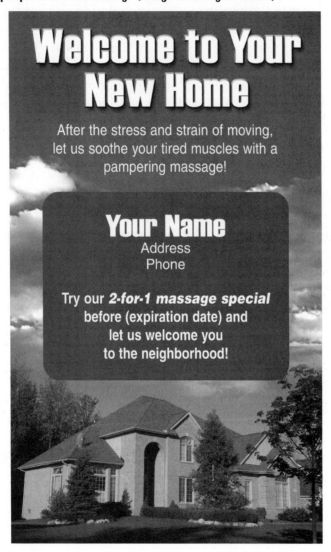

mutual marketing partner can offer, but if you want to be the first massage therapist that newcomers meet, this avenue is worth considering.

Hot Tub Dealer

Depending on your target market, a hot tub dealer can be an excellent source of referrals. The concept of relaxing in a hot tub is a good association for a massage therapist and would be a natural fit for a partnership. You can promote both businesses by offering gift certificates for outcall massages that the dealer can give to buyers to go with their first soak in their brand-new backyard hot tub. Bring a complimentary basket of fresh fruit with your card attached and really make an impression.

Cross-Selling Bonuses

If you like marketing, you can take some additional steps toward growing your practice. One way is to gather up free items, discounts on products and services, and other goodies from your partners and give them away. You can give them to your current clients as thank-you gifts, or you can use them as an enticement to help potential clients make the decision to buy.

Why would your partners give you free or discounted products and services? Because it will promote their businesses cheaply and easily to your customers. And, their promotions let them gain access to your customers without you breaching their need for privacy. To gather up bonuses to give away, consider again who you are and what you like, what your ideal clients would value, and what needs of theirs you can help serve. With those in mind, think about which businesses provide those things you and your clients value, and consider what they would be willing to give you to gain access, albeit indirectly, to your clients.

Sample Bonuses You Can Offer to Your Clients or Prospects

"Buy one, get one free" coupon for a restaurant

Free drink at the local juice bar

Certificate for organic wines

Free lesson at a local riding stable

Free month at a weight-loss clinic

Free bicycle tune-up

Free session at tanning salon

Free housecleaning

Free haircut

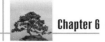

Free workout with a trainer

Free month at a gym

Free dozen roses from a florist

Free yoga classes

Free martial arts lesson

Free tai chi class

Consultation with nutritionist

Free herbal product, bath salts, or oils from bath and body shop

Discount from local health food store

$10 off on health-related book or specific title at local bookstore

Free consultation with a homeopath, naturopath, osteopath, or chiropractor

EXERCISE: USING CROSS-SELLING BONUSES

Write down five cross-selling bonuses you would enjoy giving as gifts to your current clients or using to market to new clients. If you want ideas, look in the advertising section of your phone book and think about what those businesses would be willing to give you as a way to be introduced to your clients.

_____

_____

_____

_____

_____

How to Get Cross-Selling Bonuses

There are hundreds of variations of **cross-selling bonuses** from businesses that will want to reach your clients, and many businesses will be happy to give you "freebies" or big discounts for the chance to get your clients in their doors. It is cheaper for them than advertising blindly, and if you have a strong client list, the businesses you approach will be more receptive to your ideas. Remember, just don't show them your list!

If you are smart and determined, you can gather a load of desirable bonuses that will help you get clients. You can say something like, "I'm a massage therapist, and I have wealthy, health-conscious, active clients. I want to offer them bonuses and gifts, and make them glad they're my clients. I'd like to promote your business or service to them in exchange for a discount or free introductory offer from you. Once they are in your door, you can upsell them to buying more from you, or follow up later with other offers. Since my clients fit your target market, I thought you'd be interested." If the person you are talking to can't see the value in what you are saying, try somewhere else or go higher up. A middle manager or employee may not think this is smart, but the owner who pays the advertising bill will be thrilled.

How to Use Your Bonuses

Once you get some bonuses, you can use them as incentives in more traditional marketing pieces, such as a letter to a mailing list you got from one of your partners. For example, let's say there is a wine shop near you that is trying to promote a new line of organic wines. They want to reach a clientele that would value organic wine, and your clients would more likely be interested in organic products than the average person. You could arrange a deal where you get free or deeply discounted bottles, and then you package them with a romantic Valentine's Day offer for a couple's massage that includes the free bottle of wine. Or let's say there is a new juice bar in town, and they want people to know they are now open for business. You could ask them for coupons for a free glass of juice and then give the coupons to your current clients just to keep them amazed at how wonderful you are. If you've lost contact with some former clients, your new bonuses can be a good excuse to get back in touch. It's better to open a letter with, "I just got a wonderful gift that I would love to share with you as my valued client," rather than just basically saying, "Hey, where are you?" You also can give your new bonuses to your other mutual marketing partners as thank-you gifts, incentives to remember to refer you, and just to stay in touch. After all, do you think the wine shop merchant would like your real estate agent to also know about his wine shop and maybe even tell his clients or colleagues about it?

Bonus Packages

Bonuses from multiple partners can be gathered into packages. If you have been working with a nice restaurant and a floral shop, you can create a holiday special by offering a package containing a dinner for two, a dozen red roses, and two massages. If you know how to do spa treatments, you can make the package even fancier. Your partners can advertise the package to their customers at their place of business or through a joint mailing, and you can market it to your current clients. Any expenses are shared, and you all benefit from the unique angle you have used to stand out from your competition. In exchange for a little thought and some good communication, you just may have gathered yourself enough clients from one project to start your whole practice. Beats putting up a business card in a gym, doesn't it?

Drawings

If you enjoyed working with the restaurant and florist, you can cross-refer in another way by offering giveaway prize drawings around special occasions or holidays. (See Figure 6–7.) If you have an office, each of you can put up a sign announcing a package or single-bonus giveaway to be drawn on a certain date. The sign can provide all the necessary contact information for all of the partners so, if people don't want to participate, they can at least start to associate you with your partners and the images they represent. A month or so before the drawing, you can put out a bowl to hold the business cards to be drawn. If your clients don't want their names on a list or if privacy is an issue, provide blank cards with only their first names that can go into the mix. If one is pulled, you will know who it is. Not only do you each get a long period of free advertising and recognition, but you can also follow up all of those cards with other marketing materials, if you choose.

If you want to be more strategic with your bonuses, packages, or drawings, consider your business needs and set the rules to help you the most. For example, if you want people to come in more often for a massage, you can

Figure 6–7 | Drawings let you gather valuable contact information for your target market.

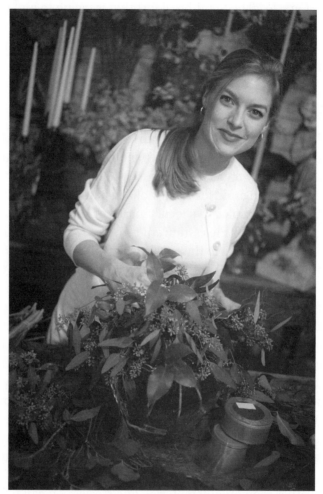

have a drawing that the client can enter each time he or she gets a massage, instead of having the client just put in one card and get one chance. If you have slow days and want more clients during those times, you can have a "Thirsty Thursday" special and only give out the coupons for the free juice bar drinks on Thursday. If you want your clients to send you more referrals, you can let them put another entry into the drawing for every new person they refer.

These may seem silly, but people love to win things, no matter how small, and they also love challenges and competition. If you have a really nice giveaway, like a free night at a local bed-and-breakfast that is trying to build business, you can build a whole practice on referrals from a few clients who are really vying to win that prize. Could they afford to buy a night there on their own? Of course they could, but it's much more fun to win it.

Media Events

If you really like marketing games and want even more exposure, team up with the restaurant and florist and any other business that fits your market, and give something away to needy people over the holidays. You can make it a public event by saying that for every holiday package sold, you will donate a set amount of money to a local charity, or you can give away your own products or services. If the restaurant provides food for a dinner at a shelter, you can give massage to the cooking staff that is pulling together dozens of dinners, or you can massage the recipients themselves. Or, if you sell products in your business, like special soaps or creams, you can either donate some yourself or ask your product manufacturer to donate them to the event. Either way, send a press release (that's covered in the next chapter) to the local media and get coverage of your donations. The media love holiday stories that are unique, touching, and different from the same old stories they ran last year, and you have a great shot at television and newspaper coverage. Since massage will be the most unusual partner in the promotion, figure out how to do an on-site or hands-on demonstration for the cameras so they can get some interesting photos or footage. Your promotion will create interest and goodwill in your target markets, and even if a resulting story or article does not directly reach your target market, it can be great for future press releases, other promotional material, and stories you can tell your clients.

Try It; You'll Like It

I realize that many of these marketing ideas are not yet commonplace in the massage profession, but they are effective tools that have been used successfully for years by other small businesses, and we should use them for our own success as well. Once you consider the possibility of using bonuses, cross-selling, and single- or multi-partner promotions, you will start to see opportunities everywhere. Now that you know how to think this way, if you are willing to get out there to try even a few of these ideas, you can build your dream practice in ways that will amaze you.

CHAPTER 6   SUMMARY

Building a practice using the bare-bones skills and tools has worked for countless therapists, but if your situation requires that you build your practice quickly, yet still maintain your safety, the muscle marketing skills become very helpful. In this chapter, we started with the skill of knowing yourself and what kind of practice, clients, setting, and work you want to have. The process of reviewing your ideal scenario is critical; otherwise, you can waste a lot of time and money going after the wrong goals for the wrong reasons. Only after we figured out what matters most to you did we then pick out a target market by identifying your ideal client profile. With those people in mind, we then worked on what specialties, additions, and benefits you would offer them so they would become your client.

Knowing whom you want to work with and what you can offer them leads you to one of the fastest and safest strategies for building a practice, which is mutual marketing. By doing cross-promotional work with other small businesses that already serve your target market, you can literally knock on one door and have it open up to your dream practice. For less involved projects that can still get you leads and access to your ideal clients, we also covered cross-selling bonuses and how even some simple contacts and projects with the right businesses and people can get you amazing and rapid access to clients.

CHAPTER 6   ACTION STEPS

Based on the information in this chapter, do the following to reach new clients:

❈ Get to know yourself and your ideal work scenario.

❈ Identify your target or niche market.

❈ Figure out which additions or products, services, or environmental enhancements would appeal to your target market.

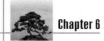
✳ Identify mutual marketing partners who already serve your target
market, and propose doing promotional projects with them.

✳ Gather cross-selling bonuses from other businesses to use in
promotions.

CHAPTER 6   KNOWLEDGE CHECK

Check your understanding of the chapter by reviewing these questions and
answers.

Q: What are the two primary benefits of muscle marketing over bare-bones
marketing?
A: Speed and control.

Q: What are the "Three Rs" of marketing?
A: Reaching, rebooking, and referrals.

Q: List three of the eight categories of additions you can use in your
practice.
A: Things clients can see, touch, hear, taste, smell, feel, learn, and act on.

Q: What are the three questions of mutual marketing?
A: Who is my target market? What small businesses already serve my
target market? What do I have to offer a business to get my hands on its
customers?

Q: Should you make your client list available to your mutual marketing
partners? Why or why not?
A: No; it breaks confidentiality.

Q: What are three primary needs that most businesses have?
A: Attract attention for new customers, stand out from competition, make a
sale, bring the customer back, upsell current customers, and get referrals.

Q: What is the benefit of a preemptive strike?
A: In a highly competitive market, a preemptive strike gives you an edge over
other therapists or massage businesses in the area because it gives you first
contact and creates loyalty.

Q: What is a cross-selling bonus?
A: A free or discounted product or service gathered from other businesses to use as promotional items or gifts for getting and keeping clients.

Q: What is a target market?
A: A profile of the type of group or individual you would enjoy and profit from working with.

Q: What is client net worth?
A: The sum of what one massage client is potentially worth to you over the lifetime of your working relationship.

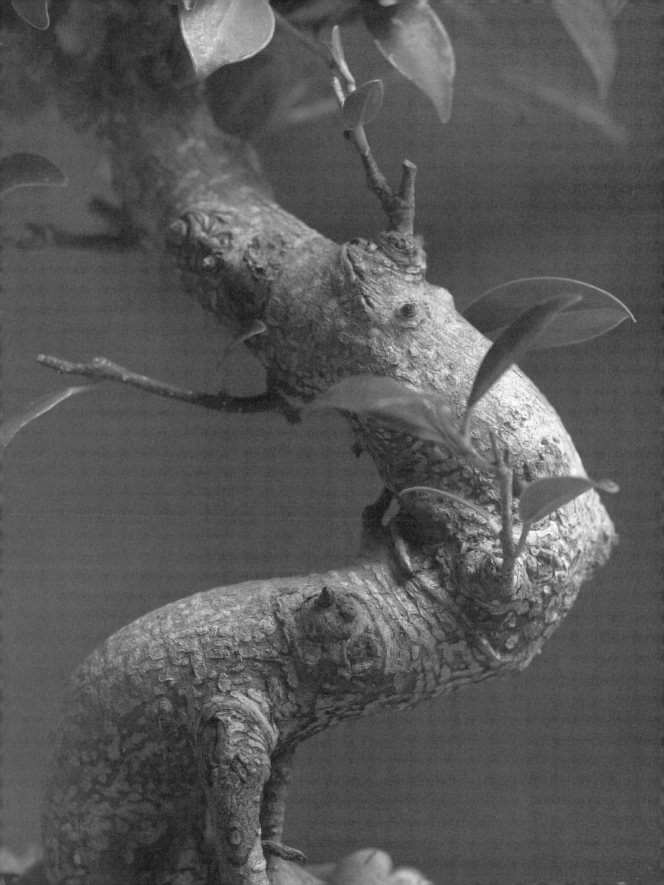

7

Reaching Tools

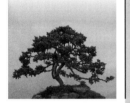

CHAPTER OBJECTIVES

After reading this chapter, you should be able to:

- Design a professional business card.
- Design a professional brochure.
- Describe three ways to distribute your brochures.
- Create a gift certificate.
- Identify uses and sources of **promotional gifts**.
- Discuss the benefits and drawbacks of having a Web site.
- Describe the difference between reference and action marketing tools.
- Explain the key elements of an action marketing piece.
- Explain the uses of postcards, letters, flyers, and surveys for reaching clients.
- Explain the benefits and methods of testing marketing products.
- Write a professional press release.

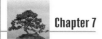

REACHING TOOLS TO BUILD YOUR DREAM PRACTICE

Building your dream practice may require more advanced marketing tools than the simple business card covered in the bare-bones section. This chapter now takes you to the next level of marketing tools, which can help you build your business rapidly. We will cover many muscle marketing tools, but there are two important factors to consider as you choose them: speed of reaching people, and control of who gets your marketing message.

I wish I didn't have to start a chapter on marketing tools with a warning, but the massage field still faces issues of safety and risk for practitioners, especially for those who work at home or do outcall, and you may need to keep tight control on who gets access to your marketing tools. The other risk therapists face in broader marketing is exposure to regulating agencies. Unfortunately, many massage therapists are forced to work without all the necessary licenses or pieces of paper required by their city or state. Getting full approval, whether from zoning laws, building requirements, or home use permits, or even just getting a business license to do massage, is still a difficult, unpleasant, expensive, and sometimes almost impossible process for many qualified practitioners in our profession. The marketing drawback to not having your pieces of paper is that faster and broader exposure through marketing tools and media becomes risky and inadvisable. If you have to pay a few hundred dollars for the continuing education units needed to maintain your state license, or need to bite the bullet and go through that annoying vice squad checkup process, then do so; it will give you the freedom to market yourself more fully, and will more than pay for itself because you will be able to reach more people, more rapidly.

That said, in this chapter, we will cover some of the fastest ways to reach new clients, but we will also keep in mind that safety may be an issue. We will aim for a balance between speed and exposure while designing marketing tools that still create trust, establish value, positively and accurately shape public perception, and motivate and guide a person to book an appointment. This will require more levels of thinking than other professionals have to deal with, but for where our field is today, it is vital that you understand the many functions your marketing materials need to serve beyond just getting your name out into the public eye.

These tools have one primary purpose: leverage. They give you the opportunity to reach new clients more effectively in person, and to reach more clients without having to be physically present. Basically, your goal is to spend your time doing massage and to let other people, businesses, organizations, mass media, promotional events, mass mailings, and other written materials build your practice while you're busy with clients.

WRITTEN REACHING TOOLS

Among your best options for marketing materials are written tools, which for most therapists are the safest leverage for the least amount of money, with the highest potential of return on investment. Written marketing tools can be broken down into two categories. The first category is **reference marketing tools**. These are passive marketing materials that educate potential clients, enhance their perception of you and massage, create a compelling reason to use your services, and provide contact information. Reference marketing tools include business cards and brochures, or educational pieces that go along with gift certificates.

The second category of written materials is **action marketing tools**. These are proactive documents that inform the reader about you and your services. However, they go an important step further by giving the reader a specific action to take, usually right away or by a specific deadline. Action marketing tools can include a package consisting of a letter, brochure, and special-offer coupon sent to mailing lists; table-tent cards; pads of tear-off-page information cards; time-limited coupons in a multi-business booklet; or classified ads in the publications your ideal clients are likely to read. I encourage you to look at direct response ads such as direct mail, infomercials, coupon books, and other marketing pieces you see around you on a daily basis. If you like them, notice what they include, especially if you've seen them before; if they have been around a while, they are probably working. Muscle marketing gives you more speed and direct control in building your dream practice, and in order to reach new clients in as many ways as possible, you should consider the following written reaching tools.

Reference Marketing Tools

- ✽ Business cards
- ✽ Brochures
- ✽ Massage menus
- ✽ Gift certificates
- ✽ Promotional gifts

✳ Resumes

✳ Articles

✳ Web site

Action Marketing Tools

✳ Coupons

✳ Direct mail—letters, postcards, surveys

✳ Flyers

✳ Business reply cards

✳ Table tents

✳ Business proposals

Both

✳ Ads—phone books, newspapers, magazines

✳ Press releases

✳ Signs

Creating any written marketing piece means thinking about, crafting, and pulling together a variety of elements that can be mixed and matched, depending on your needs, your budget, the amount of space you have, and the purpose of the tool. Whether you are writing a six-panel brochure, creating a folded business card, or designing a quarter-page phone book ad, you will want an image and message that are attractive to your market, and tell readers what they need to know to take the next step toward becoming your client. In this next section, we will cover the muscle marketing business card and the key elements of written reference and action marketing tools.

THE MUSCLE MARKETING BUSINESS CARD

The bare-bones business card covered in the first section of the book included just your name, title, and contact number. A simple card can work well if you are talking to many people yourself and simply handing it out in person. However, when your card is distributed by others, posted in public places, or

Figure 7–1 | **My business card from 1984.**

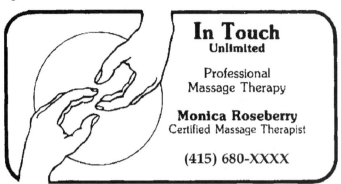

received as part of a package mailer, it needs a stronger graphic presentation that represents you and your services in your stead.

A good business card uses graphics, print fonts, color, white space, and well-crafted words to portray an image of you that is appealing to your ideal clients. (See Figure 7–1.) Bold colors and robust shapes give a much different feel than pale pastels and curlicues, and it will take some thinking and probably some expert advice to create a look that suits your style while appealing to your market. Logos, photos, type and thickness of paper, and layout all affect your professional image, and need to be chosen to create trust and value, and to shape the perception of the person who sees your card.

These points became clear to me at a meeting of professional public speakers. One woman in our group announced that she wanted to break into the $10,000 speaking bracket, which sounded very impressive. However, when we reached the point where we all exchanged business cards, I was quite surprised. Her cards were printed on her home computer's dot-matrix printer on flimsy paper, and featured bright, psychedelic colors. Her graphic representation was incongruent with the impression she was trying to create, and if I were a large company looking to pay $10,000 for a convention speaker, I would take one look at that homemade card and assume she wasn't up to the task. She may have prided herself on printing her own cards, but they were so unprofessional that they were a detriment to her business. If you are going to make one financial investment in your marketing, put it toward your business card. You use it most often, will be judged by it, and it will affect what people think of you and are willing to pay you.

Go to a graphic artist or high-quality print shop for the details that are too numerous to cover here, but consider these points before you do so. Business cards are what people use to find your information in order to contact you, so make your card easy to keep and easy to see. Avoid cards that are oversized because they are hard to store in wallets or cardholders, and usually end up getting thrown out. For your "look," stay fairly conservative. If your graphic artist wants to make a marvelous piece of wild art for you or put some esoteric or symbolic logo on your card, remind him or her that you need a practical card, not an oddity or an art piece, unless, of course, your target market is into the abstract and unusual.

Business cards can contain many elements and be laid out in numerous ways. Below are some of the many options you can consider in your text and design.

Business Card Text

Your name

Title (remember, you can make it up!)

Office or work phone number

Home phone number

Voice mail number

Toll-free phone number

Cellular phone number

Pager number

E-mail address

Street address (only if it's safe)

Business name

Slogan

Massage menu

Web site address

Fill-in appointment times

Graphic Elements

Map to your office or location

Logo

Photo

Use of color for background, print, and graphics

Choice of fonts (typefaces or styles)

Amount of white space

Paper—weight, texture, finish

Layout

Printed on one or both sides

Folded

Printed lengthwise or widthwise

The Elements of a Business Card and Other Written Tools

In the process of creating a business card, you will design and decide on many of the elements just listed that also can be used in any other written marketing tools. Therefore, let's take a close look at some of the primary elements of your card. In the first section of the book, we talked about your name, title, and access numbers, and how to handle having a business telephone in your home if you work at home or do outcall massage. Beyond the access information are some other options to consider.

Your Business Name

A business name is fun to create. It can lend an air of credibility and professional stature, and provide a creative way to promote your special work. A business name is not required for our profession, but if you are going to use one, be careful. First, you have to create one that will represent your business accurately while appealing to your target market. Second, you have to make sure no one has already registered, trademarked, or service-marked the name. Before you spend money to have cards made, you should conduct research online, including at the U.S. Patent and Trade Office Web site at http://www.uspto.gov, and at your county business registry to see if the name you want is already taken. If it's not taken locally, then file for a **fictitious business name** (FBN) with your county. Look in the front of your telephone book in the "County Government Offices" section under fictitious business names for further help. If you want to open a business bank account, have checks made, and so on, you will need an FBN document proving that you have paid for the name and had it listed in a local newspaper. When your name goes into the paper, it gives other businesses the time and right to challenge you on a name they may already be using. Don't print anything until the whole filing process is over. You'd be surprised how many people claim they are the first to use "In Touch," "Healing Hands," and other such names. Again, a business name is not necessary, but if you want one, go through the legal process before you print your cards or any other materials.

EXERCISE: CREATING A BUSINESS NAME

Use your imagination and brainstorm a list of possible business names. Play with serious-sounding names, fun names, names that use classic endings like "Inc.," or use the initials of your title. Sometimes the right name will come quickly and easily, and sometimes it takes a lot of attempts to get it just right. Try business names that use your last name, the name of the town or city where you live, the state where you live, the kind of work you offer your clients, or something special and unique to you that will draw in clients. Write up a list of words you like, and mix and match them. Write out a few names, and if you need more time, keep the list nearby and add to it later.

Your Graphic Representation

Having traveled this country with the intention of meeting massage professionals, I can tell you that I have seen more than my fair share of business cards with hands on them. I've also seen beautiful cards with abstract logos or pictures of trees, flowers, rainbows, sailing boats, and other pretty scenes. With every card, my question was, how did the logo or image help the business? My personal opinion is that logos for business cards and printed matter are nice, but they won't really help you much unless they create the right look and feel for your business. Generic logos or clip art may be cheap and simple, but if you are going to use a logo, do the work to create one that speaks to you and your prospective clients.

For example, the logo on the card from my colleague Kim Monser (see Figure 7–2) is simple but strong. The logo, layout, and light green color reflect her character and business well, and she only puts the most important information on the front of the card to avoid a cluttered look. She saves the detailed contact and appointment information for the back of the card, where it won't detract from her image. Her font choice is easy-going but clear, and it suits the clientele she aims to reach in the two towns she serves in northern California.

Since you are selling a service, what you are really selling is you, and the most memorable graphic representation you can have is a high-quality photograph of you in either a headshot or an action shot. The photo can be used as the whole background of the card with the words superimposed, or as a distinct stand-alone element.

I no longer expect that people will remember my name or much about me after I have given them my card. I have had marvelous conversations with people and have even written things on the back of their cards such as "Kate's party" or a date, but months later, the details have slipped my mind and I can't remember why I kept the card in my desk. What people will remember most is a face, and if you are going to use an image, use one that will be hard to forget. When I set out on my cross-country research trip for this book, I made a new set of cards with my cell phone number and a new photo. I had an image in mind of being seen as friendly, fun, casual, a traveler, and someone approachable, so I chose a full-body photo taken on a vacation, and it gave the relaxed yet professional feel I wanted.

Figure 7–2 | **Your logo should represent you while appealing to your target market.
(Image courtesy of Carol Lynn Coster Design,
http://www.costerdesign.com)**

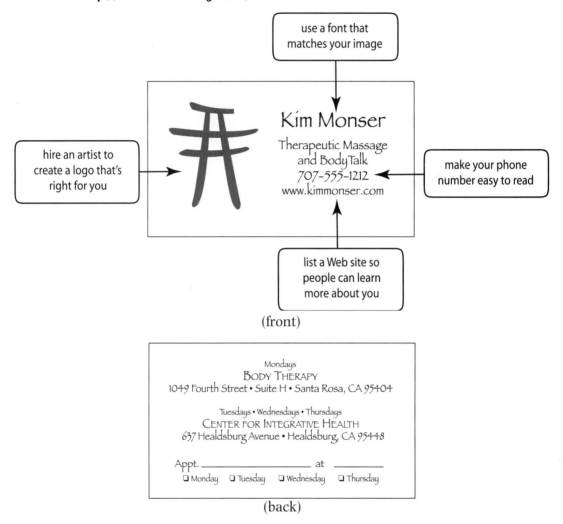

use a font that
matches your image

Kim Monser

Therapeutic Massage
and BodyTalk
707-555-1212
www.kimmonser.com

hire an artist to
create a logo that's
right for you

make your phone
number easy to read

list a Web site so
people can learn
more about you

(front)

Mondays
BODY THERAPY
1049 Fourth Street • Suite H • Santa Rosa, CA 95404

Tuesdays • Wednesdays • Thursdays
CENTER FOR INTEGRATIVE HEALTH
637 Healdsburg Avenue • Healdsburg, CA 95448

Appt. _____ at _____
❑ Monday   ❑ Tuesday   ❑ Wednesday   ❑ Thursday

(back)

(See Figure 7–3.) Because I am smiling and happy in the picture, people
have a tendency to smile when they see it, which is a great way to start
any relationship. Not only does my card stand out in any pile of papers, but
the photo reminds people instantly of who I am. I took the photo and my
contact information down to a large office supply store, selected a font,
talked with the clerk about the layout, and for $90 they put together the text
and photo, and printed 500 of them. Even nice cards don't have to be a big
hassle or expense.

Figure 7–3 | To help people remember you, use your photograph on your card.

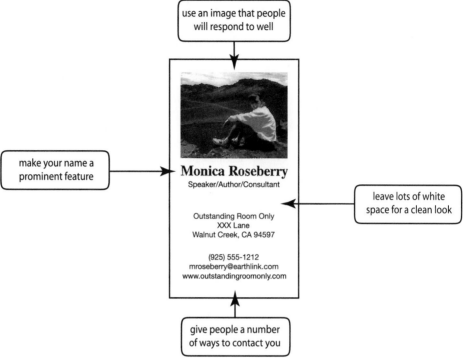

Many massage therapists do other kinds of work besides their practices. As their fields of interest grow and overlap, they can still reach multiple markets and offer different services on one card. For example, my colleague Steve Capellini offers a wide variety of services, from writing to training to spa services. His card packs in a lot of information, and the emphasis is on his name and an action-shot photo of him doing chair massage. (See Figure 7–4a and 7–4b.) Even with all this information, the card doesn't feel crowded because he uses both sides, spaces apart his graphics, and lays out his text in a triangular visual element. On a small piece of paper, Steve has managed to convey in one quick glance a lot about himself and what he does.

If you are going to use a photo taken by a professional photographer, be careful when choosing the image you want to convey. I was handed a card by a massage therapist who had gone to one of the "glamour" portrait franchises for her business-card photo. While the picture was pretty, she had been overdone with so much makeup that the photo was inappropriately seductive.

Figure 7–4 (a) An action photo plus other representations of your work make you memorable. (Image courtesy of Steve Capellini) (b) Use the back of your card to advertise your other services. (Image courtesy of Steve Capellini)

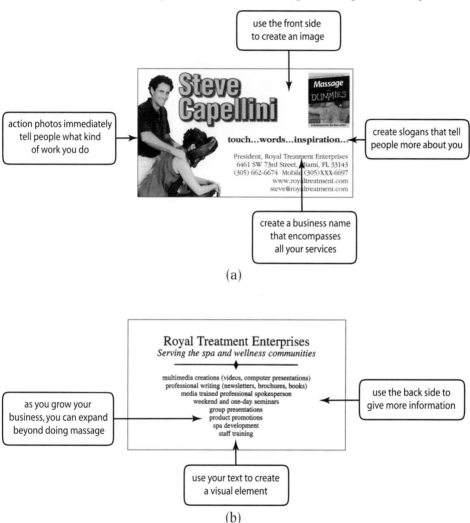

(a)

(b)

In addition, she never looked that way in "normal" life, giving a feeling of incongruity to those who met her and compared the photo to how she looked.

Whatever logo or image you use, make sure it represents you well, be consistent with it, put it on all of your written materials, and get people to become familiar with it. Repetition is important in establishing your business identity, so choose one image and stick with it.

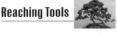

EXERCISE: CREATING YOUR GRAPHIC REPRESENTATION

The inspiration for creating your graphic representation can suddenly come clear to you if you program yourself to be looking for graphics or photos that you like. As you watch TV, read a magazine, look in the phone book, wander around a store, watch a bus drive by, surf the Internet, walk out in nature, or look through your old photos, notice what images you like. Does a box of cereal have a really cool logo, or does a magazine ad or Web site have a picture that just feels right to you? Then start collecting them. You can adapt them (don't just copy them—you will get in trouble with copyright laws) and/or show them to your graphic artist or photographer as an example of what you want your graphic representation to look or feel like.

Your Slogan

If you are going to do a lot of mass media marketing, you might consider using a slogan along with your image. Phrases such as the U.S. Army's "Be all that you can be" or Motel 6's "We'll leave the light on for you" are catchy, stick in people's minds, and give the audience a feeling or impression. If you want a slogan, there are two ways to approach creating one. You can pick a specific market or client profile you want to work with, consider the needs that market has, and address those needs directly or indirectly. If your market is comprised of people who are lonely, in pain, or stressed, or who need to relax, you can use phrases such as: "Always There for You"; "Your Weekly Vacation"; "Touch You Can Trust"; and so on. You also can create a slogan by thinking about who you are and what you want to offer. Choose a slogan that represents you and your work, and the people who want what you offer will become your market.

Personally, I am not a big fan of slogans for massage therapists. Unless you are highly specialized and have a narrow target market, you may choose a slogan that inadvertently turns away potential clients who see your materials but think you won't be right for them. For example, you may decide on a sporty theme, slogan, and look for your marketing tools, but even if you are willing to have elderly widows or pregnant women as clients, your marketing tools likely will turn them away since they don't have sporty needs.

In addition to the risk of shutting off various markets, your slogan may be misinterpreted by people who are at different levels on the Perception Continuum. My suggestion is either to create a professional but generic image for general marketing, or to have multiple cards and marketing tools specific to your various markets, and distribute them with controlled dissemination. If you are like most therapists who need to appeal to multiple target and "flanker" (or side) markets for enough people to fill your practice, be careful that your slogan does not close doors on viable clients.

Massage Menu

If you will be handing out your business card personally, what is printed on it can spark questions and conversation that give you an easy opening to tell more about yourself and your work. Having a massage menu on your card that lists the kinds of work you do can give you the chance to talk clearly about your services, whether you hand out your card yourself or someone calls who got your card elsewhere. Offering multiple options shows that you know how to do more than one rote routine, educates others that there is more to massage than their one preconceived notion, and gives more options to which people can say "yes." If you want to list more than two or three modalities, print them on the back of your card; otherwise, your text becomes too small to read and looks too crowded. This card, from my colleague Anthony Valdez, uses the back to list his menu and provide a space for an appointment time as well. He repeats the logo from the front of the card on the back of the card, using it as a black and white background image, which looks really sharp. (See Figure 7–5.)

While I highly recommend having a massage menu, keep in mind that one of the marketing mistakes massage professionals make is believing the general public has awareness of and value for a particular massage modality and specialty. Of the some six billion people on this planet, the vast majority of

Figure 7–5 A massage menu on your card can open up conversations about what kind of work you do. (Image courtesy of Anthony Valdez)

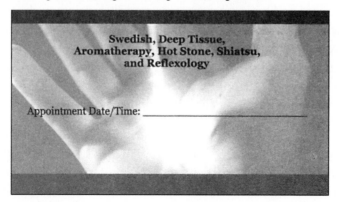

Swedish, Deep Tissue,
Aromatherapy, Hot Stone, Shiatsu,
and Reflexology

Appointment Date/Time: _____

them have no understanding of different bodywork styles. It can cost you clients if you think people will want to book an appointment for a session of a bodywork modality they have never heard of, even if you have spent thousands of dollars studying it. If you are going to list your specialties, you can put down specific bodywork modalities, but be prepared to explain them. Since education is one of the most important forms of marketing you can do, a menu gives you the opening to do so. If you have to choose between a snappy but meaningless logo and a menu, go for the menu.

If you were to have only one marketing tool, consider a folding card that can include many educational elements in a small but keepable size. It can act as a mini-brochure and be given out in any setting. Somehow, handing out brochures at a friend's party seems a bit gauche, but handing out cards is acceptable protocol. As with any marketing tool, the more you distribute, the better your leverage for building your practice. Remember, most successful therapists I interviewed used only a card to build their practices, so give this tool the respect it is due.

EXERCISE: CREATING A MINI-MENU

The back of a business card can hold a good amount of information. Write down a list of massage modalities, spa treatments, or unique facets of your business that would open a conversation or convince someone to come see you for massage. If you can teach them meditation skills, relaxation techniques, or have a unique setting or piece of equipment like a sauna or hot tub, list those to stop people from just putting away your card and instead get them to start talking to you.

For example, the back or fold of a card could say: "Specialist in Swedish, Spa Treatments and Stress Reduction. Beautiful office in forest setting with hot tub and secluded outdoor spa treatment arena."

Take a moment to write a mini-menu for the back of your card.

_____

_____

_____

_____

_____

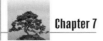

BROCHURES

A brochure is a common staple for many small businesses and can be an effective tool for building your practice. Brochures can educate your clients about your services, further develop your business image, say things about you that you wouldn't say yourself, and give an air of professionalism to your practice. Even if a brochure won't necessarily close a deal or convince someone to buy your services, having it around can create a feeling of trust in you. However, before you decide to spend the time and money on a brochure, consider first how you will distribute it. Where and how you distribute your brochure will determine its content, so let's consider a few possible uses for this marketing tool.

Ways to Use Your Brochure

Distributed directly by you to a new prospect

> Give out at promotional events—health fairs, expos, partner projects

> Give out at speaking engagements—demonstrations, classes, seminars

Distributed directly by those who know you

> Include with gift certificates—given by clients, family, friends, mutual partners

> Give to mutual marketing partners to distribute at place of business

> Have in massage room for clients to pick up and give to personal referrals

> Give out at networking meetings

Distributed indirectly

> Mail to mutual marketing list along with letter

> Mail to clients, either for them to have or to distribute for you

> Put in public places

Depending upon where your brochures are distributed, they will either be picked up by someone who has no other concept of you, or someone else will broaden the receiver's view of you by speaking further on your behalf. If most of your brochures will be given out by you or by those who know you, the factor of trust is much easier to establish. This lets you focus your brochure's content on establishing your value and leading the reader to the decision to buy from you.

In this kind of scenario, imagine that one of your friends or clients hands your brochure to a friend and says, "She's great! You have to get a massage from her!" The friend looks down at your brochure, opens her mind to the possibility of getting a massage because of the strong recommendation, and then starts to do a quick once-over of the page. How does your brochure need to look to make her want to read it thoroughly, and what can you say about yourself and your work that will convince her to call you? Let's consider some options.

Designing Your Brochure

The space available on a brochure may tempt you to include many more elements than appear on your business card, but resist. Your brochure's primary purpose is not to tell your whole story but to act as an engaging introduction to get the reader to the next step of the buying process: to contact you. Just as a resume is designed to create enough interest to get to the interview stage, your brochure needs to capture the reader's imagination with enough information to go forward but without bogging him or her down with too many details. As with your business card, you can consider the following factors to include in your brochure, along with a few new elements.

Contact Information

    Name

    Title

    Telephone numbers

    E-mail address

    Street address

    Business name

    Web site address

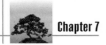

Marketing Message

    Slogan

    Headline

    Services—massage menu, description of modalities, special offerings

    Benefits

    Testimonials

Graphic Elements

    Map to your office or location

    Logo

    Photos or illustrations—photo of you, charts, graphs, anatomical illustrations

    Use of color for background, print, and graphics

    Choice of fonts—variety, print size, bullet points

    Amount of white space

    Paper—weight, texture, finish

Layout

    Size—page size, number of panels, panel size

The Look of Your Brochure

Playing a song on a piano requires you to play notes in a particular order. What makes those notes sound beautiful or chaotic is the amount of space left in between the notes, and it is the silences in the piece that create the flow, emotion, and movement of the song. Run all the notes together and you have noise; separate them too far apart and the song is lost. Laying out your brochure and business card follows the rules of music. The printed elements have movement and flow because of the empty space around them, and the placement of the words and artwork gives the piece a visual rhythm.

If you want some ideas for your brochure's "look," go to the bookstore and look at the magazines that your target market is likely to read. Look at the advertisements and see what advertisers to your market have done to draw in the reader. Notice the amount of empty space, the placement of elements, and the imagery used, and pay attention to which ads capture your eye. Even though ads are used more to invoke feelings and use more imagery than a brochure might, you can learn a lot about choosing the look of your brochure from them. Whether you use a sheet of colored paper photocopied and folded, or an 11 × 17 glossy foldout with gorgeous photographs, consider your business image and your target market's preferences before you choose your look.

EXERCISE: RESEARCHING YOUR MARKETING MATERIALS' "LOOK"

Imagine your target market and think about what kinds of marketing materials and advertisements they see on a regular basis. What magazines do they read, Web sites do they visit, or TV shows do they watch? Then gather advertisements that have been designed for your target market from a variety of magazines, Web sites, and other media. Analyze what elements are being used to appeal to your market and see if any of them would work in your marketing materials. If you are in a group, bring the materials you have gathered and explain the key marketing elements in them to your class. In a prior exercise you collected items for what you'd like to use as a graphic representation, and in this exercise we take it a step further and include your target market in the process.

Creating Your Marketing Message

Beyond the elements covered with the business card, brochures allow room for more text to inform your potential clients of how and why they should book with you. When people are reading your text, they are deciding whether or not to "buy" from you, and there are three common frames of reference from which they make their buying decisions.

A "people person" typically makes buying decisions based on what other people will think, and he or she has a high need for external approval. These are the "me-too" buyers who will jump on the nearest bandwagon, fashion, or trend. One way to begin marketing to these people is to think about what they wish they had when they were in high school. They wanted to be popular, to be liked, to be in the in-crowd, and to belong. Many of their buying decisions today are based on trying to get what they never got in high school. For these "me too"-ers, feeling connected and trusting is important. They search for chemistry and a relationship based on mutual good feelings. Your words need to let these buyers know that you are accepting and welcoming, yet exclusive. You can offer them an opening to belong to your small group of clients or even to your personal mission.

Another type of buyer is the "scientist." These people make many of their buying decisions on a subconscious, emotional basis, but consciously they want to have logical rationales to back up or justify their decisions. While "people persons" usually work in service jobs, the "scientists" usually work with things. As our profession conducts research and studies on the benefits and efficacy of massage, we gather the evidence these people need to consider including massage in their lives. If your primary market is made up of "scientists," your marketing will need to address their desire for rational, logical data before they choose to get massage from you. Your words need to be concrete, specific, and results oriented. Even your graphics can be scientific, with official-looking charts and graphs or anatomical illustrations.

A third type of buyer is the "WIIFM" buyer. Their buying decisions are based on the "what's in it for me?" principle. Control of any situation is important to them, and, often, they are entrepreneurs. They don't care about what other people think of them, and scientific data isn't that important to them either. What matters is what you and your massage can do for them. Pay careful attention to the benefits and advantages that you offer WIIFM buyers because this is what they care about. If you work with a lot of entrepreneurs, choose words that will convey clearly how much you can do for them.

If you know what type of buyer your ideal client is, you can use slogans, words, graphics, and other elements in your brochure to engage that personality type. If you don't know what draws your target market, cover all the angles by either taking a generic approach in your brochure or appealing to all three types in the different panels or pages.

Besides having different ways of making buying decisions, your brochure readers are also on different levels of the Perception Continuum. Within the Continuum are two primary stages that affect which words you choose to answer the silent questions and concerns in their minds. One stage is known as "product acceptance." In this stage, the reader is in the lower levels of the

Continuum, and needs to be educated about massage and its value and benefits before even considering booking with you. The second stage is called "brand recognition." In this stage, your readers want a massage, but they don't know or trust you personally. In this case, your brochure needs to give the details about you and your massage skills so they can decide whether or not they will choose you over your competition.

Mixing these factors together, you can figure out what you need to say to convince your readers to call or book an appointment. If you are not sure which category your prospects fall into, use the space allotted in your brochure to appeal to all three categories and buying stages. One paragraph can emphasize the growing popularity of massage; another can emphasize that massage has been around for centuries and its methods are tried and true; and a third can emphasize to the WIIFM buyers that they can design the session according to their needs. Introduce the value, benefits, and descriptions of your massage to the uninitiated, and introduce yourself almost as if you are writing a resume so that the readers can become familiar with you and choose you as their massage therapist.

Answering the Unspoken, Frequently Asked Questions (FAQs)

Besides taking into consideration the buyer types and stages of acceptance before choosing your words, consider using your brochure to answer questions that your prospective clients may have. Questions may range from, "Do I have to take off all my clothes?" to "Are you going to turn me black and blue like that person up at the mud baths did?" After hearing many questions over the span of my practice, I still am surprised at some of the misperceptions people have about massage, and what interesting fears they have.

As a rule, never assume that a prospective client has the slightest idea about what to expect from his or her first session. In the first year of my practice, I would leave the room while clients got on the table, and I would come back to find people lying down on the table fully clothed, lying buck-naked on top of the blanket, or lying face up with the backs of their heads falling through the face-rest hole. I learned quickly that I could not assume anything about what people know about getting a massage. Many people would like to try a massage, but they have many unspoken questions that prevent them from ever doing so. If you can identify and answer their unspoken questions and fears in your marketing material, you are more likely to be seeing them soon as your clients.

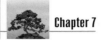

Common FAQs

Trust Questions

> Do I have to get undressed?
>
> Is this therapist safe?
>
> Does massage hurt?
>
> Will I be too relaxed?
>
> What if I get "hooked" on massage?

Value Questions

> Is this worth my time and money?
>
> What can I expect for this fee?
>
> What if I don't like their work?
>
> Will this fix my problems?
>
> How long do the benefits last?

Convenience Questions

> Is this going to be worth the hassle?
>
> How much time is this going to take?
>
> How frequently do I have to get massage for it to do any good?
>
> If I'm oily, will that ruin my clothes?

Establishing Your Benefits and Advantages

As you look at the prior questions, keep in mind that one way to answer them is to provide information about the many benefits you offer. Even if you don't answer every question, if you give your brochure readers really good reasons to come see you, they at least can make the decision to talk to you personally, or book an appointment and get the rest of their questions answered later. Massage professionals can offer many benefits, and we can distinguish ourselves from other therapists and services with unique advantages that will help convince the reader to get a massage, and to get it from you. Consider these possible categories of advantages as enticements for your brochure reader.

❋ Your background, training, experience, specialties, massage modalities

❋ The advantages you offer that are different from your competition's

❋ The benefits your clients will gain by seeing you

❋ The problems your clients will avoid by getting regular massage from you

❋ Your unique character and gifts

More specifically, the benefits and advantages you list in your brochure may include some or all of the following points.

1. You cost less than . . .

2. You cost more, but here's why . . .

3. You have a higher quality of . . .

4. You offer better customer service.

5. You offer education with your service.

6. You offer a 100-percent money-back guarantee.

7. You offer bonuses.

8. You give long sessions.

9. You specialize in a particular area (neck, lower back).

10. You specialize in a problem (TMJ, fibromyalgia, sports injuries).

11. You incorporate a non-massage skill (hypnosis, crystals, stress management).

12. You have a specialized background (nursing, physical therapy, athletics).

13. You help a specialty category (overweight, clean and sober, survivors, phobic).

14. You do outcall.

15. Your location is easy to find, with ample parking.

16. You work more hours, late hours, early hours, and weekends.

17. You offer a full list of referrals for a particular specialty or need.

18. You cater to a specific group and draw on your interests or background to service the frail and elderly, active and elderly, children with diseases, people with AIDS, executives, women in menopause, telecommuters, infants, soccer moms, tennis players, and so on.

19. You have worked with famous people.

20. You arrive on time.

21. You reverse the limitations of aging.

22. You change how people feel or you affect some kind of change.

23. You are a Nationally Certified, licensed, 1000-hour graduate.

24. You have a bodywork specialty.

25. You promise performance enhancement of different types.

Your Services

Educating your reader about your different services gives them valuable information about why they should book with you. You can use your brochure to tell people about how your massage is applied, what each modality is designed to do, what results can be expected from each service, and how your services can be combined in various ways. The massage menu from your business card can be expanded to tell more about the value and application of aromatherapy, Reiki, reflexology, deep tissue, acupressure, spa treatments, assisted stretching, postural assessment, or whatever else you offer.

Testimonials

Somewhere along the line of establishing your value in other's minds, there comes a point where you risk having your marketing sound unpleasantly like bragging. While clients want the best available, we have an odd cultural rule that talking too well about ourselves or "tooting our own horn" too loudly is not a good thing. We love athletes who break records and wow crowds, but too much hot air, taunting, or arrogance will cause us to turn our backs. To be able to further explain your benefits and expertise without turning people off, use an age-old marketing tool, the **testimonial**. Having other people say nice things about you is totally acceptable, and readers usually are more inclined to believe a claim if a group of strangers make positive statements agreeing with it. You can get testimonials from current clients, family, friends, fellow massage students, colleagues, or anyone to whom you give massage. Here are some sample testimonials, just for fun.

- ✳ "I've thrown away my crutches! Monica is a miracle worker!"

- ✳ "I've never felt better! Monica knows just how to fix my aches and pains!"

- ✳ "No one could help my nagging back pain until I found Monica. In three sessions she had me back out on the dance floor."

- ✳ "Bending down to pick up my grandkids used to hurt so much I had to stop. After a few weeks of massage, I'm hurling them around like a sack of potatoes."

Photographs or Illustrations

When a person first looks at your brochure, the artwork is usually the most eye-catching element. What people see in your photographs, drawings, and illustrations can intrigue them enough to read further. Your artwork needs to capture and maintain interest, introduce you and your work, establish your image, and build trust in you. Gaining trust may or may not be difficult, given your target market, but understanding how to build trust with images is important. One of the tenets of marketing is called the "law of familiarity." The gist of this law is that people trust what is familiar to them and distrust what is unfamiliar. The most common perception of massage is what people see in **advertising** for resorts, hotels, and other products or services that use massage to associate the product with being part of the good life. Television ads abound that use the image of massage to sell candy, trucks, chicken, auto financing, and pizza. Typically, the image of massage is conveyed either by a person lying on a table receiving some form of work that looks like traditional Swedish massage, or the person is getting a seated massage. Even more typically, the image shows a massage client with his or her face turned to the camera, even if a face-rest is available. People just don't seem to like the image of others with their faces covered up or in a place where breathing may be impaired, so even if you use a face-rest, take your photos with a happy, face-forward client.

Your modality or specialty may be quite different in intention and application from Swedish, but since the law of familiarity states that people buy what is familiar, you might consider using a photograph or illustration of yourself working with a Swedish-style application, or using a non-action photo. If you are selling to an uneducated market, it becomes even more important to use images they are already familiar with and probably have good feelings about. Once your brochure reader has made contact with you to learn more about your work, when the law of familiarity is less critical, you can further educate him or her about your specialty.

If you are marketing to a more educated buyer who knows about different types of massage, choose imagery that emphasizes your differences from other, more common massages. Being different, exotic, or artistic can be important when you face a great deal of competition and your market is in the latter part of the brand recognition stage. This is when people become the bored "been there, done that" buyers, and they want something exciting and new to try, and to tell their friends about. There is a growing percentage of people who are in this "tried it all, now what?" category, but unless you are working directly with many clients who are very experienced in receiving many types of massage, stick with the familiar to build that all-important trust.

Producing a Brochure

Brochures can range from simple and inexpensive information pieces to elaborate, graphically stunning works of art. If you are on a tight budget, create and print a brochure on your home computer using a simple graphic layout program and beautiful, preprinted paper stock. Or trade massage with a graphic designer and printer to get a beautiful end product. If you are new to a practice, I highly recommend that you buy preprinted massage brochures sold by companies like Information for People. (See Figure 7–6.) (Check "Marketing Tools" in the "Resources" section for other providers of premade brochures.) This gives you a quick, quality brochure with your contact information on it, and later, when your practice is more developed, you can produce your own if you choose to.

If you can't make a high-quality brochure, it is better to not have one at all. A poorly designed and unattractive brochure with misspellings and bad grammar can drive away business just as a good-looking and informative brochure can help create business. Your talent and abilities as a massage professional are judged by your representation on a piece of paper, and if you can't afford a quality representation, stick with your cards and direct contacts until you can make a brochure worthy of your practice. Think of your brochure as an investment. It will cost you money up front, but it can pay for itself quickly and has the potential for creating profit well beyond what it

Figure 7–6 | Brochures let you introduce yourself and tell people how you can meet their needs.

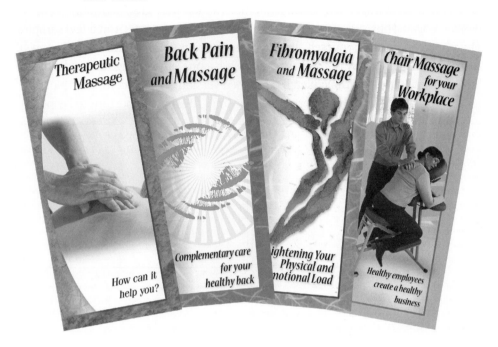

initially costs. Your brochure can be a valuable form of leverage, so take the time to do it right.

Phone Book Ads

All the work you have done to design your card and brochure, up to this point, can be condensed into one piece that reaches many people with your carefully crafted image or message. This is a mini-advertisement in the business section of the phone book, or what many people call a Yellow Pages® ad. You can just list your name and phone number, pay increasingly higher prices for bigger print, color, and more space around your name or ad, or buy large, full-page ads.

EXERCISE: CREATING A PHONE BOOK AD

Get out your local phone book (or go to the library for phone books from all over the country) and look in the advertising section for "Massage Therapy." Notice which ads you like or don't like, and try to figure out what affected your perception of the ads. Do the ads make sense, do their graphics fit with their message, and do they seem legitimate? Notice the big ads (if there are any) and look at how they use color, white space, fonts, graphics, logos, photos, maps, and other visual elements. Then notice what information they give, including contact details, slogans, business names, and anything else in the text. Draft a few samples of a phone book ad for yourself that includes the elements you think would appeal to your ideal clients. Lay out a quarter-page ad, a one-eighth-page ad, and a three-line ad, using either a simple sketch or a typed version on your computer. Notice, as the ad gets smaller, what information becomes the most important to keep!

Gift Certificates

Gift certificates are powerful muscle marketing tools. Unlike other pieces of paper you use to market, gift certificates have real value in the mind of the holder, and they are not likely to be lost, misplaced, or thrown away. Getting gift certificates into your prospective clients' hands can be done quickly through your mutual marketing partners, current clients, family, and friends. If you want to build your practice quickly, give a lot away. If speed is not important, distribute them more slowly through direct sales. Gift certificates can come in many shapes and sizes, but they need a few elements for them to work well. Since the odds are good that some of them will be mailed to gift recipients, you should have your printer create pieces that can fit inside a standard-size greeting card, or create an envelope and certificate package that the gift-giver would be proud to send. You can buy a box of nice envelopes, measure one, and have your printer set your insert paper size to fit inside.

Use your gift certificate as an educational piece. If the receiver has some reservations about getting massage, which is more common than you'd think, print some of your other marketing elements on the back of the certificate to coax him or her to call and set up an appointment. While some people have unscrupulously exploited this knowledge and sold certificates knowing they won't be used, this is a shortsighted view of how to make a living with massage. Solid practices are built by happy clients returning and referring others, and the more people who come in to get a massage from you, the faster you can rebook them. Due to abuses of gift certificates, it is now illegal in many places to put expiration dates on them, and scams that involve selling certificates with fast expirations are not only unethical but also illegal in a growing number of states.

Your certificate needs to include these elements.

> To: (the name of the recipient)
>
> For: (a one-hour massage, a hot stone treatment, an aromatherapy wrap)
>
> From: (the person giving the gift)
>
> Date: (the date you sold the certificate)
>
> With: (your name and title)
>
> Your contact information: (business name, address, phone)

Beyond that, you can include any of the elements from your other marketing pieces to get recipients to call. If it is illegal in your area to use an expiration date, entice the gift certificate recipient to call quickly by offering a special incentive if he or she books by a certain date. You can give away extra time, a promotional gift, or a product or service from one of your mutual marketing partners. If your certificate is being given out by one of your partners, or through a promotional ad or coupon, put a code on the certificate so you know which of your marketing ventures are working and are worth your time and effort for future projects.

Reaching new clients with discounted or giveaway gift certificates can be one of the fastest, least expensive, and most effective forms of marketing you can do. Gift certificates remove the whole issue of the decision to buy, and let you prove your value and create trust the best way possible: by putting your hands on your new client.

You can quickly and easily get gift certificates by buying beautiful premade gift certificates from companies like Sharper Cards or Massage Warehouse (see "Resources" section), or you can make your own with a little imagination. (See Figure 7–7a and Figure 7–7b.)

EXERCISE: CREATING A GIFT CERTIFICATE

Working freehand or on a computer, lay out a sample gift certificate including all of the elements just covered. Do you want a pretty picture in the background that you print the words over? What would the picture be? Who will most likely buy your gift certificates, and to whom are they giving them? If most of your buyers are men, but they are buying gifts for women, do you make the certificate look more masculine or feminine? (Hint: design it for the receiver.) If you can, go to an office supply store and look at their types of paper or card stock that would work well for your gift certificate. Finally, see if they have matching envelopes or at least envelopes that your certificate can fit into, because people will need to mail them! If you are ready, have a bunch printed up and start giving them out or selling them to let people know you are in business! Even if you decide to buy preprinted gift certificates, this exercise will get you to think about what kind of certificates you would want.

Promotional Gifts

Reaching new clients through the printed word does not have to be limited to a paper medium. Muscle marketing is designed to get you into people's awareness, and to give them reasons and ways to contact you. Since paper can

Figure 7-7 | Gift certificates can be a powerful tool for building a practice.

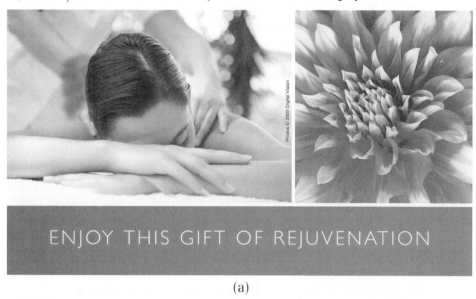

(a)

(b)

be easy to lose or throw away, putting your name and contact information on novelty items or promotional gifts greatly increases your odds that someone will be able to find your telephone number easily, even months later. For example, if you had a booth at a health fair, and a man picked up a free mug you had on display, he might realize months after meeting you that buying a massage gift certificate for a coworker would be the perfect gift. Surprise, your number is on the coffee mug, and your contact information is right there in his kitchen cupboard. Cost of mug: negligible. Value to you: the price of one massage, and the ability to rebook and gain referrals from your new client. Now that's a good return on your investment!

Depending on your target market and what's appropriate, you can give out sample bottles of massage oil with your label on them, bath beads or soaps in containers with your name on them, candles, incense, crystals, meditation books, inflatable travel neck pillows, those plastic maps you gave to the real estate agent, coffee mugs, golf visors, massage tools, or anything else that will make people think of you when they look at it every day. Of course, if you have a mutual marketing partner with products that you can put your name and number on and give away, you have the opportunity to cross-promote both of you.

A wonderful promotional gift to give away is one that people will play with and keep on their desks. Therapeutic toys like squeeze balls, or, my favorite, the Tangle®, let people reduce their stress and help keep their hands working well, all while seeing your name and number on a regular basis. (See Figure 7–8.)

Figure 7–8 | **Promotional items keep your name and contact information in front of people.**

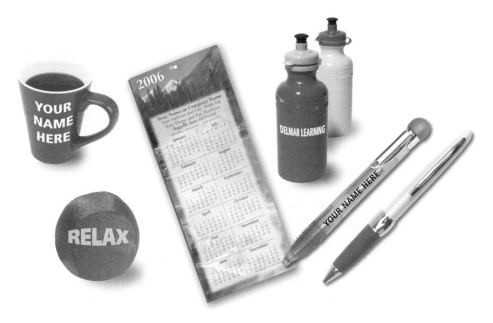

Small Promotional Items

If bigger gifts cost more than you can afford in the beginning, use pens, bookmarks, restaurant tip cards, laminated reflexology cards, preprinted sticky notes, memo pads, coasters, jar openers, refrigerator magnets, key fobs, golf tees, and other promotional items. (See Figure 7–8.) If these promotional items mean you get a new client, book one additional massage, or create a referral because your client had your telephone number handy, these freebies more than pay for themselves. Find companies specializing in premium or promotional items by looking in the phone book and online under "Advertising Specialties." (Look in the "Resources" section, too.) Visit their stores or get their catalogs, and let your mind run wild with great ways of keeping yourself at the forefront of your prospects' or clients' minds.

The Walking, Talking Billboard

With the growing acceptance of massage taking place across the country, many people are suspended between the stages of wanting to get a massage and not knowing from whom to get one. Of all the ways to get yourself recognized by those looking for you, wearing clothing that indicates you do massage can be one of your most effective forms of marketing. You can design your own T-shirt, polo shirt, denim long-sleeve shirt, baseball cap, tote bag, or other wearable item that can lead to seemingly miraculous and coincidental moments when people ask you if you do massage. Even if you buy predesigned shirts from companies such as Stress Away Systems (see "Resources" section), you should use this inexpensive and fun form of marketing. (See Figure 7–9.) You can introduce yourself in any setting with your wearable message, and, for goodness sake, have your business cards with you to give to those who want to talk to you.

Resumes

Reference marketing tools sometimes only have an audience or target market of one. If you want to cultivate relationships with massage colleagues, medical and health practitioners, joint venture partners, or other individuals who can be a valid source of referrals, it may be appropriate for you to give them your professional resume or curriculum vitae. If you want to teach a class, speak for a group, get a booth at a health fair, or otherwise show your massage

Figure 7–9 | Clothing with the word "massage" on it can start conversations with potential clients.

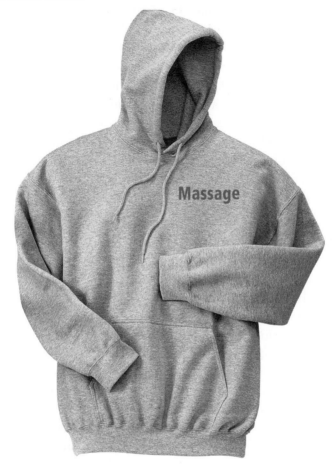

background, you most likely will need a resume as part of the package you submit. Writing a resume takes thought and effort, but having a good resume in reserve means you can get it out quickly when opportunities come your way. Many books cover the details of writing a resume, and the first chapter of this book goes into extensive detail about writing a massage-based resume.

Web Site

An Internet Web site promoting your business can be a good form of marketing, or it can be pretty useless. The first drawback is that while the Internet is highly touted for its many benefits, it is frequently used for pornography, and you must make it very clear on your Web site that the type of massage you are advertising is nonsexual. If you want to give out a telephone number for people who have visited your Web site to use, get a voice-mail number to screen your potential clientele. A number of my colleagues with phone book ads that say "professional therapeutic massage—nonsexual only" still get harassing calls. If callers can't understand that an ad actually means what it says in the phone book, they probably won't pay attention to what you say on your Web site either.

The second drawback to a Web site is that it is a fairly passive marketing tool for reaching new clients. It is great for current clients or partners to use as a reference when telling their referrals more about you, but it is not usually an active marketing tool for a one-person massage practice. In other words, don't think that just putting up a Web site will get you tons of new customers. Anyone doing a blind search for a new massage therapist on the Internet will have to wade through numerous pornography sites, and if trust is an issue, it will be very hard to convey your professionalism when your site comes up sandwiched between "Lovely Girls' Massage" and sex toys. It is unfortunate, and it makes the Internet a somewhat inhospitable place for advertising a massage practice.

In addition, most people don't look online for personal service professionals such as hairstylists or psychologists. They want direct personal referrals from people they trust, and the same applies to massage therapists. If you do want to use the Web, consider setting yourself apart from the crowd by getting pay-per-click placement on sites such as Google and Yahoo!, and be listed in a separate area from all the other sites that show up in a general search. You can also work with Google, Yahoo!, and other search engines very easily and affordably by using ads targeted toward people with specific interests and area codes.

That said, if you choose to have a Web site, you also can use it for the rebooking and referral stages of marketing. All of the elements that go into your brochure and resume can go on your site in an expanded version, since page space is not an issue. You can include your massage menu, information about yourself and your background or training, information about your work, client testimonials, more photos, and links to your marketing partners' sites. Then, when you give out your card at a party, speak on a radio show, or talk to someone in line, you can point out that anything else they want to know about you is on your Web site, which is easy to find because your URL is printed on your card. In addition to your card, brochure, gift certificate, or promotional gift, a Web site gives another air of legitimacy to your practice and lets people research you if they want further evidence of your value and trustworthiness.

For the rebooking function of marketing, your Web site can have an on-screen calendar with time slots open for appointments, letting your current clients book with you online. Your client can see what's open, book the time slot or request it by e-mail, and get a response back as often as you check your site. You can answer at any time of day without having to consider your clients' phone availability.

For a more interactive Web site, you can have viewers sign up for an electronic newsletter, leave information on how you can reach them to talk to them in person, or fill in an electronic survey of their opinions and preferences about what kind of massage benefits they want. They can take a guided photo tour of your office, watch a video of you working, listen to audio or video testimonials, study an anatomy lesson about how massage affects muscles or relieves pain, or do anything else you can think of that would engage your Web visitors and convince them that they should call you for an appointment. If you have the ability to take credit card payments, which can be set up easily with companies like PayPal, you can also sell gift certificates, which the person can then print with a simple click.

ACTION MARKETING TOOLS

Reaching out to new clients is, for most therapists, a fairly well-controlled process. Reference tools such as cards, brochures, gift certificates, and promotional items are given out primarily by you or those who know you. These are your safest tools to use to build your practice and may be all the tools you need. Reference tools remind people of you and give them direct access to reaching you, but they have some drawbacks if time is of the essence for you. The first drawback is that the tools can take a lot of time for you to disseminate. The second is that they provide little or no incentive for the recipient to make the buying decision faster.

To leap these two tall buildings in a single bound, we can employ action marketing tools. Action tools are various forms of marketing that are distributed rapidly to larger groups of people through means such as direct mail or e-mail. They include time limitations and, often, a bonus or discount for responding within that set time period.

The purpose of action marketing is to get a potential client to take some form of action upon seeing your marketing tool. That action can be to call a telephone number for a free gift, schedule a free consultation, book an appointment, write in for a coupon, go on your Web site and download a coupon, come by your office, or pick up a gift certificate from one of the places you are holding a promotional.

If your target market includes people who are in the product acceptance stage, the action they will feel most comfortable taking is to learn about the value of massage. It may take you a number of small, safe steps to educate them before they are ready to book. If most of your target market already accept massage and are simply looking for a trustworthy practitioner, you can skip some of the small "wooing" steps and be more direct in your approach toward the goal of booking their first appointment.

Types of Action Marketing

Numerous ways exist to reach your market with some form of action marketing. Simple flyers with tear-off telephone numbers on the bottom can be posted in select locations; postcards can be sent to a large number of people on a rented mailing list; or elaborate, multipage promotional kits can be sent to a select group of people referred by a marketing partner. Regardless of the cost, length, or sophistication of your marketing materials, some basic elements should be included in every marketing piece. These include the:

- ❈ Headline
- ❈ Body copy
- ❈ Call to action
- ❈ Closing

Headline

The first part of any action piece is your headline. Your headline is what draws readers in and convinces them to read further. A weak headline means your piece gets discarded, while a strong headline captures enough interest to have your offer considered. Your headline must convey a powerful, self-serving, desirable benefit for your reader. It can focus on what the person wants, doesn't want, or wants to avoid. For example, if your market is getting older, you can focus on what they want (to feel young again), what they don't want (to feel the effects of aging), or want to avoid (the limiting symptoms of aging). Your headline can motivate the reader to take action due to the promise of pleasure, the easing of pain, or both. The headline should be educational and provide information that will lead to a result they want, and it should promise that if they continue to read, there will be a payoff for their time and attention. Essentially, you need to write a headline so that the reader can't help but want to know more.

Given the current state of massage during this time of transition, your headline and the rest of your material would better interest and educate your reader by being informative, logical, pragmatic, objective, definitive, scientific, analytical, measurable, and strategic. Since you are trying to present yourself as a trustworthy professional, don't be vague, cute, ethereal, or obscure. What may work for marketing more established products or services doesn't apply to massage yet, so stick to the basics.

Body Copy

Following the headline are the opening paragraph and body copy that provide the payoff promised in the headline. Much of the work you have already done on your reference marketing tools can be used directly in your body copy here. We will go over a few new elements, and you can mix and match your own reference elements and the following elements, depending on your goals and the amount of space you have. Your body copy can include:

- A promise
- Clear and detailed facts about you, your work, your advantages, and so forth
- Explicit benefits and reasons for buying
- How you will take away their risk by providing guarantees
- Endorsements or testimonials
- Gifts, bonuses, deals, or discounts for acting by a specific time
- All the necessary information to make a decision
- What action to take now

These elements are important in selling any service business and are especially important when selling massage. By including these elements, you clear the way for a faster and easier decision from the reader.

Promises

Promises are attention grabbers. However, very few people take the act of making a promise seriously, so when someone does make a promise to us, we stop for a moment to consider whether they actually will fulfill it. With so much mistrust between the public and advertisers, anyone willing to stick their neck out and make a promise will get attention. Since trust is one of the main barriers between massage therapists and our potential clients, making a promise may be a potent way to make a case for your trustworthiness.

Specific and Measurable Results

You don't have to make any kind of promise, but if you choose to do so, you can strengthen it further by making it measurable as well as desirable. If your target market includes elderly women golfers, don't just say you'll improve their game or help them feel better: say you'll add 10 yards to their tee shot and then tell them how. Tell them that massage can help them have better range of motion in their hips or improve their energy to last a full 18 holes because of better posture, improved breathing skills, stress management tools, and the like. Use your promise as a way to educate, or if you feel you can't back your promise, just educate. If you do make a strong promise, provide a money-back guarantee and be ready to back it.

If your clients are executives, don't just promise them they'll be more productive. Tell them they will be able to make faster, smarter decisions with better mental clarity due to improved blood flow to the brain because you will release the compressing muscles in the shoulders and neck. Describe how your stress management techniques or the relaxation audiotape you'll give them as an added bonus may help aid sleep at night so they will have two extra productive hours each workday.

While these are just examples, if you know your target markets, you can make similar types of claims. Just don't exaggerate. If you don't know your target markets well enough to make such specific promises, then read magazines and trade journals, join associations, search the Internet, or interview people in that market to learn what their needs are, and start with more generic claims. You can make an educated guess, but if you are wrong about what your market needs and you sell a solution to a problem they don't have, you'll waste valuable time and resources by marketing the wrong message.

I made the mistake of trying to sell to high-level executives by telling them I could reduce their stress. It seemed logical and valuable to me, but I wasn't having much luck. I finally decided to ask a friend and powerful executive why my marketing message wasn't working. "If I let go of my stress," he said, "I'd fall apart. My stress is the only thing that holds me together, so I'm afraid to let go of it." The thought of a long, luxurious, stress-reducing massage had no appeal to him, and he guessed it probably wouldn't appeal to his colleagues, either. So, if he were to get a massage, I asked, what would he want and why? It turns out what he really wanted was a quick, energizing, oil-free massage that could let him work more hours. So much for that assumption!

If you want to save yourself money and time, do some research first; then you will know what your market wants and needs, and you can make a compelling offer to meet those needs.

Guarantees

Of all the things that will make your marketing stand out from other massage therapists, I recommend that you offer a guarantee so powerful that all risk is removed for your prospect when booking a massage. Many people have had bad experiences or heard horror stories about a heavy-handed massage therapist who beat his clients black and blue, or they've suffered through listening to their massage therapist, a talkative divorcee, go on about her ex-husband for the whole session. These prospective clients are worried that you may not be worth their time or money, and that worry may stop them from booking an appointment. Whatever new clients may be wary of, dispel their fears by assuring them that you will give them their money back if they aren't happy for any reason. Your guarantee relaxes and relieves them, and they will be impressed that you are that confident in your work. If you are willing to provide a guarantee, make it a prominent feature in your marketing piece. It will be novel, unexpected, and very welcome. The purpose of a guarantee is to reduce the risk in the decision to buy and to give you leverage in convincing someone to try your work. A guarantee helps establish trust. Even if your prospects are not initially convinced of the value of your work, you can take away their risk until you can prove it.

Protecting Yourself from Guarantee Abuse

A guarantee takes away the risk of the buying decision for your client, but it puts you at risk of wasting your time with a scammer. There are ways to protect yourself, however, so do not hesitate to use guarantees. After all, if offering a guarantee doubles or triples your client base, and two or three people scam you for a massage over the years, are those lost three hours worth all those new clients with their net worth, plus their referrals? Of course they are! No marketing or advertising program is going to be effective 100 percent of the time, so don't be tight, cheap, greedy, or come from a feeling of scarcity with your guarantee. Instead, come from a feeling of abundance, be a service and quality fanatic, make every facet of your work be top of the line, let your clients know what you are doing for them, and, if your work is good, your guarantee will pay off big for you.

Your written guarantee in your marketing materials can bring clients in the door, and to protect yourself and provide good customer service, you should review your guarantee during your pre-massage conversation with the client. This gives your client, as well as you, an "out" on the guarantee. You can state that you provide a money-back guarantee, and, if after the first half-hour the client is not happy, he or she can leave without paying. Then, at the half-hour mark, ask the client if he or she is happy with your work and would like to continue the massage. In that way, if the client really doesn't like your work, he or she can simply get up and go. Or if the person is scamming you, he or she won't really be able change his or her mind at the end of the session. In the best-case scenario, your client can give you feedback on what would make him or her happier. Either way, you have protected some of your time, and if you learn quickly what makes your new client happy, you will be able to do better work.

Endorsements and Testimonials

Having other people promote you is often a more effective way to lead people to action than by having the words come from you. Somehow, it is more acceptable to have a client or marketing partner say, "Jane Doe is the best massage therapist ever! Run, don't walk, to get a terrific massage from her!" Endorsements have a bit more push to them than a testimonial. Usually a testimonial just says that you're great or provides examples of how you help, but an endorsement tells the reader that he or she should take some sort of action. It's a subtle difference, but having your endorsers tell your potential client what to do next can make the difference between just informing someone and getting him or her to take action.

Who endorses you may or may not be a factor in your marketing. Endorsement statements can be followed by data ranging from "Mary C., California" to full names, job descriptions, and photos. The more information you can give about your endorsers, the more legitimate they seem. If you are aiming for a narrow target market such as horseback riders and competitive show jumpers, then you want endorsements from like-minded people, preferably those who have won a few ribbons or are notables in the sport. People trust people who are like them, and who face their same problems and needs, so pick your endorsers to match the market you want to reach.

Offers

Before you make offers to bring in new clients, think about the purpose of your offers. If you have a long-term strategy and want to have clients come back on a regular basis, then you want a multi-massage package offer that demonstrates the cumulative value of your work. If you need larger sums of money to buy a washing machine and dryer, then create a multi-massage package offer asking for payment up front with a discount for each session, or have the client buy a package of 10 sessions and get one free. If you want to get people in the habit of referring their friends to you, make an offer that allows them to buy a massage for themselves and receive a gift certificate to give away. We will cover a number of options for creating offers, but first you have to think about what you need most so your offer really can help your business.

Factors to consider include money, time, repetition (number of sessions), frequency of sessions, your needs, and the clients' needs. Let's look at these factors further.

Package Deals

Money and time are two pieces of your offer strategy. If you don't have a lot of time to build a practice, then make lower-price offers to get new clients in the door. If time is not a factor, your offers don't have to give as heavy a discount. The next factor in your strategy is the repetition or number of sessions purchased. Package deals mix and match money, time, and repetition in a variety of ways, depending on the desires and needs of you and your market. For example, if your need is to create long-term, repeat clients, one of the best strategies you can use is to offer discounted package deals that bring in clients for at least three massages. This gives them a price break and the experience of the cumulative effects of massage, generates value in their minds, and proves your benefits.

Years ago, my mother ran a package deal in a local coupon book offering three massages for $99, paid up front. The coupon ad ran once and it gave her enough clients to fill out her practice. She traded massage with the woman who created the coupon books so no money was spent, and when she gave me one client who needed deeper work than she could do, I built a big part of my practice on that person's referrals. Mom did a lot of $33 massages initially, which was hard for her, but enough clients stayed with her after their initial three massages to make the promotional offer more than worth it. Honestly, given the amount of money most businesses spend advertising, the fact that we get paid to advertise (which is what a package deal ultimately amounts to) should make us clap our hands with joy.

You can do all sorts of variations on this, ranging from simple two-for-one offers to selling a set time slot for an annual up-front fee with good discounts. For example, say a person agrees to massages every Monday at 2:00 p.m. If the client can't be there, he or she can send someone else. If no one shows up, you get the hour off but keep the fee you charged up front.

Time Bonuses

Another offer element—time—can be used as a low-cost, high-value bonus. Again, consider your needs first. If you want people to value your price but you want to get them in the door, you can send out coupons, mailers, or ads offering a free, extra half-hour for the price of one hour. You can offer one free massage when they buy four up front at your full price, or, if they don't have that kind of money, you can offer a free massage after they've had 10 full-price massages in a row. If you want your clients to come in with a particular frequency, you can offer a time bonus of a free half-hour if they get four massages within a month. If you have slow days or times, you can offer an extra 15 minutes for massages on Tuesdays, or between the hours of 11:00 a.m. and 2:00 p.m., for example. A different take, if you want referrals, is to offer a free gift certificate to your client to give to a friend after he or she has come in for four sessions. As you can see, the possibilities are almost endless.

You can mix and match these factors to get needed cash up front, keep customers for the long term, train them with regard to how frequently to get massage, get them familiar with and ready to pay your full price, or whatever else it takes to build your dream practice. Anytime you consider making an offer, ask yourself what you want and to what your market will be drawn. People may differ in their opinions on this topic, but in my research, it seems more beneficial than not to be generous with your time up front. Time is a flexible asset. It is your cheapest, most effective benefit to offer, and it can pay off handsomely.

Combining Guarantees, Bonuses, and Gifts

The most desirable and irresistible combination to buyers is a totally risk-free trial proposition or guarantee, along with a bonus or gift just for trying you out. For example, you can offer a money-back guaranteed, three-massage package deal, offered at a discount, along with a free consultation from a feng shui expert, a personal trainer, or a nutritionist. Packages such as these can separate you from competing therapists, lead someone in your direction, or remove a barrier that is keeping a person from making a commitment to massage. Your guarantee removes that person's risk; your offer or deal moves him or her closer to a decision; and your marketing partners' bonuses or gifts create a tremendous advantage, link you positively with people or businesses already known and trusted, and create a high perceived value with little or no cost to you. If you want a strategy more effective than standing around at a networking meeting handing out brochures, this combination is hard to beat.

Deadlines

What makes your action marketing tool effective in bringing people to you rapidly is a deadline by when they will lose the opportunity to take advantage of your deal or offer. Busy people often procrastinate about getting to things, even things they want to do. Creating a deadline moves your offer into a more active part of their awareness, with a conscious or unconscious time clock ticking down to move them to action. After all, if it weren't for deadlines, taxes would never be paid, tulip bulbs wouldn't get planted, and books would never get finished. The possibility of losing out on your good offer is one of the most powerful forms of leverage you can use to get your buyer to call you. Make sure you have a clearly stated deadline to your offer, and put it in a big enough font that people will see it, even if they are just quickly scanning your marketing piece.

How to Close Your Action Marketing Tool

The final element of an action marketing tool is a closing that has the purpose of "opening" a potential relationship. One of the biggest mistakes marketers make is that they don't treat their ad, coupon, or letter like a sales call, and don't close the piece by asking the prospect to take some kind of action. If you make a call, send a letter, or leave a flyer, conclude the process by taking your prospects by the hand and leading them to some kind of action.

For example, imagine that you are talking to a woman who got your name as a referral and has called you to ask about your work. At the end of the conversation, after you've explained your benefits, type of work, and the like, would you just hang up? Of course not. You'd move to the natural completion of the conversation by asking for the opportunity to work with her, and inquiring whether she would like to book an appointment or take some other kind of action. If you treat your marketing tools like a sales conversation, you need to close with the call to action, telling your readers explicitly what to do.

Possible Actions for Prospects to Take

Depending on the level of trust or value your readers have in you, your marketing tool can lead them directly to booking an appointment, or toward a smaller, less committed step. You can ask them to visit your Web site, drop by your office to meet you for a free consultation, or pick up a free gift, coupon, or certificate. You can ask them to attend a speech or seminar, or ask them to take a less risky, more educational step like e-mailing or calling you for a brochure, questionnaire, newsletter, resume, or free tape you offer about massage or a related topic. Whatever action you ask for, do what you can to get them to respond right now, before they put down your ad, letter, or whatever you sent, and forget about your great offer.

This final element of asking the person to make a decision is where marketing becomes selling, and it is also where the process can become the most uncomfortable. Images of used-car salesmen and other negative selling stereotypes often are associated with getting a person to make a decision to buy. If those images make you uncomfortable or resistant, you will need to call on your higher self, or your greater purpose or mission, to remind you of why you are marketing massage in the first place.

Going back to the first attribute, the desire to serve, you can remind yourself in moments of self-doubt, fear, or discomfort that you have an incredible gift to offer, and you can endure a few minutes of conversation or lines of type to get to the joy of helping others with your touch.

As human beings, all of us face the fear of rejection, and at the closing moment of any marketing or selling point, we have to look someone in the eye or hear a voice on the phone saying "yes" or "no" to the personal gift being offered. If we were selling tires or refrigerators and people did not like them, the rejection would not be personal. However, with massage, we are selling our touch, and ourselves, and being rejected can feel personal and painful. If you never ask a person to make a decision to get a massage from you, you will never be rejected or have to feel that pain, but the odds are high you also will do very little massage, which can be even more painful. All of your marketing culminates in the final act of giving a massage, and since that is the backbone of your dream practice, using the more direct action marketing tools will help build your practice quickly.

PUTTING IT ALL TOGETHER

Creating a marketing tool of any type takes knowing the purpose and goals of the piece, and combining the many elements we have covered into a viable piece. Depending on your needs, budget, skills, or the skills of those who help you, you may decide to create coupons, postcards, letters, surveys, newsletters, flyers, or other types of tools to reach out to new clients. Let's review these tools in more detail.

Postcards

The primary benefits of postcards are that they are not as intimidating to write as long letters because of their limited space, and they are relatively cheap to print and mail. Since your recipients don't have to open an envelope, there is also a higher likelihood that they will at least turn the postcard over and read your eye-popping headline. Postcards also give you the benefit of doing three or four mailings in a row to the same recipients. This makes them more effective, since your mailer or advertisement message often doesn't even register in a person's consciousness until about the third or fourth time it is seen. Beautiful or eye-catching postcards made specifically for massage therapists can let you select the look you want for minimal expense, leaving you to focus your time and energy on your message that will appear on the back side. (See Figures 7–10a, b, and c)

Figure 7–10 | Postcards are a quick and inexpensive way to stay in touch with clients. (Image courtesy of Lynn Johnston postcard)

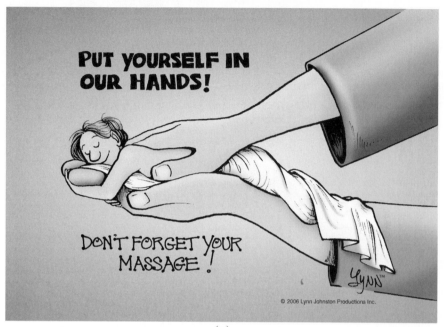

(a)

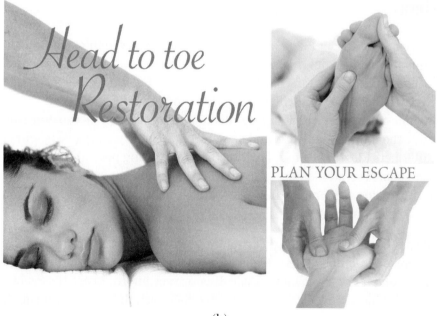

(b)

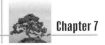
Figure 7–10 | (continued)

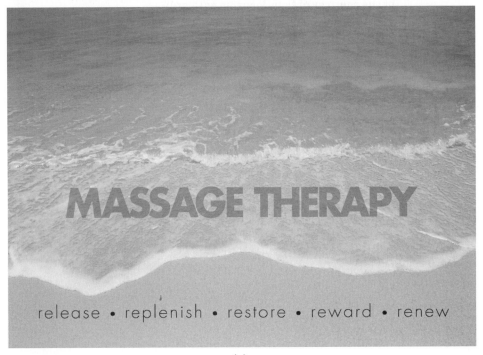

MASSAGE THERAPY

release • replenish • restore • reward • renew

(c)

Letters

Letters can range from a simple one-sided sheet of paper to thick, multipage documents that resemble magazines. Letters can have pages of text and use various means to attract the reader's attention, including circling important words with red ink, using yellow sticky notes to highlight sections, inserting small note cards that fall out of large documents, and so on. If you ever want to study the ultimate in letters and mailers, take a look at the packets sent out by Publishers Clearing House. Their tactics of including postcards to mail, stickers to lick, scratch-off dots, highlighted lines, and personalized photos with your name written on a big check, are all elaborate, clever, and obviously very effective marketing tools.

While postcards are good as quick attention-grabbers, letters are better if the recipient is actually interested in massage. A letter can provide enough information on its own to make a sale. If your very informative letter reaches a person who has been looking for a massage therapist, the amount and quality of information you give can build enough trust to inspire them to call and book an appointment.

To create an effective letter, use the elements we've covered, have a unique look and message, present your most important material early, in case your readers only give you a few seconds to catch their interest, and tell them what to do once they are done reading.

Letters can be enhanced by their envelopes, and how your envelope looks will probably determine whether or not your letter will be opened. Handwritten addresses make your letter look more personalized, and you can print your offer and deadline on the envelope so recipients will see it clearly as they sort through their piles of mail.

Letters Sent Through Mutual Marketing Partner Mailing Lists

Before you create a mailer, learn as much as you can about who you are sending it to. You will have a much better chance of understanding who your recipients are if you send your mailer to your mutual marketing partners' mailing lists rather than to a blind or rented list. Whether you pay, trade for, or are given mailing lists, do your best to get your partner's endorsement to personalize your letter.

Golf Pro Example

Let's go back to the example in the "Mutual Marketing" section, and imagine that there is a golf pro who already has a large clientele of students that matches your target market. However, when you ask him to be part of the process of contacting his student list, he balks a little bit because he "hates selling anything." Since he doesn't want to "sell" golf, ask if you can sell massage and offer a free golf lesson as a bonus for signing up for a certain number of massages. (See Figure 7–11.) In this way, you can benefit from your association with him and establish yourself as a golf massage specialist. You can offer a free half-hour lesson to those who book and pay for a set number of massages, and you then either pay the pro nothing, or a discounted or full price for that lesson.

The true benefit to the pro is that he gets the opportunity to regain contact with former students and sell them a series of lessons if their free half-hour lesson shows them how rusty their golf games have become. If he has been out of touch with many of the people on his mailing list, your direct mail letter is a way for him to get back in contact with former customers without having to pay a dime. All he has to do is give you his mailing list, provide a few free

Figure 7–11 | Partnering with a golf professional can open many doors to potential clients. (Image courtesy of Getty Images)

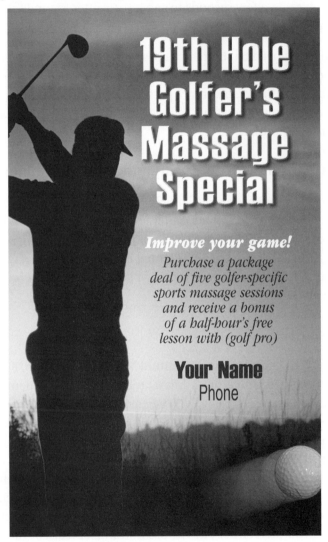

lessons (unless it actually is worth it for you to pay for them), and turn those free lessons back into paying clients.

If you want to turn your letter into a more far-reaching piece, go to a golf club salesman and ask for some discount coupons for equipment to include in your mailer. In fact, you can ask the golf store or salesman to cover the cost of your printing and mailing since the golf pro's list of people includes his or her target market too. If the club where your pro works is experiencing slow sales, you can include coupons for their greens fees in your direct mail piece. With the pro's permission, you can ask the club to give you their mailing list, along with discount coupons for their greens fees, restaurant and bar, or clothing items from their pro shop. Now the club salesman will really want to pay for your mailing because you have access to a whole new list of golfers. And your golf pro has a whole slew of potential prospects you've rounded up. Send out your mailer and, as extra insurance, post your flyer, card, or brochure prominently at the club, give a bunch to the golf pro and the golf club proprietor, and you've pinpointed and reached your exact target market for nothing except some creative thought, good communication, a few telephone calls, and the time spent writing your direct mail piece. I could go on and on with variations of just this example, but you get the idea of what this one direct mail letter can do for your practice.

Flyers

The purpose of flyers, comprised of many if not all of the elements of action marketing, is to get your prospects' attention, create interest, and lead to some form of action. Flyers can be easy to make, cheap to print, and fast to distribute. If you have a home office or do outcall, flyers are not advised, since they can't screen people. If you have an office or workspace where other people are around, then flyers can be a safe and effective tool. They can be given to mutual marketers, sent to a mailing list, or posted in a place frequented by your target market. Since your flyers will be seen by a large number of people, it is important to make it good looking, eye catching, and professional. Changing it often means that people will see it and not be as likely to overlook it.

The drawback to flyers is that because they are inexpensive to make and can be put together quickly on a home computer, they don't have the same cache or image as other forms of advertising. For example, you wouldn't see a flyer posted for a doctor, dentist, psychologist, or physical therapist advertising those professionals' services. However, it is more common to see flyers for manicurists and hairstylists since flyers are acceptable for many service businesses. Since massage can be both a personal and professional service, you will need to determine who your market is and what you are offering to determine whether or not a flyer would be congruent with your target market's perception of your services.

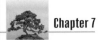

Surveys

Another possible way to market is to use surveys. One use of surveys is the more traditional method of sending questionnaires to current and past clients to get information that can be used in testimonials or for research about how to improve your practice. However, a second use is to send surveys to prospective clients, using them as a marketing tool. Instead of telling your prospects what you do, ask them what they would want from a massage experience. You can say something along the lines of "I am a new massage therapist in town and want to know what you want and expect, or like or dislike, about massage." The people who take the time to answer your survey or questionnaire are good candidates for further marketing pieces, and, of course, you can learn a lot from what they tell you. If you are new at massage, this is a fast way to gather information about your target market, and it replaces guessing with knowledge of what people want so that you can create more effective marketing material. Even if your recipients don't respond to your survey, it lets them know of your existence, and that may be all you need to make a sale. In addition, the fact that you have marketed with a survey tells them you actually care what they think, and that customer service and value are important to you.

A word of caution here: don't believe everything people say in response to your survey. Studies in the marketing and advertising world have shown repeatedly that what people say they want is often different from what they are willing to spend money on. However, surveys are a great way to start your marketing research and can teach you a lot about your market.

Distributing Your Marketing Tools

Since the purpose of marketing tools is to give you leverage in reaching more people quickly, it makes sense that the more places your tools are distributed, the better your leverage will be. There are almost endless ways to distribute your marketing, so look at the world around you and see where you can spread your message of massage.

Getting Mailing Lists of Your Target Market

If you are going to be mailing marketing tools to potential clients, gather mailing lists from various sources and then edit them so you don't waste time and money sending materials to people who live too far away, or the like. You can rent lists, borrow lists, trade massages for lists, or do your research and create your own list. Lists can be obtained from:

❊ Mutual marketers

❊ Associations/clubs/organizations

❊ Magazines

❊ List brokers (look for advertisements in the phone book or online under "mailing lists")

❊ Library (ask the reference librarian for the SRDS mailing list directory; then call and ask for free catalogs to see what scope of lists they offer so you can tightly narrow your search to reach your target market)

❊ Yellow Pages or other phone book listings by profession

❊ Create your own list (buy contact management software to document names and addresses, and make notations about which direct response ad was sent)

Advertisements

Most of the marketing tools covered in this part are designed to be educational, informative, and persuasive. These tools are going to be distributed mostly by you, those fairly closely connected to you, or to narrowly targeted markets. In combining your needs for safety, speed, low cost, and reaching your target market as accurately as possible, we have stayed away from the more expensive, risky, and uncontrolled tool of advertising. Because of where the profession exists at this time in the general public's perception, advertising to mass audiences has been a less common tool for building a practice. This is now changing, and if you are in an area where massage is well accepted and competition is high, you might find value in traditional mass media advertising.

Designing a mass media ad requires many of the thoughts and elements with which you are now becoming familiar. The difference will be that your message now has more exposure. Whether you are creating a phone book advertisement or a television infomercial, you still need to get attention, create interest, offer the audience something they want, and give them the reasons and information needed to contact you. You won't need much help making a phone book ad, but if you are going into television, radio, the Internet, magazines, and other more

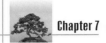

expensive media, you'll want to get professional help specific to any medium with which you are unfamiliar. Mistakes can be costly.

Again, before you begin any marketing, start with the end in mind: set clear goals of what you want for your practice, what markets you want to serve, and what to say to introduce prospective clients to your touch.

Testing Your Marketing Factors

After all is said and done with regard to creating an effective marketing tool, how do you know if it will work? The only way to really know is to test it using definitive and measurable means. Testing will show you which headline is effective, what offers or bonuses appeal to your market, what graphics catch people's eye, or what tools people actually read and keep. Before you invest in any marketing medium, verbally test out elements such as your slogan, headlines, or key phrases on everyone you can. Watch people closely to see how they respond. If they look confused at your message or offer, go back and streamline your words. Continue to practice your material and get feedback until you think you are onto a message to which your market will respond. Then, and only then, should you put forth the time and money required for marketing tools.

We have introduced many elements you can include in your marketing tools, and if you use a tool more than once (which you may not need to!), you should test those elements individually. Factors to test include your price, your slogan, your offers, your rationale of why the public should buy, your benefits, and your guarantees. If you use presentations or public speeches, test different elements on a live audience; if you use printed materials, experiment with your packaging, look, and message. Don't assume anything about your marketing. Let your clients tell you what they want. You can test printed materials not only for content but also for the frequency and timing of distribution.

Depending on your goals, finances, and time, you can conduct a mail or e-mail campaign one time a week for three months, send out a monthly mailing featuring different offers, or mail a quarterly newsletter with advice or health tips, coupons for a massage series, various offers, and anything else that will help them become familiar with you.

If you will be doing frequent marketing, you will have more opportunities to test your factors, but, if at all possible, test one factor at a time. Testing may not sound like a lot of fun, and most businesses never actually test their marketing. So why should you test? First of all, you'll never have to deal with failure, being wrong, being disappointed, or looking bad. It may be less ego damaging to guess what will work with your market, but if you are going to put any significant time and money into marketing tools and projects, you should test them to see if you are on the right path.

When I was new to my practice, I got a referral to a woman who lived in a very small, wealthy community. After driving through the tree-lined streets past stunning mansions and manicured lawns, I decided I wanted to have more clients in this gated community. I figured that since they had their own private post office, I could make up a flyer and give it to the postmaster, and he would put it in their mailboxes. Being a bit cash-strapped at the time, I cheerily made up my own hand-drawn flyer with a goofy-looking cartoon character giving a massage as a way to announce my services. Needless to say, I got no clients from that marketing endeavor. However, I learned a few lessons, including that my "look" needed to be more in line with what other ads for their upscale market looked like.

Another lesson from this uncovers a basic rule of marketing and life: successful people fail much of the time; the difference between them and everyone else is that they just get back up and keep on trying. In that instance, I failed to get clients, but I learned a lot that helped in the future, so it wasn't wasted effort. Be careful how you define failure, even with marketing projects that get a small response. If a flyer or coupon only gets one or two new clients, the response could be viewed as a failure. However, as I found in my research, one or two key clients can become the foundation of a practice that goes on to long-term success.

Have no ego attached to your marketing, and don't presume to know what will draw in clients, keep them coming back, or make them leave. Our industry is so new that we don't have the luxury to look back on successful marketing campaigns or myriad books of examples and data the way other professions can. We still don't even have national consensus on what to call ourselves as a profession, so we have a long way to go in fully understanding how to market this field.

Even with my college degree in public relations and advertising, and with all the studies I have done, none of what I talk about here is "the truth" about marketing. The best you and I can do is to talk to people, do our research, make educated guesses about why people buy massage, and use that knowledge to appeal to them through some form of marketing. Why people buy massage in Florida may be very different from why they buy it in California or France. With that in mind, the only way you can really know what marketing will work for your target market in your corner of the world is to: establish a goal for your projects and tools; test them out; observe your results; notice what works and what doesn't work; make changes; and try again until you get it right. Maybe that's why a massage business is called a "practice."

Public Relations and Publicity

Reaching out to new clients can be done through one of the best forms of exposure money can't buy: public relations. Having the press, media, magazines, or television tell your story or talk about your massage work is priceless coverage. Stories about you and your work simultaneously give you the three fundamentals of marketing: creating trust, establishing value, and shaping perception. A half-page newspaper story on the massages you did at a local fundraiser or soup kitchen can tell thousands of people you're legitimate, you're available, you're good enough to make the papers, and you're working at a specific location.

While your direct marketing is done for the purpose of booking an appointment, the primary purpose of public relations is to gain credibility or credentials, and create a reputation, name recognition, and legitimization. Good public relations can direct people toward you and toward the final action of booking clients, but you won't always be able to control what a journalist says or whether your contact information will be included in the story.

Even if a story does not lead directly to sales, you still can make good use of it by using reprints of the piece for sales letters, ads, newsletters, handouts, to hang on your office wall, or to put on your Web site. Since most everyone likes to have a brush with celebrity, no matter how local, send copies of the story to your current clients to validate their own choice of you as their massage therapist. If you want new clients, you can include, along with the copy of the article, a special deal that for every two or three referrals your clients bring in during the next month, you'll give your current client an extra half hour, a free massage, a bouquet of roses, a nice dinner out at your marketing partner's restaurant, or whatever else you can offer to take advantage of your public relations story.

What Media Reach Your Target Market

Even in an area as broad as publicity, you still can aim directly at your target market. If you have a fairly good idea of who your target market is, you can start to research or even just guess which newspapers, magazines, or newsletters your clients read; what radio stations they listen to; or what television stations or shows they watch. When you have identified those media, narrow down your target further by aiming at the sections of those newspapers, magazines or stations that would be interested in your story. Massage is not hard, front-page, or breaking news, but it can go into the lifestyle section, business section, sports page, or anywhere you can slant a story.

The Purpose of Articles

When I started writing magazine articles, I had a meeting early on with one of my publishers who told me a secret that changed my writing style forever. He was kind of a brusque and short-tempered guy, but he knew what he was talking about, so I listened. "Do you know what the purpose of your articles is?" he asked me, fixing me with a hard stare. "Um, to inform the readers?" I guessed, trying to sound logical. "No," he said, "that's not the reason we publish your stories. The only reason we run good stories is to keep the reader on the page long enough to see the advertisements around your article. Your job is to make sure people see the advertisements."

When you approach any form of media for publicity, you will be light years ahead of others if you know up front that the main reason you will get a feature story or air time is because you have a story that will keep the audience's attention long enough to see the ads. The reason a publication will print a story about you, or a television station will send out a crew, is because you have a story that is novel, unusual, interesting, informative, or entertaining. The media do not publish stories for your sake or income: they do it to sell toothpaste. You can resent this idea or you can use it. You can shun publicity or you can learn to think like a news producer facing a boring lineup of stories that needs a kick to grab the audience's attention. Massage is still a very novel topic, and a clever marketer, which you are becoming, can get tons of free publicity by coming up with great story angles to promote to the media.

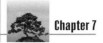

What Makes a Good Story

To get free publicity, determine what makes your work interesting, different, unique, or remarkable. Do you have a touching story about working with elderly shut-ins? Have you done chair massage at a disaster site? Are you doing on-site work at a business that is in the news, or working on volunteers at a local political campaign? Are you giving massage to the local high school or college sports team? Have you donated free massage as a raffle prize for a prominent local charity? Have you invented a new massage product or style, written a book, or done a research project on the benefits of massage on lowering blood pressure? Do you use a hot, new item, offer spa treatments, or work with crystal gemstones? Did one of your clients drop 10 strokes off his golf game or hit a hole-in-one the day after your massage? Ask if you can tell the story and then share the glory!

Local Community Angles

Editors in local newspapers and magazines love to get new and uncustomary stories, and since many people are curious about massage, you could be the perfect antidote for a boring news day. One of your easiest ways to get through the door is with a local community angle. Did you get the first massage license in your city? Do you have a photo of yourself doing an on-site massage on that city's chief of police? Have you hit an anniversary of serving your community, whether massage related or not? Are you and a marketing partner doing a marathon massage giveaway where every customer who comes in gets a free chair massage, and every customer who buys your partner's product results in a $100 donation toward building a local library, school, animal shelter, or firehouse? If you read your local paper and see what local issues you can do a promotion in conjunction with, you can land yourself stories that will make you and the editors mighty happy.

Industry Spokesperson Angle

One way to get a steady flow of publicity is to consider declaring yourself an industry spokesperson. Craft a story about the history of massage in your town, or become a futurist and create a piece on the role of massage and holistic health in the future. Follow news stories and debates on hot topics, and offer slants from your industry's perspective. Will health coverage include massage? How many doctors now offer massage as one of their services? Does massage help diabetes or asthma, or relieve the pain of arthritis in the aging population? If you offer enough story ideas, even if they aren't all used, after a while the paper will start calling on you as the local expert when massage shows up in a story that is making news.

Trend Angles

Newspapers like scoops and trends, and they can turn around a story idea a lot faster than magazines, which sometimes have lead times of six months or more. Angles on consumer-related stories are often of interest, so use them. Have you helped a client that an HMO turned away? Do you work with women with breast cancer undergoing chemotherapy, and is breast cancer a growing concern in your area? Do you help stressed-out employees who have been downsized from a large local company? Are your neighborhood soccer moms' kids getting knee injuries and concussions? Do you cater to an ethnic minority new to your community? Or are you facing discrimination in getting a business license because you do massage? Go to the paper, tell your story, and get help and community support.

Keep Your Eyes Open and Let Others Do the Writing

If you are not a great writer, that's okay. Publicity stories are usually written by journalists and professional writers—not by you—so don't let writing stop you. You just have to keep your eyes and mind open, and figure out how you can slant your massage practice to almost any topic for a good story. Fortunately, massage is so versatile and multifaceted that your story options are myriad. Submit story ideas, and don't let "no" stop you. If one story doesn't capture the imagination of the editor, send in a different story with another angle. Even if you never get a story published or told, you will have learned to think like a marketer, and that can be invaluable.

The Elements of Writing a Press Release

If you have a hot or newsworthy item, call an editor in charge of the department in which you think your story would fit. Or, if it's not a rush, write him or her a press release and mail or e-mail it in. Most media have submission standards listed on their Web sites, so check to see if there are specific ways they want you to write or submit your story. Whether you want to be interviewed on a local radio show, have a television news crew do a shoot, or have a writer come out and talk with you, you should send out a professional press release. A press release is easy to write and not intimidating if you follow these simple, logical steps.

1. Write in a simple, uncomplicated style. Make your story idea clear and easy to understand.

2. Double-space your lines, and use a large, easy-to-read font. If your page looks too crowded or hard to read, an editor will toss it.

3. Make no mistakes. If you don't write or spell well, get help. A friend may help you or you can go down to the local college and put up a notice for a writer, journalist, English major, or the like to help you out.

4. Make your press release look good. Print it on good paper with a good printer. If you don't have a good printer, take your disc or USB drive to a photocopying store, or a friend or marketing partner's office, and print it there.

5. Use white paper with black ink. The editor may want to send your release to some other department that can follow up on your story or make copies for a committee that reviews story ideas. Colored paper looks gray and murky when photocopied, so stay with white.

6. List a contact name and telephone number where your editor or assigned writer can call you. Answer your telephone professionally, using your name, and have a message machine with a professional outgoing message.

7. Put a dateline at the top of the page with the date you mailed your press release and the city from which you mailed it. Sometimes a story idea may sit around for a while, and if an editor comes across one without a date, he or she won't know if it's two years old or brand new, and into the trash it goes.

8. Even if you don't have formal stationery, use a professional letterhead format that includes your name and address, and type the word "NEWS" at the top of the page.

9. Start with your most important information. Grab the editor's attention quickly by using some of your tactics from your other marketing tools. Leave less relevant information for the end of the release.

10. At the bottom of each page, put in a page number. If there are more pages to follow, type in the word "More" beside the number so that the receiver knows all the pages have made it, especially if the press release is faxed. At the end of the last page, type in ### to indicate it is the end of the piece.

11. Don't overhype your story. Give real information: who, what, when, where, and why. Don't use a lot of adjectives such as "great," "the best," "superlative" service, and the like. Provide facts the editor can use, especially if he or she has to convince other people to run your story.

12. Write a short, simple, respectful note to go with your release. It can say something like, "Dear X: I thought you might be interested in the enclosed. Sincerely, (your name)."

13. Send your press release.

14. Wait a few days, then follow up with a one-minute telephone call to the editor. You only need to say who you are and that you are confirming that he received your release. If you sent your release via e-mail, send a brief e-mail to request confirmation.

15. If the paper, magazine, or station runs your story, send a thank-you note. Most people don't, and being an editor can feel like a pretty thankless job. Continue your standard of going the extra mile and giving outstanding service, even with news editors.

Press Releases for Television Coverage

If you want television coverage, entice the targeted show's producer with visual elements and images he or she can show the viewers. If possible, send photos with your release that give the producer an idea of what the cameras would see. Can you get a camera crew into the locker room of the local sports arena for a demonstration on one of your professional athlete clients, or do you work with your county's only isolation tank? Do you have an unusual setting such as an outside garden, work for the circus, or have a client whom you've helped recover from an accident that dominated the headlines a year ago? Are you doing on-site massage at your client's office as a Christmas gift to the employees? The media always need new holiday stories, so give them a great piece that they can do with you in advance. Television shows and newspapers are now including more soft pieces with feel-good stories, so you might as well be in one.

If you plan to use publicity to promote your practice, there are a few factors to keep in mind. One, since we still have to consider the privacy of clients and those we touch, only do stories with people who are willing to be seen on camera. Two, you may need to educate your producer about the issue of legitimacy. There is still some titillation to the word "massage," so be clear with the news producer that you don't want any double entendres or sexual overtones. And three, we still need to promote massage as a profession. Publicity may or may not bring you clients directly the way other marketing methods do, but remember that every time you make the news or reach the public with regard to the many great benefits of massage, you continue to shift thousands of people up the Perception Continuum. Many of us are able to practice today because of the work other therapists have done to pave the way for the growing acceptance we now enjoy, so keep in mind that publicity represents and benefits not only you but also the rest of the profession.

Sources for Press Releases

The best place to go to get your story told is to publications you know and read, or to radio and television stations you listen to or watch. Pay attention to the types of stories they run, and the tone or attitude of the writer or producer, and custom tailor your story for that individual. I got my very first magazine article accepted, sight unseen, in a two-minute conversation with the publisher because I had studied his magazines for many months until I found a story angle I knew he couldn't resist. That one story led to a column and many more articles, and it started because I understood what the publisher wanted. Find columnists, writers, or television shows you like, create a good story that matches their style, and then make your pitch.

If you want media coverage but don't know where or to whom to send your press release, go to your local library and look up the *Bacon's Publicity Checker* book. This tells you where to send releases for all categories of story takers. It includes information on newspapers, editors, columnists, wire services, magazines, and trade publications. You also can look in the book entitled *Working Press of the Nation* for other sources. Staff changes at newspapers and magazines can happen without notice, so make one final call to the front desk beforehand to make sure you have the correct information, name, spelling, and address for where to send your press release. Don't be afraid to try this great form of marketing. Publishers always need good stories, so introduce yourself, pitch an angle, and see what develops.

Public Speaking

According to statistics, public speaking is the number one fear Americans face. More people are afraid of speaking than they are of dying. If you don't like public speaking, then don't use it as a means of marketing. You'd be better served doing a promotional project at a local fundraiser or the local fire station where you can let your hands do the talking. However, if you have good presentation skills and enjoy the spotlight or the stage, consider using public speaking as a form of marketing. The mere act of standing up in front of others helps to build trust and shape positive perception, regardless of your message. (See Figure 7–12.)

You can approach speaking in a number of ways. If you have a topic you love talking about, then craft a speech and promote that topic. If you want to speak but aren't sure what to talk about, call the groups you want to speak for, tell them who you are and what you do, and tell them you would be interested in speaking during one of their regular meetings. Since you want to tailor your talk to the specific needs of the group, you need to know what the group would like to know about massage, and if they have an interest in holistic

Figure 7–12 | **Public speaking can introduce you to potential clients quickly and easily.**

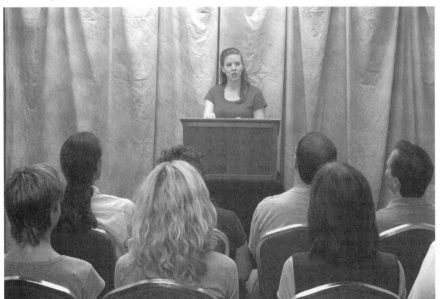

health, alternative or complementary medicine, stress education, meditation, or another topic you can address. The contact person you speak with may not have a good topic idea at the moment, so be prepared with a generic backup one, such as how massage can benefit this tennis club, philanthropy group, service group, or whatever.

Friends, family, and even clients who belong to groups such as the Soroptimists, Lions Club, and Rotary Club can get you in the door and help you design your speech for the group. Even if you don't know anyone in a group to approach, realize that if the group holds regular meetings that need a speaker, the person in charge of getting speakers is often desperate to find somebody for the next meeting.

The art of writing and delivering a speech is too broad for this book, but if you want to be a speaker, give seminars, or teach, think about:

- ✳ Who you are and what you enjoy talking about
- ✳ What your audience wants to know to improve their lives and/or entertain them
- ✳ What purpose you have in giving a speech
- ✳ How to get new clients from the group without your speech sounding like a sales pitch

Be forewarned: public speaking can be addictive. It is fun, engaging, and challenging. If you find yourself enjoying telling people about yourself and your work from the stage, public speaking can be your ticket to a full practice, and maybe even a career path toward teaching and seminars.

Ethernet

Finally, in addition to all the marvelous marketing tools for reaching clients we have covered so far, this one is my favorite. I call it the "Ethernet" because this form of marketing is about getting your communications and messages to your current and future clients through the invisible, mysterious ether. Ethernet marketing has no form or substance, no concrete tools.

Basically, your message is carried only by the power of your intention. The research on the effect of intention, belief, focus of thought, and more has shown again and again that thought changes things. Wayne Dyer, a cutting-edge thinker, wrote a book called *The Power of Intention*, which I highly recommend if you want to develop this level of application to building your practice. Even the research on quantum physics has demonstrated that our connections to others through thought are beyond our understanding, so perhaps this section should be called "Quantum Marketing." On a smaller scale, I have experimented with the power of intention for a very long time, and I am amazed by its force. If I need time off but am totally booked, clients magically call to cancel. If I need extra clients for my car registration fee, I just put the request out there in the Ethernet and the telephone starts ringing with people I have never heard of calling for an appointment. The more I use the Ethernet, the more I learn to trust it.

Sow Your Seeds

There are two points I want to make about using the Ethernet. One is that you must have done your homework and laid your groundwork for it to succeed. When I send out my intentions or requests and people call in, they say things like they got my card from a friend, saw me in a class, or met me at an event. I have been sowing the seeds of success for a long time and only after that do I get to reap the harvest.

Have Clear Intentions

The second element of tapping into the Ethernet is to have very clear and specific intentions about what you want. Simply saying you want to have a lot of clients doesn't work. Saying that you want to have 15 clients a week programs the Ethernet to go out and get you what you want. If you have ever done a search on the Internet, you know that the more specific you are, the more quickly and easily you can find what you are looking for. Type in the word "book" as a search word and the system isn't very helpful. Type in the book's title, though, and what you need shows up almost instantly. As we close this section on how to reach your new clients, remind yourself again of who you are, what you want, and why you want to serve people.

The Ethernet works in ways I do not understand fully, but I do know that you can jam the power of the Ethernet by sending out mixed messages or unclear intentions. The old saying, "Be careful what you ask for; you may get it," holds true on the Ethernet as well. If you are ambivalent about success or are afraid to get out there and try your hand at life, you can put out all the slick brochures and ads you want, and people won't call. Success comes when you can handle it, so the more you practice success with visualizations, affirmations, or role modeling, the more the Ethernet can connect you with the target market that wants and needs you.

CHAPTER 7   SUMMARY

Reaching a large number of people quickly can be leveraged with marketing tools. In this chapter we went over how to design, produce, and distribute marketing tools intended to reach a wide audience. We covered what to say in brochures, letters, and postcards, on Web sites, in press releases, and more. To make your marketing tools more visually appealing, we went over graphics, layout, logos, and photos, which are your best graphic representation. For text decisions, we distinguished between reference and action marketing tools and how they could answer people's questions about trust, value, and convenience, while getting them to understand the many benefits you offer and how and when they should take some form of action. The value of publicity and how to obtain it was reviewed, and we went through the points of a professional press release. In the end, though, of all the tools possible, your business cards and gift certificates should be your first investment. Print a lot of cards and hand out stacks to others to give away for you, and give or sell at deep discount a lot of gift certificates because, really, your best marketing is your touch. Once people feel your hands, they will rebook and refer, which is the easiest and most effective marketing of all.

CHAPTER 7   ACTION STEPS

Based on the information in this chapter, do the following to reach new clients:

- ✶ Create your business card, if you don't have one yet.
- ✶ Get a stack of gift certificates, either to sell or give away.
- ✶ Create a massage menu of the services you offer. Choose a variety of services at different price points and durations.
- ✶ Research other marketing or advertising aimed at your target market to assess what "look" you might use in your marketing tools.
- ✶ Gather elements for marketing materials such as FAQs and testimonials.

- Get a few items of clothing that say "massage" somewhere on them.
- Create projects and promotions that can get you publicity.

CHAPTER 7 KNOWLEDGE CHECK

Check your understanding of the chapter by reviewing these questions and answers.

Q: What are two factors that are important in developing marketing tools?
A: Speed of reaching people and control over who gets your marketing message.

Q: What is the primary purpose of marketing tools?
A: Leverage.

Q: What are the two categories of written marketing tools?
A: Reference marketing tools and action marketing tools.

Q: What is the primary difference between a reference and action marketing tool?
A: The action marketing tool includes a specific action to take.

Q: What is the best graphic representation you can use on printed material?
A: Your photograph.

Q: What are the three types of buyers you can design your marketing message for?
A: The people person, the scientist, and the WIIFM buyer.

Q: Is having a brochure necessary for building a practice?
A: No.

Q: What is the purpose of an action marketing tool?
A: To get a person to take action upon seeing it.

Q: What are the four basic elements of an action marketing piece?
A: Headline, body copy, call to action, and closing.

Q: Should press releases be sent in to publications or other media professionals on brightly colored paper?
A: No (they don't photocopy well).

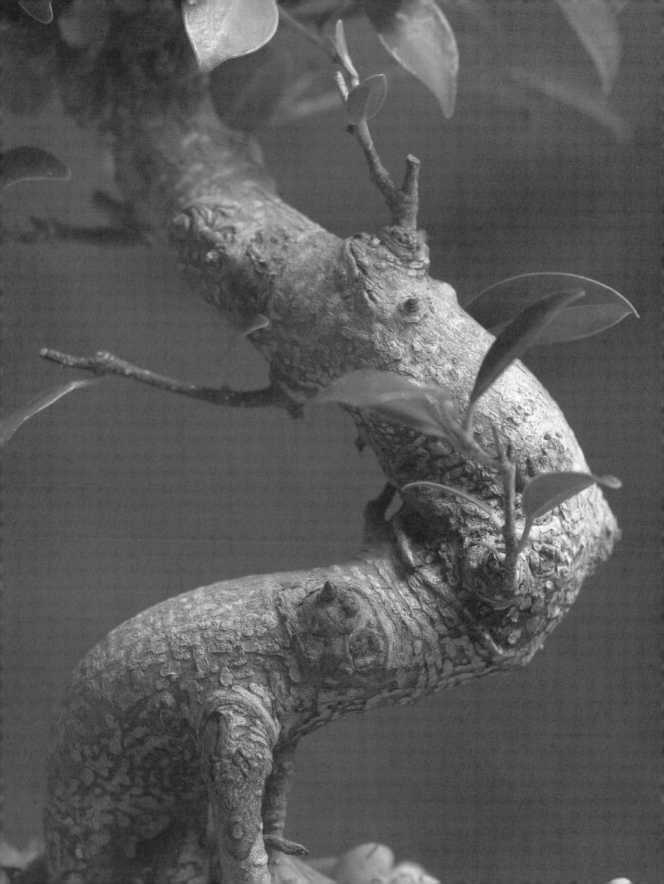

8 Rebooking Skills and Tools

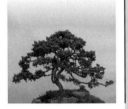

CHAPTER OBJECTIVES

After reading this chapter, you should be able to:

✻ Identify the five **moments of decision** for rebooking clients.

✻ Describe four factors of personal presentation that can affect rebooking.

✻ Deliver pre-massage instructions to a new client.

✻ Discuss the importance of managing boundaries.

✻ Describe four elements to ask about during verbal check-ins.

✻ Explain the importance of handling a drape properly.

✻ Describe seven moments of transition during massage.

✻ Explain the six levels of client participation during massage.

✻ Describe how to handle the separation stage of a session.

✻ Describe how to deal with a dissatisfied client.

✻ Explain the value of a welcome letter and suggestion lists.

✻ Create a client file.

✻ Describe how to use various marketing tools to manage or encourage a rebooking.

✻ Describe ways to stay in contact with clients on a regular basis.

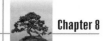

REBOOKING SKILLS TO BUILD YOUR DREAM PRACTICE

Marketing for a massage practice has two primary functions. The first is to get new clients; the second is to keep them. Successful practitioners know that the true secret to a long-term career in private practice lies in the second function of marketing, which centers around rebooking current clients. The practitioners who had to give up their dream of a long-term massage practice probably made the unfortunate but common mistake of assuming that once a client was in the door, their marketing was done. Nothing could be further from the truth. All the work that was done prior to getting a new client onto the table is only a small percentage of the true marketing that builds and maintains a satisfying and financially successful practice.

The majority of your marketing is done during your session, and the following pages will take you step by step through the key elements of what it takes to serve your clients in such a way that they not only rebook but also refer. As you may have noticed in the prior chapters, marketing to reach new clients takes time, effort, and money, and the less you need to focus on that function of marketing, the better. It is far easier to keep a client coming back than to get a new one, but it takes a conscious and concerted effort to do so.

THE FIVE MOMENTS OF DECISION FOR REBOOKING

The marketing strategies for rebooking current clients utilize the same basic principles as those we have covered for reaching new clients. In both cases, your marketing is designed to continually shape your clients' perceptions about you and massage, instill value that your massage is worth their time and money, and prove that you are trustworthy to touch them.

Once a person has booked an appointment, a number of instances occur that provide you with key opportunities to market. These instances are what I call the "Five Moments of Decision." They are the times during your whole encounter with new clients when they are most likely to evaluate you and your work, and when they make conscious and subconscious decisions about whether or not to rebook. While every minute with your client is important, you need to be especially mindful of what to do and say during:

❋ Moment 1: Before your new client arrives

❋ Moment 2: The moment of arrival

✳ Moment 3: During the massage

✳ Moment 4: At the end of the massage

✳ Moment 5: After the client has gone

Rebooking Moment 1: Before Your New Client Arrives

Getting new clients in the door is the first step to rebooking them. This may sound obvious, but having a booked appointment is no guarantee that your new clients will show up. This is especially true if they have received gift certificates for a massage but have doubts or fears about getting one. Your new clients may have made an initial decision to book an appointment with you, but sometimes it may take a little extra effort to get them in the door.

Marketing before a new client arrives centers around building trust, and setting accurate and appropriate expectations for the massage. If you have enough lead time before your new client arrives for his or her first session, there are many ways you can demonstrate your professionalism and let the client feel good or safe about the decision to get a massage from you. If you sense hesitation during your initial conversation, it is your job to figure out what their concerns are and dispel them. Your new clients may be afraid of nudity or touch, have had a prior bad massage experience, have body issues such as scars or deformities, feel fat, feel intimidated, or worry about a host of other concerns you never may have considered. Creating trust at this moment should be your first priority.

To help ensure that your clients show up for their appointments, you can:

✳ Send a welcoming note with a confirmation card and a map to your office

✳ Telephone the day before with a confirmation call, and ask if they have any questions

✳ Send your intake form and **policy form** to demonstrate your professionalism, and let them accurately and totally fill in the forms without rushing or feeling like they are wasting massage time filling in paperwork

✳ Send a suggestion list for how to prepare for their first massage, including an explanation of what to expect, how to make the most of their massage, and so on

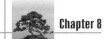

- Send your brochure, a copy of a newsletter (if you have one), copies of articles about the benefits of massage, or whatever you can think of to help build value and trust
- Send a coupon for a free gift with your confirmation card, especially those mentioned in earlier chapters

There are other ways to stay in touch before the first appointment but, in short, make your new clients glad they are working with you before you ever touch them. Obviously, most people who book an appointment are willing and ready to be under your hands, but it is wise to be prepared for a little extra marketing, just in case. If all goes well, at the appointed day and time, you will get the opportunity to market again, this time for the second moment of decision, the moment of arrival.

Rebooking Moment 2: The Moment of Arrival

The second moment of decision in rebooking occurs when your new clients show up for the first session. Impressions made at this point are especially important in establishing trust. If your new clients have never met you before and have only talked with you on the telephone, they already have some impression of you. The first time they see you, they will quickly reevaluate their first impression and start to solidify their second impression. You have about one minute to make the second, more lasting impression, and your job is to make it a good one. To rebook these clients, it is important for you to shape their future decisions now, because once a person's mind is made up about you, other data that may be contrary to the initial impression may not be considered or even noticed.

Two of the most important factors you will be judged on are your personal presentation and your environment, if a client is coming to see you at your home or office. In the section discussing professionalism, we talked about what you can wear and how you can present yourself in order to make your new clients feel comfortable and at ease. We covered what people see visually when they meet you, and in this chapter, we will go a step further and review how people use their other senses to evaluate you and your space.

What Your Clients Hear in Your Personal Presentation

Sight is probably the primary sense your clients will use to judge you upon their arrival. After that, what they hear, smell, and feel will make an impact with varying degrees depending upon which senses are more attuned and sensitive. With regard to sound, we are first evaluated on our voice and our words. Volume, pitch, rate of speed, accent, speech patterns, grammar, choice of words, and other elements of verbal communication are all part of what your new clients hear when they first meet you. However, unlike our physical appearance, judgments that affect trust and value aren't as rapid or as strong, but there are still some points to consider in verbal communication.

At the moment of arrival, how you greet and talk with your new clients can either set them on edge or relax them in preparation for the session. The basic rules are to speak professionally and clearly, refrain from foul language or slang, don't use bodywork jargon or acronyms, and use your voice to show you are happy they are there.

Above all, your job at this moment of arrival is to make your clients feel safe and welcome. Perhaps one of the best ways to do that in your opening minutes together is to let your clients hear the sound of their own voices, not yours. Nervous chatter, trying to tell your life story in the first few minutes, or needing to demonstrate your massage prowess by telling them how great you are just don't set a good precedent or create the right atmosphere.

When you do all the talking, it tells your clients that the upcoming session will be about you, not about them. People take the time and pay the money for massage so that someone will take care of them for at least one hour out of their lives, so ease their minds immediately and let them know that they are the focus of attention. Of all the complaints I have heard from clients about their massage experience, having massage therapists who talk the whole time about themselves and their lives tops the list. To be head and shoulders above your massage competition, let your hands do the talking, not your mouth. Clients who want to rest and relax will appreciate this immeasurably, and if they are happy, they are more likely to rebook and refer others to you.

What Your Clients Smell in Your Personal Presentation

As a teacher, I was surprised again and again at how unaware students could be of the importance of smell. While it would seem common sense that a professional show up for work clean and bathed, with brushed teeth, and basically smelling fresh, not everyone did so. This wouldn't be crucial if our work required us to sit alone in front of a computer, but a massage therapist is often mere inches from a client's nose. As a touch professional, you are expected by your clients to show up clean and neat, and while this was covered before in the professionalism section, it bears repeating here.

Along similar lines, wash your hands before each massage. As a teacher, even though I stressed hygiene in class, I sent more than a few students back to wash their hands when I happened to be outside the school's bathroom door, heard the toilet flush, and then saw the student immediately emerge without my hearing the water running in the sink. Ick! Beyond the obvious issues of cleanliness and hygiene, this is a marketing book, and if your clients are within earshot of your bathroom and/or sink, they may be listening to hear if you are scrubbing up well. Clients have every sense attuned to whether or not they will be safe with you, so it is tantamount that they know they can rely on your hands being clean. If your clients somehow figure out that you start your massage without washing your hands, especially after you've been to the restroom, I can guarantee they won't rebook. Would you?

Another sense of smell clients encounter when they first meet you is your breath. As best you can, keep your breath smelling fresh. If you can't, don't breathe heavily on your clients. I had the unfortunate experience of receiving a massage from a person who seemed to have a great fondness for garlic. While this may not have been so bad, she insisted on taking deep cleansing breaths and blowing her garlic breath all over my face, especially during her opening grounding at my head. Did she do good work, help my sore muscles, or ease my pain? I have no idea. All I remember is that garlic breath, and I vowed I would never go back.

If you have an office or work at home, keep mouthwash, a toothbrush, and toothpaste handy. If you do outcall and can't brush, sugar-free gum or breath mints are the next best things. Americans have been trained by advertisers to believe it is natural to smell "minty fresh," so if you want Americans as your paying clients, know that this is important to them.

Perfumes, colognes, strong aromatherapy oils, pet odors, cigarette smoke, and other such smells are a final factor to consider from your clients' perspective. Given how close you are to your client's nose, much care needs to be taken around scents, and it is best that you have a scent-free body. That way, you don't have to deal with people's allergies, scent sensitivities, and preferences. If you really like certain scents, you can have them in the form of incense, room sprays, or in your massage oils, and you can use them if your client is okay with it. Headaches, migraines, and allergic reactions are not uncommon with perfumes and synthetic air fresheners, so leave them out of your practice. Your goal is have clients come back, and since individual smelling preferences vary so much, keep yourself neutral and everyone else happy.

What Your Clients Feel Externally About Your Personal Presentation

The sense of touch and the primary kinesthetic sensations your clients will experience at the moment of arrival will occur during your greeting, and there are definitely a few factors to consider. The first factor is how you touch new clients when greeting them. In the beginning, a professional handshake is recommended. People evaluate others based on their handshakes, so be prepared. Have clean, oil-free hands, and when you take your client's hand to shake it, hold it firmly but not too hard. You can demonstrate your amazing hand strength later when you dig that big muscle spasm out of the levator scapula, but don't give it your all in a handshake. The best way to apply pressure is by pressing your thumb into the hand, not squeezing with your fingers from the bottom. A firm grasp with solid pressure tells your new clients that you have confidence, whereas the proverbial "dead fish" handshake can make some people's hair stand on end. Somewhere between the dead fish and the vise grip is a nice, welcoming handshake that can quickly help build trust and rapport.

A handshake should be the extent of your physical greeting for new clients. Even if you enjoy giving hugs, this may not be right for a new client. Not everyone is comfortable with hugs, and people who are standoffish may be very uncomfortable receiving a hug from you. Despite the natural inclination to do so, hugs are not something to do without permission. Maybe after you've seen a client for a while, a hug would be an appropriate and wonderful gesture, but for the first-timers, keep your touch to a handshake at the outset or respond in kind if they go to hug you first.

EXERCISE: SHAKING HANDS

If you are in a class or group, practice shaking hands with everyone. Experiment with different handshakes and how it feels to give and get them. Discuss with your group what you felt and noticed. If you are reading this book on your own, try to shake hands with as many people as you can in your

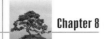

daily life and notice what you feel. Pay attention to how people respond to you and how you respond to them because of their handshakes.

What Your Clients Feel Internally About Your Personal Presentation

Finally, your personal presentation culminates in how your clients feel emotionally, or internally, about you. All of your hard work preparing for that first moment together should shape your clients' internal feelings that they made the right choice coming to see you. If you have thought ahead about what will make your new clients feel comfortable, at ease, and safe with you, you will have done extraordinary marketing. If you can see yourself from your new clients' eyes, hear yourself with their ears, and otherwise imagine what it might be like for someone to come to a massage therapist for the first time, you will have compassion and insight into their hopes and fears about who you will be. Presenting yourself as a professional, and radiating a loving, caring attitude during your very first moments together, will set the stage for the rest of your first session and, hopefully, for many more to come.

Gaining Rapport

Beyond presenting yourself with confidence and competence, there is a more interesting but complex way of presenting yourself so your clients feel safe and sure about working with you. It is a concept I first learned in a seminar on Ericksonian Hypnosis, which I then added to with material from the book *Unlimited Power* by Anthony Robbins. The concept is called **matching and mirroring,** combined with pacing and leading. The gist is that if you want someone to really feel at ease with you, you should match or imitate their posture, movements, gestures, words, and the like. The more you act like someone, the more he or she will like you. It is a natural instinct to be drawn to people to whom we are similar, and if you want to gain incredible rapport and trust with your clients, make a few subtle changes in your self-presentation so that they feel you are similar to them. Matching and mirroring creates a sense of familiarity and connection because most people think they are pretty wonderful, and, if you are like them, you're wonderful too.

This doesn't mean you should give up your personality or mimic people. It means you should pay attention to them, notice how they stand, move, talk, laugh, dress, maintain eye contact, and so on, and then just be a bit more like them. When you greet your new clients, shake their hands with close to the same amount of pressure they exert, move at the speed they are walking, and talk at about the speed they are talking. If this concept makes you uncomfortable, you don't have to use it, but if you actually pay attention to how you are with your friends and family, you will see that you probably already match and mirror others. It is a natural human behavior, and if you learn to use it consciously, you can quickly help your clients feel at ease.

The concept of pacing and leading is a little different. Its premise is that humans can lead each other more easily if they are already in step with one another. If you have taken a walk with a friend, you probably ended up walking with the same basic speed and direction, and maybe even ended up in step with each other. If one of you veered a little in one direction, the other person most likely followed that subtle change.

This is important when you are encountering your new clients for the first time, and you want to lead them to a relaxed and peaceful state. If you have a client who sat in traffic for an hour while driving to your office, and he is now agitated, waving his arms while he talks, speaking rapidly, and breathing quickly, be prepared to change. If he encounters you all mellow and relaxed from the massage you just gave, there will be a subtle form of friction between you. If your behaviors and states are too different, it will be much harder for you to lead him to a relaxed state. In this case, your job is to pick up your pace a little, speak at about the same speed, move your hands (not quite so fast or wide), and otherwise copy or pace him. Once you are in sync with him, you can start leading him into a more relaxed state using small changes. Slowly soften your voice, deepen your breathing, and reduce the size of your movements. If you are in sync, he is likely to follow your lead. Again, we do pacing and leading all the time as well, but having conscious knowledge of it allows it to be a powerful tool. It helps reduce friction and mistrust between people, and creates a great beginning connection during the second moment of decision.

EXERCISE: PACING AND LEADING BEFORE A SESSION

Pair off into groups of two and choose a Partner A and Partner B.

Partner A acts as the client, coming in from a hard day of work, talking loudly, waving arms, and complaining about the traffic and a stiff neck.

Partner B acts as the therapist. Partner B welcomes Partner A with a greeting of similar volume and expression. The two talk animatedly about Partner A's day and about the upcoming massage. Slowly, over the course of a few minutes, Partner B starts to lower the volume, speak more slowly, make smaller movements, and otherwise gradually guide the client into a state more conducive to massage.

The partners then switch roles and repeat the exercise.

Your Massage Space and Surroundings

Rebooking clients also requires that they feel safe and comfortable, not just with you, but in your massage space. It doesn't have to be fancy, but it must feel safe. If you have an office at home, or in another establishment or building, shape your clients' perceptions and gain trust by being impeccable in your cleanliness, order, and ambiance. (See Figure 8–1.) You want to portray your professionalism in your surroundings, and part of that is done by removing

Figure 8–1 | Prepare your massage setting to be comfortable, clean, and restful.

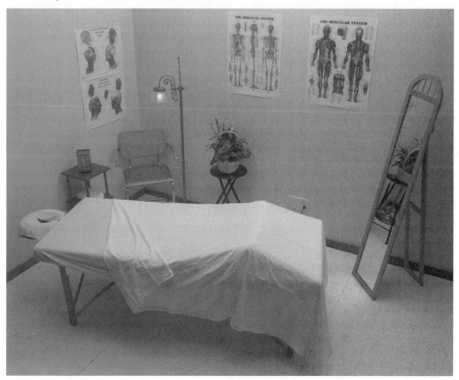

anything that might create a sense of incongruence with your image as a professional. Your new clients are taking in every detail of your environment to determine if it is going to be safe for you to touch them. One detail overlooked by you could create a distrust that you will have to overcome, if you can.

Are your sheets threadbare or frayed? Are there mascara stains on the face-rest cover? Does the table squeak? Is your laundry basket overflowing? Is there cat hair all over your pants? Do you have a dirty coffee cup on the counter? Is the bathroom dirty, out of toilet paper, or have a burned-out light? I've seen this and heard about worse; otherwise, I wouldn't mention it. You need to know that your new clients will transfer everything about the hygiene and cleanliness in your environment to your work whether you deserve it or not, so be meticulous.

You could have done all that work to cross-sell to another business in order to get new clients, but because there was a hair on the pillow or your blanket smelled stale, those new clients won't be back. If you're lucky, they won't tell the person who referred them and damage other potential clients from that source. Unfortunately, you won't know to whom hygiene matters until they leave and never come back. Or, even if they do return, they may not refer others because, even if your setting is tolerable to them, they know their friends with allergies won't enjoy having your pet dog in the room or whatever it is that borders on questionable. Again, think from your clients' point of view. Imagine what it is like to come into your environment, and ask yourself if they will feel like it's an environment they can enjoy, come back to, and send their friends to experience as well.

Today your environment will be compared to increasingly glamorous and sophisticated day spas and resort destination spas that put a premium on posh surroundings and luxury amenities. While you don't have to compete at that level with a home office or outcall business, or even a regular therapy office, take the opportunity to go to local day spas or tour destination spas to see what clients are experiencing and to what they will be comparing your environment.

Marketing at the Intake

The initial face-to-face contact with new clients will be a critical time in your marketing strategy. If a person is a referral, create a common bond by mentioning the person who gave the referral, saying you will be sure to send a thank-you card. This strengthens your association to the referrer, enhancing

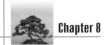

trust, and telling your new client you know you are accountable to someone else for your behavior. In the other direction, it also makes the client accountable to that person. Since you will be in contact with the referrer, the new client is more likely to be on good behavior.

Your Verbal Intake

Before your clients get on the table, you need to do a **verbal intake**. If you had a chance to send them your **written intake** form before they arrived for the session, this can save you time and give them the opportunity to have thought carefully about what it is they want from you. If they have not yet filled out a written intake form, have them fill it out before you begin your verbal intake. You also can fill it out for them as you talk, so you get a complete history.

The purpose of your verbal intake is to establish a match between what your clients want and what you offer. If you do this as an initial free consultation, it will give you something else to give away. Also, it gets the client to talk freely without rushing the conversation, since they won't be worrying that the talking is taking time away from the paid massage. The verbal intake makes sure it is safe for you to work on each person and lets you gather more information about what your clients want.

Above all, the verbal intake is a time for you to help each client feel special, understood, and known. You are establishing a relationship with each person, and your intake time gives you the opportunity to see each as an individual, and to introduce yourself as a person as well as a practitioner. If they are coming to you because of some kind of physical pain their doctors could not help them with, this is important to know. Many people have had doctors' appointments where they felt that no one listened or cared enough to really help. They were treated as symptoms, not as people. Unfortunately, because of limitations that insurance companies place on medical professionals, doctors and other caregivers have limited time to develop rapport, offer comfort, or get to know a patient well. Fortunately, when you work for yourself in your own private practice, you can take the time to listen and demonstrate that the person, as well as the client, is important to you.

The Written Intake

Before you start your session, you need to take notes during the time your client is talking to you. If you are filling out intake forms for insurance purposes or because you are working on a doctor's referral, follow their

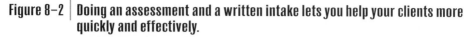

Figure 8–2 | Doing an assessment and a written intake lets you help your clients more quickly and effectively.

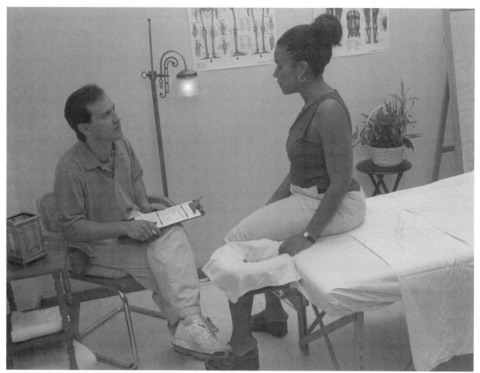

protocols. Your written notes can guide you and remind you about your clients' complaints and problem areas, and assist you if you are making notes for a lawyer when working on an accident case. Notes also give you a place to document improvements, detail which techniques you have tried, and otherwise let you work in a professional manner. (See Figure 8–2.)

While all of these are important reasons to take notes, this is a marketing book. When you take notes, you demonstrate that you are paying attention to this individual's needs and you are behaving in a manner that matches his or her perception of what a professional should do. When you fulfill people's expectations, they are going to rebook and refer.

Give Your Clients What They Want

As we discussed earlier in the section on setting client expectations, you can find out what your clients want and expect by asking them. You can use a marketing questionnaire to ask about their goals for the session, and what they want you to focus on or accomplish. (See Figure 8–3.) Ask if there is anything that they liked in previous massages, or that they don't want you to do. If they want to just relax and forget their day, don't spend 10 minutes trying to dig that knot out of a calf muscle. That's not why they are there. If they tell you their lower back is bothersome, address the area immediately so they feel heard. In other words, listen closely to what your clients want and GIVE IT TO THEM.

Educate Your Clients

Much of marketing is really educating, and as you listen to what your clients want, educate them in what you do and what you offer based on what they need. Your education also can reveal if they have misconceptions, unrealistic expectations, or false notions about what you do or how they think you should work. For example, if a big guy has a sore lower back and wants you to spend a whole hour using brute force to dig into the few muscles that hurt, you will disappoint him unless you educate him about a better strategy for working out lower back pain. Tell him you would hurt him by working too deeply, too quickly, and for too long in such a small area. Teach him how the body works holistically, and explain that the problem may be starting from somewhere else, such as an injured ankle or tight hamstrings that are making him compensate with his quadratus lumborum or psoas. Point to a muscle chart and talk about his body in intelligent, clear terms, and you will be doing some of the best marketing you can ever imagine.

Why You Do What You Do

Explaining to your client what you are doing, and why, is marketing gold. If you went to a school with a short program and didn't get much anatomy training, or it has been years since you've been in an anatomy class, take the time and effort to become facile and conversant in anatomy. As I used to tell my students when I taught our 100-hour anatomy program, the American culture associates anatomical knowledge with medical professionals. If you can speak the language of anatomy, your listener often will give you the credibility and esteem usually reserved for doctors. This is not so you can diagnose, treat, or prescribe. You should know the body well enough to educate your clients about the anatomical principles behind your strategies and applications, and to name the muscles on which you are working. Educate

Figure 8–3 | In addition to a regular intake form, consider filling out a marketing questionnaire for each client. They can fill out the form themselves, or you can do so while asking each question.

MARKETING QUESTIONNAIRE FOR NEW CLIENTS

Date: _____

Name: _____

Address: _____

City/State/Zip: _____

Home Telephone/Work Telephone: _____

Birthday/Age/Sex/Marital Status: _____

Education: _____

Occupation: _____

How did you learn about me?_____

_____

_____

Have you had a professional massage before?   _____Yes _____No

If yes,

    How long ago?_____

    How frequently did you receive massage?_____

    How many massages have you had? _____

    What kind of massage did you receive?_____

    What kind of massage do you want now? _____

    How often would you like to receive massage?_____

    Why did you leave your last therapist?_____

If no, what made you decide to get a massage now?

_____

_____

What are your primary reasons for receiving a massage?

_____

_____

What would you like me to know so that I can best serve your massage needs?

_____

_____

The above client information is strictly confidential. It is used only by me to better understand and serve the needs of my clients.

your clients, not only so they can understand what you are doing and why—and, therefore, value your work more—but also so they have a better idea of how to help themselves. Being able to talk about what you do, and why, in clear, anatomical terms can be mighty impressive.

What You Can't Do

Occasionally, you will need to educate your clients about what you can do and what you can't do. If your new clients want massage you are not strong enough for, trained enough for, or qualified to do, tell them that what they are asking is beyond your strength, skill, or qualifications. Tell them what you can do, and offer them other options to get the same results they're looking for. If they want to go, let them leave without charging them. I have had clients who truly believe that "no pain, no gain" is the only kind of massage to get, and since that is not the kind of work that I choose to do, it is better for both of us that I let them go. As a marketer, I also do this because, ultimately, they would be unsatisfied and unhappy. And, really, who wants an unhappy client?

What You Shouldn't Do

If there is something clients don't want done, don't do it. I have heard stories where clients have explicitly told a massage therapist they don't want their feet done, their face touched, or their hairdo messed up, only to have the therapist do exactly what they were told not to do. In one particular story, a client told her therapist not to work on her feet. His response was, "Oh, I do great feet work, and I know you'll love it." Then, in spite of her protests, he proceeded to work on her feet, unleashing unpleasant memories and flashbacks. That experience was bad for her and she became very distrustful of all massage therapists because of this man's ego. She originally came to me because she had been given a gift certificate for a massage from one of my clients, and it took a great deal of promising on my part before she believed I would not work on her feet or otherwise trample on her boundaries. Ask and listen to learn about pressure preferences, how to communicate during the session, and what signals to use in case of discomfort, and learn from the start what will make your clients ecstatic that they've found you.

The Pre-Massage Conversation

The purpose of your pre-massage conversation is to instill trust, relieve fears, and set appropriate expectations. This conversation will vary depending on each client's experience with massage, but regardless of what they already know, you will want to prepare them for the experience they are about to have with you. Even if you have learned intake skills in other classes, you also need to view this process through the eyes of marketing. Tell clients who have never had a massage before about your process, from beginning to end, so they will know what to anticipate and what to do at each step. This preparation may seem obvious, but it can alleviate a great deal of anxiety and enhance the massage experience by letting them drift a bit more than they would if they did not know what to expect next.

If your clients have been to other massage therapists, their expectations will be different. They will have a preconceived notion of what you will do and how the session will go. Even if you do a good job, they might not enjoy the experience because something did not match their presumptions. On the other hand, if they had a bad experience with a previous therapist, they might be bracing themselves in case your work also won't be of good quality. Tell your new clients you give a 100-percent money-back guarantee and that you do a reevaluation partway through, which alleviates their fear of being trapped. I have heard stories of clients who endured terrible, painful, or unpleasant massages, but when I asked them why they didn't just leave, they basically said, "I didn't want to hurt the therapist's feelings. I didn't want to be rude and I kept hoping it would get better." Giving clients the option to just walk away not only alleviates a host of different fears but also demonstrates your confidence in your own work, and confidence is catching.

Getting on the Table

Once the pre-massage conversation has concluded, expectations have been spoken, and questions answered, refamiliarize your client with your massage process. To do that, say something like, "I am going to leave the room now to wash up, and while I'm gone you can go ahead and get on the table. I'd like to start you face down (or face up), and if you'd like, you can use this face-rest so that you don't have to twist your neck. Most of my clients prefer to use the face-rest, but if you don't want to, that's fine. Being comfortable is what's most important. It may take us a couple of tries until you are totally comfortable, but once we've got that figured out, you'll be set. If at some point you need to turn, scratch your nose, change a pillow position, or go to the bathroom, just let me know; my goal is to make this massage perfect for you, and I want you to be comfortable at all times. I work best if you don't leave any clothes on, and you will be covered by this top sheet the whole time, but if you want to leave anything on, that's fine. When I come back, I'll stand outside the door and call out to ask if you are ready; when you answer me, I'll come back in."

Throughout the conversation, demonstrate what you are talking about. Demonstrate putting your face in the face-rest, and lift the corner of the top sheet and point underneath. If this is a person's first massage, the image the person may have is based on what he or she has seen in magazine ads, which often show the models lying face down with their hands folded under the chin, so don't be surprised if every so often someone still ends up lying down on the top sheet. Your clients may have no idea what a face-rest is or how to use it, so explain it beforehand so you don't have to make them move too much when you come back into the room.

Also during this initial conversation, be careful not to use words that sound like commands; instead, give explanations. You don't know what this person has been through before, especially with the issue of undressing, so don't push the panic button with poor choices of words. I was working with a group of some 20 other massage therapists at a Palm Springs "ladies' day of beauty" convention event where the massage tables were crammed into a large room and were separated only by cloth curtains. Of all the conversations I overheard, ringing out over the top of all of them was a loud voice from a nearby therapist giving the command, "Just get naked and hop on up here." That pearl ranks right up there with such phrases as "Strip on down to nothing," or "Take it all off and I'll be back in a minute." Given that millions of people have been molested, you do not know what phrases their perpetrator used, so it is paramount that you craft a phrase for this moment in the massage process that is pretty much guaranteed not to bring back bad memories. This may sound a bit overboard to some people, but it is a reality I learned about in painful depth from many of my massage students, and it has created a sensitivity and awareness I had not considered until I heard their stories.

Clear communication is so important at this pre-massage juncture. Assume your new clients know nothing about massage, guide them through every obvious step of the way so they remain comfortable, and let them know your every move so they can trust that you won't walk in on them while they are undressed. Marketing includes all the little things you do to get and keep customers, and part of that is being sensitive to and tolerant of your clients' issues about nudity. For the clients I have worked with who have left other therapists because the therapist just stood there and talked while the client undressed, or the therapist mishandled the drape or otherwise exposed them, this may be the one significant piece that makes or breaks a positive, long-term relationship.

If you work in a spa or other type of establishment, the facility may have a policy that you must help the client onto and off of the table. While the purpose of this is to ensure that the client doesn't fall off the table and file a subsequent lawsuit, this can be a good or bad experience for the client, depending on how you handle it. Clients who have received massage from a practitioner who leaves the room while they undress and get on the table may feel uncomfortable with this more "hands-on" approach. Your job is to make them feel safe and cared for, and to position this step as a "special treatment" for the facilities' guests. This may seem odd, since once they are lying down you will see and touch much of the body, but being seen naked standing up is somehow quite different to most people. So regardless of your own comfort with nudity, be respectful of others' need for modesty.

Rebooking Moment 3: During the Massage

Once your clients are safely on the table and comfortable, the massage comes down to two things: what you do and what you say. We are first going to cover a few key points about the application of massage, then thoroughly review what to say during this moment of decision.

Universal Massage Skills

It is mind-boggling how many different types of bodywork are available on the market today. Despite their differences, there are some universal factors that apply to almost all forms of bodywork, and understanding their importance can make a huge difference in whether or not clients rebook. These factors are:

- Your **opening ritual**
- Types of touch
- Transitions
- Client participation
- Results of the session

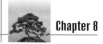

Your Opening Ritual

Opening rituals create a marvelous transition from your intake process to the actual hands-on work. An opening ritual demarcates the beginning of the session with the pomp, flourish, or focus befitting the moment. You are taking your client onto a magical journey into the body, and the moment deserves special recognition. An opening ritual can be anything you want it to be. Depending on your personality and that of your clients, it can be very subtle and short, or a time of great ceremony.

I have met some very successful therapists who put on quite an opening display, including smudging the room with burning sage, waving owl feathers, ringing chimes, laying out crystals, and other such rituals that are a big part of why people come to see them. These actions have their own value, but they also are quite theatrical and some clients just love it. It is not my intention to take away from the sacredness of more spiritually based rituals; they serve wonderful purposes, but they are also fascinating to the uninitiated and can be a big part of your draw. Create an opening ritual that suits you and your clients, and then stick with it. After a few sessions, the very act of your opening ritual is enough to trigger their relaxation response, and they'll relax much more quickly. Many spas have tapped into the importance of ritual, sacred time, and setting the tone with elaborate processes, and you can do the same.

My ritual serves multiple purposes. It includes an opening grounding where I rest my hands on the back or feet, followed by running my hands lightly over the sheet to bring awareness to the body from head to toe. This prepares me energetically and focuses me emotionally, all the while introducing my touch and creating trust from the first impression that my touch is safe. I tell my new clients I am introducing my hands to their body to build trust, sort of like a full-body handshake, and that I am feeling for temperature variances and subtle tension patterns. This, I explain, lets me know where to look first for possible problem spots, then strategize where I should concentrate my time. By revealing this as my intention, it tells them that I care enough to pay attention to their individual needs and that I will make the most of their time. I highlight these two points because I have dealt with many clients who felt their prior therapist only did a routine massage and didn't spend time in the areas with the highest need. This simple ritual and explanation sets the tone that my intention is to meet their needs and shows that I have some skills behind that intention. This ritual also gives me a chance to gain an energetic "permission" to work with the client, which relaxes them faster and more deeply than if I were to just start in quickly.

EXERCISE: CREATE AN OPENING RITUAL

Write down a description of your ideal opening ritual. Start with the purposes of the ritual, such as what you need to do to create more trust, demonstrate your intention, or impress your client. Think about how you can convey your purposes with your touch, words, and movements. Run a few scenarios through your head, find one you like, and write it down. If you are in a group, have a few people share or demonstrate their opening rituals.

_____

_____

_____

_____

_____

Types of Touch

Once the opening ritual is complete, give the first strokes of your massage. Your first movements are probably your most important strokes because they create the final piece of your clients' first impression. Up to this point, they have heard your voice, listened to your thought process, sized up your environment, experienced your opening ritual, and evaluated you based on a million different little judgments. All of those impressions are changeable at this point. If your first strokes feel loving, compassionate, competent, professional, or whatever it is they are looking for, you may be forgiven a host of oversights because your "proof is in the pudding."

Pressure

Your massage and bodywork classes will cover much about touch and stroke skills. However, viewing a few key elements from the marketing perspective can make the difference between a thriving practice and wondering why people aren't rebooking. Of all the variables of bodywork, the amount of pressure is the one most likely to determine the satisfaction level of your clients. Pressure is not a variable about which to make guesses. Stereotypes that big guys like heavy pressure and little ladies want light, fluffy work are dangerous to your return rate. The right pressure takes work to find and entails getting feedback, both from what your clients say and what your hands feel. In addition, your pressure needs to be adjusted constantly from body part to body part and from session to session. Too much pressure is painful or injurious, and too little pressure is frustrating and irritating.

Some therapists think they should magically know the perfect amount of pressure to use, or believe they will lose face or client trust if they admit they don't know the right pressure to use. To get feedback without losing face or trust, I tell my clients I'm not psychic, and while I am very good at figuring out the right amount of pressure, I cannot feel what they are feeling, so they need to let me know when my pressure is too heavy or too light. Feedback about pressure takes a bit of work to get out of some clients, and I have learned not to ask questions that can be answered with the word "fine." Questions that actually give you valuable feedback need to be specific. "Would you like more pressure?" or "It feels like you're tightening up; do I need to lighten up?" can teach you, over time, to trust your hands to the point where you will have to ask for verbal feedback less often.

The opposite of the mute, lie-there-and-take-it client is the over-directing, micro-managing client. If you have clients who demand heavier pressure, but you can feel the tissue resisting under your hands, be aware that they probably have so little body awareness that you could push through to the other side and they would say it's still not enough pressure. Many people are out of touch with how they feel, and they need more stimulation than normal to the tissue and nervous system before it registers that they have even felt your touch.

Be careful with clients like these, especially if they are new to massage. Since they aren't able to feel pressure accurately, they will demand more pressure. If you comply, you will most likely hurt them. Having fallen into this "more-pressure" trap a number of times to please a client in the moment, I have learned that the aftereffects are not worth the act of giving in to an insistent client. Education is the best way out of this bind. You need to tell people that you understand they want more pressure, but your hands are telling you that you have gone as deeply as the tissue allows without tightening up and, if you work deeper, you will hurt them. If you are fairly new to massage and don't yet have the hand sensitivity that comes with years of practice, be careful with too much repetition in one place or forced pressure in any areas. You can hurt people that way, and that's not why we got into the profession.

Do your education up front instead of waiting for a comment about pressure. Tell your new clients that it takes some time to get familiar with their tissue and to figure out what their normal muscle tone feels like compared to areas of tension. Explain that while you are getting familiar with them, you will be using a lighter pressure than they might expect at the outset. Explain that once you have gained their body's trust, their muscles will relax more and you can work deeper without hurting them. This alleviates your need to prove anything in the first few minutes, which can be easy to feel with new clients. When their tissue has relaxed, point it out and then say that you can now go deeper if they would like you to. If they do, gradually start adding pressure, asking for feedback as you go.

If you do the above but clients keep telling you they want more pressure, you will need to make some decisions. You can make a concerted effort to strengthen yourself, refer your clients elsewhere, or consider using or learning a modality that is effective without clients expecting heavy pressure. Whatever you choose, don't let clients bully you into doing work deeper than you can physically handle. Building a dream practice means you should avoid as many hand, wrist, and body injuries as you can, and how you handle pressure will either lead to problems or to a long and fulfilling career.

Transitions

During the massage, you are touching your clients in ways different from your massage strokes. The other types of touch that impact rebooking are the non-massaging touches of moving the client around and handling the drape.

Repositioning Clients

Moving or repositioning your client is a skill that often does not get the attention or practice time it deserves. Picking up a client's arm to do a range-of-motion (ROM) exercise or move it under the drape can be a graceful and unnoticed motion, or a startling disruption, depending on how it is carried out. Moving a leg onto a bolster or placing a pillow under the neck needs to be done with the same smoothness and speed as the rest of your work; otherwise, it can be a disturbing and disconcerting experience. It is one thing to have a massage therapist press into tissue; it is quite another to have limbs picked up and maneuvered. Many clients probably will be fine with being moved around, but it can be disconcerting to others for a host of reasons. Before you do much range-of-motion work or a significant amount of repositioning, ask permission or notify them before you do so. Then your clients won't resist or reflexively try to help.

Even if you are given permission, move people with the same amount of caring and regard that you use for the rest of your work. One client I spoke with had gone to see a massage therapist who used to be a nurse. The client was greeted brusquely and, as she soon discovered, was handled brusquely as well. Using maneuvers and efficiency no doubt developed with hospital patients, this ex-nurse whipped the client around like a rag doll, rolling her sideways in the sheet to get to a bolster and stuffing pillows around with jolting vigor. Never was the client asked if the pillows were comfortable or wanted. Hospital patients may not know they have a say in being comfortable, but massage clients do, and, surprise, comfort matters. Need I say that the client didn't rebook?

Handling a Drape

Handling a drape is also a much bigger deal than many people would think. Clients are watching you for every sign of whether they can trust you, and if, before the session, you are jerking on the sheet edges, slapping on the blanket to smooth it, or jamming pillows around, you will probably see them involuntarily flinch. How you handle inanimate objects around you may not be how you touch your clients during the massage, but they don't know that. Once the massage has started, and the client is under the sheet or towel that you are adjusting, you should handle the drape the way you would handle the client. Don't toss aside blankets, yank off sheets, or drop pillows on the floor. Small but crucial bits of trust can be lost when you mishandle a drape, so be conscious of how you move it.

For the sake of your clients' comfort, don't wad the drape up into a big lump and jam it under a thigh, shoulder, or, as I once saw done by a new student, rolled up and neatly tucked into the gluteal cleft. Visually it looked quite neat and tidy to the therapist, but for the client who proceeded to reach up and extract it, it looked very uncomfortable. Please, do not trade neatness that only you see for comfort that your client feels.

Draping is a topic about which there are many varied and conflicting opinions, but what matters most is, does it work well for your clients? Some clients may love being wrapped mummy-like in a tight cocoon of blankets, but do that to a client with even mild claustrophobia and you've got a big problem on your hands. The purpose of the drape is to help the client stay warm, maintain modesty and privacy, and feel safe that he or she is not in any way exposed. That said, I have seen professional demonstrations of draping that were supposed to make the client feel safe, but the movements were so invasive and close to the genitals that they bordered on indiscretion. Unless you are doing a lot of deep massage into the inner thigh and are going to be doing big ranges of motion, there is no reason in the world your hand needs to come anywhere near the genitals to shove the sheet under the thigh. You must weigh which is of more concern to your client: that you are somehow peeking if you use a fairly loose drape, or that your hands are going way too close to places they shouldn't be.

Beyond these points, the mere act of disturbing a client floating in a relaxed state just to rearrange sheets in a particular manner is not worth it. On the financial side, ask yourself whether lots of tight, neat draping is what your clients want to be spending their money on. If you charge $60 an hour, or $1.00 per minute, one minute of fussing with the sheet per limb on both sides equals blowing their money in ways they will resent. Clients come to you for a good massage, not for good draping. The bottom line is that you should keep your clients draped appropriately for modesty and warmth, and not disturb them or waste their time and money for what should be an invisible part of the massage.

Amount of Time Spent in One Area

Another hands-on variable to consider during the massage is the amount of time you spend working on one area of the body. Rebooking a client requires you address the needs they came in with, and how you spend your time affects how well you are able to address those needs. I learned this lesson the hard way by making the mistake of taking too much time doing massage work in areas the client had not come to see me about. In particular, I remember a woman, early in my career, who had come to me because of her sore neck. Being a firm believer in the value of full-body massage, I began my routine the usual way, starting at the feet and working my way up. Unfortunately, I kept finding trouble spots elsewhere, got involved in working those out, and, by the time I got to her neck, I had run out of time for what mattered most. Having booked my appointments too closely together, since I hadn't quite learned that lesson yet, I had no extra time to do the work necessary on her neck. I had done good work, but not in the right place. The woman didn't feel like giving me a second chance and, frankly, I don't blame her.

Client Participation

Keeping clients happy enough to have them rebook also means paying attention to what level of participation they want to have in the session. Some people think the ultimate massage means not moving a muscle and wishing you had a giant pancake turner to flip them over. Others expect to be fully engaged with range-of-motion work, muscle testing, and constant feedback. Needs for rest and relaxation usually involve less participation, while needs for injury recovery or performance enhancement require the client to be awake and active. Mixing up these needs can leave clients frustrated.

If a stressed-out executive just got to the dozing stage and you insist on rousing him with your regular routine of range of motion for the hips, complete with the involved draping, he will resentfully change his state to accommodate your routine, but he probably won't be happy. If a marathon runner with tight hamstrings wants help with muscle lengthening and strengthening, and your basic routine doesn't incorporate even passive range-of-motion work, her needs will not be met and the odds of rebooking diminish greatly.

To know what level of participation your clients want, ask them. Tell them during the intake time that you want to serve their needs, but you need to know how awake or involved they want to be. Clients can participate at varying levels, including:

- Actively participating—ROM, resistance, involved feedback, working with breath
- Partially participating—giving feedback, maybe some passive ROM
- Awake and talking—general conversation with minimal feedback
- Awake and silent
- Floating in alpha state
- Sleeping

When working with clients who want to actively participate, be careful how you lead them through their exercises, tell them how to breathe, or ask for feedback. Be patient with people and give guidance, not commands. Instructions on anything from taking a breath to assisted stretches can elicit resistance or cooperation, depending upon how they are given. Old dictating-style communication models from football coaches and drill sergeants may work in other settings, but not for massage clients.

New clients who have never had massage before also may find that their limbs and body don't cooperate the way they want them to. The more a client participates, the more apparent it may become that range of motion has been lost, muscle control has diminished, and strength has evaporated. Tears of frustration or anger have been part of the process for a number of my clients trying to regain fine-motor control lost in an injury. Commanding someone to relax an arm he or she is holding stiffly rarely works; providing instructions to imagine it being warm and heavy or falling into your hand makes more sense, and creates less embarrassment over uncooperative limbs.

So what does this have to do with marketing? Everything. Clients who are given education, gently guided through stubborn holding patterns, and treated as the intelligent adults they are will appreciate and respect your methods of handling them, and they will be more likely to rebook and refer. Clients who are treated with exasperation because they won't relax on command like a dog being told to sit (and I've seen it!) will not be back. When clients don't come back, you have to go back to finding new clients, and the dream practice stays out of reach. Subtle points such as those we have covered here matter a great deal to clients, and the more you consider and try them, the faster you will succeed.

Results of the Session

Ultimately, many clients rebook based on the results they get from your work. I've met clients who put up with their therapist having a pack of dogs lounging around the treatment table because they got the results they wanted Unraveling blankets and rooms reeking of patchouli oil have been forgiven for therapists who have gotten great results or offered genuine and heartfelt caring and compassion.

Results of a session are measured a number of different ways, and understanding how clients measure success gives you a greater advantage in reaching it. The success of your work is evaluated based on your clients':

❋ Experience during the session

❋ Short-term results of the session

- ❋ Long-term results of the session
- ❋ Cumulative results of multiple sessions
- ❋ Ability to maintain improvements by helping themselves

For many people, getting a massage is about having an "experience." They just want a grand and royal pampering, and the stated purpose of their visit can seem rather vague. Massage has become a significant symbol of the good life, and some people just want the glitz and glamour of the moment, reveling in the thought that they are getting the treatment usually associated with the rich and famous. Recognizing clients with this mindset is crucial; it means that their results are measured solely by the moments during the massage, and being king or queen for the day is what is expected. Pain relief, joint mobility, or open chakras are not the goal; bragging and having stories to tell others later are.

Confusing clients who want a glamour massage with clients who want real help can be frustrating to both client types. People who want pain relief, stress reduction, posture reeducation, or performance enhancement will be judging your results very quickly, and what they decide may bring them back or not. Fast-food drive-through windows and Internet "e-tailers" have taught our culture that wants and needs can be met instantaneously, and drug companies make promises of pain relief in a matter of minutes with magical pills.

However, the body, as marvelous as it is, sometimes takes a while to repair itself, and you will need to educate your results-oriented clients about what to expect from one session. Interviewing your clients during the intake session can reveal their expectations, informing you about whether or not you can meet their desired results in one or more sessions, or at all.

Motivated clients who want to participate in their own healing will want genuine help and guidance from you. Often, they are some of the most gratifying clients to work with because they will push you to learn more, work smarter, and be more effective with your time. Results-oriented clients will come back to you if they know you are thinking and strategizing about how to help them. Patience is available for you if your clients know what to expect realistically. On-the-table education using pressure, stretches, or other feedback tools can demonstrate that you are taking steps, large or small, toward helping them, and they can measure your success with valid sensations of improvement. Giving motivated clients at-home exercises, stretches, or self-massage routines to do also can put you up another notch in the trust and value columns, and if homework increases the benefits of your work, rebookings are virtually assured.

What You Say During the Massage

The second primary element of the third moment of decision is what you say during the massage. In short, what you say and talk about can have a great deal of impact on whether or not your clients come back. Since many of my interviews with massage clients across the country revealed that talking and poor communication skills were some of the main reasons they left their therapists, we are going to thoroughly and, some may think, exhaustively cover the art of communication during your massage session. However, the purpose of this book is to help massage therapists be successful, and if what follows helps you get one client to come back for one more session, it will be worth the price of this book.

The Art of Conversation

Talking and conversation during a massage is a highly individual matter. Some clients just grunt, get on the table, and that's the end of that, whereas others want to talk the whole time. Some clients will talk only when they are face up and some will talk only when face down. Some talk for the first 10 minutes, then fall silent; others suddenly get chatty right before it is time to end the session. Clients talk out of nervousness, loneliness, interest, and curiosity about you and your work. They ask questions about their symptoms and many other topics. You can let them lead the conversation and respond, or you can let them know they might relax more if they are quiet. Some clients are afraid of silence and being quiet might be more than they can bear, so let them chat until you feel them drift.

Depending on your type of work and target market, your primary service may not be your massage, but your ability to talk or listen. My contingency of elderly widows talked from the moment I walked in the door to the time I closed my car door and drove away, as they waved good-bye. I was offered, and accepted, more than a few tuna casserole luncheons, knowing I was the only visitor coming by that week. Of course, I helped their aches and pains, but they rebooked to talk. And that was fine with me.

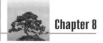

On-the-Table Education

Although some massages may be totally quiet, if you and your client are going to talk, take time during the massage to tell your clients what you are doing and why. This creates immense value for them in their impression of you and in their understanding of the benefits of massage. Once into a session, tell your clients what you discover about tension or compensation patterns, temperature variations, muscle spasms, involuntary reflexes, or whatever else you notice.

On-the-table education is one of the best forms of marketing you can do. You can tell new clients the purpose of the stroke you are using and how it affects their muscles, nervous system, blood flow, and the like. Since new clients often are nervous to some degree, this gives them something to focus on. However, once you feel them start to float away, be quiet. In addition to general education, you can provide specific information about their bodies, especially if anything your hands feel is unclear or confusing to you. Tell them what you notice, including your thought processes, hunches, or suppositions. Explain how a stubbed toe can lead to lower back pain or how a tight neck can lead to tennis elbow. If you cover holistic principles about how the body works, you can create a genuine partnership with your client, working as a team, with you offering your observations, asking questions, and striving to solve the problem for which they came to see you.

Managing Boundaries

Once your clients are relaxed and your work is under way, your responsibilities during the massage come down to two things: taking care of yourself and taking care of your clients. Taking care of yourself means protecting yourself physically, emotionally, and energetically. In this respect, your highest need is for yourself. The boundaries you set with regard to how much you will push yourself physically, how much you will reveal about yourself or allow your clients to reveal about themselves, and how connected you will allow yourself to become are of utmost importance to a long-term career. Poor boundary skills can lead to injuries, pain, and drained energy for you, and this, ultimately, doesn't serve you or your clients well.

Beyond these boundaries of self-protection, though, the clients need to receive the highest priority. It is their turn to tell stories, to be silent if they choose, to set the temperature, choose the music, select the oil scent, give feedback on your work and pressure, and otherwise control the many elements of the

Figure 8–4 | Listening can be one of the most important benefits you offer your clients.

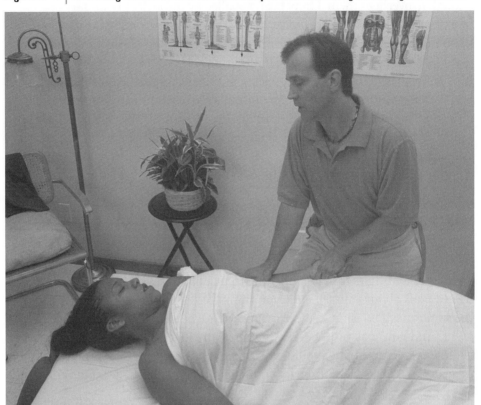

massage for which they are paying. They are not paying to listen to your problems, hear your stories, or offer you counsel, sympathy, or advice. They are paying you to listen to them. (See Figure 8–4.)

I remember a particular story during my cross-country interviews from a woman who had gone to a spa for a dual massage where she and her husband were to receive simultaneous sessions, side by side in the same room, to celebrate their anniversary. While this sounded wonderful and romantic in the fancy spa brochure, in reality, the two therapists talked between themselves the whole time they were working, chatting away about their own lives as if the clients weren't even there. It wasn't quite the experience these poor clients were hoping for, and their disappointment was evident. No rebooking there, that's for sure!

When I have worked in settings with other therapists in rooms with walls thin enough to overhear them, I have been appalled by the lack of boundaries, inappropriateness of subject topics, and barraging monologue from the therapist upon the poor client helplessly lying there trying to relax. This doesn't mean you don't talk while you work; I've had many enjoyable conversations with clients, but I let them lead the conversation, choose the topic, or just be silent. Depending on your target market, you may have formal relationships with your clients, or more informal interactions and conversations. Regardless, beyond your self-protection, put your clients first and have your time together be about them.

Responding During a Massage Conversation

The most appropriate time for you to make conversation is when you respond to what your client has said or asked. When a person asks you a question about your day, your weekend, or some other facet of your life, you certainly can respond with an answer. However, questions such as these often are a polite way for others to get an opening to talk about themselves. If you don't want to talk about yourself, or if you think this a lead-in for you to ask them the same question, simply say, My X (weekend, boyfriend, girlfriend, etc.) is great. And how was your weekend? Then settle in for a long story while you get to work on that tight shoulder. In normal life, conversation is a give and take, but in a massage setting, let your client do most of the talking.

In addition, when you are responding to their stories, do not try to top them. If your client was stranded at the airport for four hours, don't launch into how you were stuck for eight hours. If your client is excited because of finally taking a bike ride of 10 miles, don't cut off the story to talk about your bike ride across Canada. Turn over the spotlight, and let your clients revel in the horror or glory of it all. Remember, they are there to take care of themselves, and the more your responses turn the attention back to them, the more your value will increase as both a massage professional and a listening ear. When it comes time to rebook, and multiple needs have been met beyond the massage, the appointment book is much more likely to get filled in.

Verbal Check-Ins

One of the most important things you can do during a session, in order to have clients who rebook, is to make sure they are happy. During your first session, it is important to conduct verbal check-ins and to ask on a regular but not disruptive basis if this is what they had expected, if there is anything you should change, or if there is any way you can make it better. Ask about sound, heat, pressure, or room scents. If they are squirming, ask if they need to change positions. Don't ask with a sense of fear or lack of confidence—your work is good; you just want it perfect. If they are not happy with something, you can change it instantly. However, if you can't change it, and it's a big deal to the client, you can end the session and give a refund.

If your verbal check-ins frequently result in curt responses such as "I'm fine!" then take notice. Either everything is fine and they are annoyed at being disturbed from their reverie, or they don't know they are allowed to have the massage the way they want it. Many clients make the wrong assumption that getting on a massage therapist's table is like getting on a doctor's table. They expect it to be uncomfortable and don't know they are "allowed" to ask you to change anything that may be causing them discomfort. Most of them have experienced hard, crinkly, paper-lined tables, cold doctor's instruments, rooms that smell like rubbing alcohol, and scratchy paper dressing gowns. Why would they think a massage session, especially if it's more therapeutic in nature, would be different than a visit to the doctor? You'd be surprised what people think!

I talked with a woman who got a massage on a cruise ship, and she was so badly manhandled that she was bruised and hurting for days. When I asked her why she didn't tell the therapist the pressure was too heavy, her response was, "I thought he knew what he was doing, so I let him do it." Her programming told her that you just put up with what the doctor does to you, and it resulted in a bad massage for her. For the therapist who wasn't paying enough attention to the fact that she was probably stiff and tense, or flinching under his hands, she would not be a repeat client. Unfortunately, this young man by now has probably hurt hundreds of first-time clients who didn't know any better. When those clients come ashore, they probably will never get a massage from you or me, and they'll tell all their friends about how painful massage is when they show off their bruise-tinged tans. Verbal check-ins can prevent such stories, keep you on track, and let your clients know you are paying attention and care about how they feel.

Creating Awareness, Especially of Improvements

Besides not hurting people, one of the other good reasons to talk with clients is so you can point out their improvements. You can tell them when you feel muscles relaxing, energy releasing, flexibility improving, and so on. To enhance the improvement, give directive yet unobtrusive feedback, especially by using the word "good." Softly repeat to yourself "good, good, good" as you feel muscles let go. This focuses clients on where you are working and trains them to gain sensitivity to small improvements. The word "good" also serves another function. While there may be exceptions, most clients will want their massage therapists to like them. When you say "good," they know they are performing well, and your praise can give them the feeling that you approve of them. I have been testing the effect of the word "good" for many years on my clients and students, and while it is a simple word, millions of people long to hear it and feel the approval that goes with it.

Creating awareness of improvements also can be done by asking questions, but be careful: how you ask is important. Always state your question in the positive. Don't ask, "Does that still hurt?" This question starts the mind on a search for pain, which it will most likely find, and since they are now noticing the pain, they will think your massage is not working, even if you have felt improvement. Instead, ask something simple such as, "Does that feel better?" The mind will now scan for improvements, and when they say "yes," they are recognizing benefits they hadn't noticed until you asked.

Another important reason for them to acknowledge improvement is that many people have a psychological belief that their problems are permanent and unchangeable. By admitting to you that they feel better, they begin to break the psychological chain that often holds a pain pattern in place.

If they say it doesn't feel better, you may be on the wrong track, so tell them you are going to try a different technique. Switch modalities or tactics, and tell them what you're doing and why. For example, I may be trying a cross-fiber friction move, or using trigger point therapy, but if the muscle isn't responding, I will stop and say, "This muscle isn't relaxing the way I thought it would using this technique. I'm going to switch to a totally different strategy and see if this is more of a nervous system issue and try this other technique." Then I can explain how that technique works, try it, and ask if they can feel the difference. There is nothing more fascinating to people than themselves, so talk about them and what you are doing to them as a way to increase their awareness and demonstrate your efforts to get results.

Handling an Emotional Release During the Massage

Paying attention and doing verbal check-ins are important for emotional shifts as well as physical ones. If your clients feel the trust, silence, and safety to experience what is going on for them both physically and emotionally, there is the possibility that they will have some form of emotional release. While this may not happen often or at all, you should be prepared to handle it so that your client will feel secure enough to rebook a return visit. If clients suddenly start to cry, laugh, twitch, or release emotions, they may be afraid of what you will think; some people may think they should end the session and leave. Let them know the release is temporary, it will subside, and it's a good way to let go of built-up energy. Emotional-release massage is a skill well beyond the scope of this book, but how you handle an emotional release can make the difference between whether clients stay and, especially, whether they come back.

For example, if I notice a client is crying and breathing in such a way that it is apparent to both of us that I have recognized it, I will say something like, "I can see that something has come up for you. If you want to talk about it, I'm here, but you don't have to. I can stop the massage if you'd like; otherwise, I'll just keep working." This simple statement is unobtrusive, gives the client permission to experience whatever he or she is feeling, and lets the client know that he or she is in charge of the situation. It also removes the burden of the client feeling like he or she has to explain anything to me, and it prevents me from getting in over my head if the emotion is more properly handled by a trained psychologist or mental health professional.

Letting people cry can be very freeing for them. Don't interrupt them to hand over a tissue; just lay one near their hand, and don't stop the massage in the middle of a stroke. Shift your work to more gentle and soothing strokes or energy work, send the powerful intention of your love and caring, and let the emotions release. Be present and caring, ride it out, and listen quietly. Your client most likely will be very grateful, and most likely will also be back.

Music During the Massage

Music during the massage can enhance or detract from the experience. Many clients enjoy having music on in the background while you work. While your preferences in music may be different from those of your clients, having music you enjoy and can work to, with consistent volume, rhythm, and flow, is important. That said, it can be a good idea to ask if your client is enjoying your selection or would prefer silence. Play different tapes or CDs, find out which ones they like, or show them your selection and let them choose one. Unless your music is the focal point of the massage, keep the volume down. This is especially helpful when the type of client who likes to talk in the face-down position decides to tell you about his weekend trip while his face is deep in the headrest. If your clients don't like music, you can get a white noise machine and play a babbling brook or rainy day sounds. Just make sure it is a sound your client likes.

Whatever background sound you choose, get feedback on it, and, unless it is a specific part of your treatment, leave out the spoken-word tapes. I talked with a woman whose new therapist was playing a talking tape by the Ayurvedic doctor, Deepak Chopra, when she first arrived for her appointment. The client didn't think much of it at first, but throughout the whole intake time and the first few minutes of the session, Deepak's voice and words played over their conversation. Finally, after lying there listening to him talk while she was trying to relax, she asked the therapist to turn off the tape. The therapist was greatly surprised that the tape was bothering her client, and even though she immediately turned it off, that minor incident made the client wary about other ways the therapist wasn't paying attention or considering her needs. A precedent had been set with a simple oversight. And, you guessed it, no rebooking followed.

Silence

Finally, in the art of conversation, there is time for silence. Sometimes, silence truly is golden, both for your client and yourself. Let your new clients know up front that you don't expect them to talk. Teach them that they can relax better when they focus on the work being done and how they feel. It is almost as if you have to give some people permission to be still. If they want to talk but suddenly fall silent mid-word or sentence when their energy shifts, stop talking yourself; otherwise, conversation can be quite jarring and wake them up.

You also will have to weigh the value of the silence against the need to give instructions, ask for feedback, or ask background information about what your hands are picking up in the muscles. If a client is coming to you primarily to relax, then silence is the better choice. However, if you are working on a specific problem or need that is the main reason for the appointment, get feedback or provide instructions when necessary.

Interrupting the silence to have a client turn over is probably my least favorite part of massage, and it needs to be done gently. If I need to wake a client to turn over, I go through my wake-up ritual by covering them fully with the sheet, running my hands the length of the body, stopping my movements, resting my hands, and gently rocking. The stillness usually wakes them. If that fails, I quietly ask, "How are you doing?" and take it from there.

Even at the end of the massage, I am careful how I break the silence. During the pre-massage instructions, I tell all my new clients that I have a closing ritual at the end of the massage. When they hear the word "ta-da" somewhere in the far reaches of their alpha state, they will know I'm done. There is little worse than doing a great session and then having your client look up, confused, and say, "Is that it?" This closing ritual lets them know they can drift away, and that you will take care of them while they are gone and bring them back safely.

Waking Up a Sleeping Client

A predetermined wake-up ritual also keeps you from scaring your clients if they've fallen asleep. If you do have to wake them, stand near their waist and shoulder, gently rock them, and ask, "How are you doing?" This wakes them up but also lets them be in charge. It may sound odd, but when I used to ask, "Are you awake?" or say, "Time to wake up," my clients had a tendency to deny they were asleep, even if they had rattled the windows with their snoring. If they don't want to admit they dozed off, fine, but I have learned from vehement denials that some people think there's something wrong with falling asleep on the table. Maybe it has something to do with thinking they were vulnerable or out of control, but whatever the reason, I have found repeatedly that people don't like to be told they were asleep. To get past this hurdle, ask, "How are you doing?" and be in view so they can focus on you easily when they open their eyes. Don't put your face down close to theirs because when they come to, they may not know where they are or who the stranger is towering over them. It will startle them, which is no way to end a session.

I have a client who sometimes falls asleep at the end of the session. When he doesn't rouse with my usual closing ritual, I leave him snoring peacefully, wash up, read a magazine, or look out the window until he comes to on his own. Since I don't book my sessions close together, especially around his session, I can do this. That extra time for snoozing seems quite valuable to him, and not only does he always rebook but he also keeps giving me raises without my asking. In this case, silence truly is golden.

Rebooking Moment 4: At the End of the Massage

Once the hands-on part of the session is over, and your clients are up and dressed, take a moment to ask them how they are, listen to their responses, and answer any questions they may have. If they set any specific goals or had clear expectations, review those and point out improvements you have noticed. Graciously accept their compliments, which may take some practice for you, and let them bask in the glow of their massage.

Use this time to prepare them for the next few days. If they have never had a massage before, they will not know how to interpret how they feel and may think something is wrong. Depending on the kind of work you do, if they are going to be sore, spacey, emotional, or anything like that in the next day or two, let them know what to expect without setting them up for self-fulfilling prophecies. To talk safely during this impressionable time, use qualifying words such as "may," "might," "can," "some people experience," or "if you notice," then describe the symptom they may experience. In that way, if they do experience soreness or tenderness, they won't think something is wrong or that you didn't know what you were doing. If they don't experience those symptoms, they won't think anything is wrong since you only said they "might" have those symptoms.

Trust needs to be maintained even when they are not in your presence, and giving them appropriate expectations for the days following their massage will let them maintain that trust. You may even go so far as to give them a sheet of paper with instructions for the next day. You can advise them to drink more water than usual, provide them with instructions on how to apply ice or heat, or give them stretches, exercises, or self-applied massage techniques to do in order to gain the most benefit from their investment. Even if they never do any of what you suggest, going this extra step continues to build their perception of your professional skills and personal caring. Of course, if you're a smart marketer, you'll have all your contact information on that piece of paper so if they lose your card but keep this instruction form, they can rebook or refer later.

Last Impressions

Your last few minutes with your clients are critical to rebooking. Your clients now have been connected to you closely for the last hour or so, and, if you did good work, they will be warm and open. Besides being hazy and relaxed, they are looking at you with new eyes, and you can see them almost looking at you for the first time as they reevaluate their first impressions. They are watching you closely, now that the session is over, to create their next impression of you.

It is important that you maintain the loving spirit you demonstrated during the massage throughout the rest of your experience with them. In essence, your client is in a hypnotic trance. If, during the close of the session, you suddenly start moving faster and talking noticeably louder in a way that is markedly different than what was used during the session, it is both jarring and confusing to clients. Your goal is to maintain a sense of safety, trust, and connection from the moment they walk in the door until they walk out, so how you handle yourself between the end of the massage and when they leave needs to be given just as much import as when they arrive for the first time.

I remember the first time I really saw this concept in action. I had a student who was a large, muscular man trained in the martial arts, and who dressed like a biker, complete with large tattoos decorating both of his arms from his shoulders to his wrists. He was intimidating to most people, but when he centered himself using his martial arts background to prepare to do massage, a marvelous, gentle spirit emerged and his work was like a beautiful dance. However, the second he was finished working, he would pop out of that gentle state, smack his fellow student on the back, and announce loudly, "You're done!" I am happy to say that after a few coaching sessions, he realized the importance of maintaining his state throughout his entire contact time, and he did so with a grace and power that became his more permanent persona.

Handling the Separation Stage

In addition to good feelings created by maintaining the spirit of the massage throughout your contact time, your last few minutes are important for a number of other reasons. Whether spoken aloud or not, some clients go through moments of separation anxiety, fear of abandonment, and pain of loss. I have heard everything from "Don't stop," "Don't leave," "Can't this go on forever," all the way up to, "If I won the lottery, I'd build you a house out back so you wouldn't have to go." While I realize these are ways people give compliments, there is also a grain of truth in what they say. After all, who else has lavished such love and attention on them in recent years? While it may seem illogical, for some people your leaving can be a moment of betrayal.

How you handle this moment is critical. If you briskly pack up, whip sheets off the table while they are dressing, move much more rapidly than during your massage, talk louder and faster, and look at the clock, you indicate nonverbally that the client is "dismissed." The ensuing feelings can seem irrational, but some people will leap to the conclusion that you really don't care, you're just in this for the money, you're abandoning them, or that this isn't really a relationship, it's just another job for you. After all, their unconscious reasoning goes, you felt so loving and caring just a moment before and now you're giving them the brush-off.

While this mental/emotional scenario may sound overanalytical or overblown, I think it must be given credence. Massage is different than just about any other profession or service. Because of the amount of touch, type of touch, extent of touch, nudity, and length of contact time, massage can create an intimate practitioner–client connection. Due to this connection, your clients may feel incredibly vulnerable at this point for a host of reasons. Some clients have been feeling their body, maybe for the first time in years, and others may have been going through a whole host of emotions and old memories. Maybe no one touches them this way anymore, if ever, and their massage experience exposes the lack of this most basic of human needs. If your client is a single, working mother, the odds are high that it has been years since anyone has devoted time and energy to her. If your clients have had negative experiences with touch, a whole range of emotions may be swirling. If your clients think they are unattractive or unlovely, which millions in our country do, having someone touch them with caring and compassion can be emotionally wrenching.

Since you don't know what is going on in your clients' heads at the end of the massage, treat them as you did during your session to help them transition back into their "real world." Keep your voice and movements close to your massage level, act as if they're the only person in the world (even if you are running late), and keep your energy open to them until you or they are out the door. No one wants to be treated like they are one more body coming down the conveyor belt. During those last few minutes when your clients are most vulnerable, be gentle, be present, and keep your energy consistent. This is so subtle but so important, especially at the beginning of your relationship, for keeping and rebooking clients.

Booking the Next Appointment

During this final time together, you have your best opportunity to rebook your new clients. They are happy, feel good, and have immediate experience with your work. You can say something like, "If you'd like another massage, we can book one now, or if you're not sure right now, you can call me later." This relieves the pressure they may have been expecting and removes resistance. The last thing you want to do is make them feel awkward, guilty, or pressured into rebooking.

Even if you don't have full confidence in your work, you must not let that show at this time. Do not give any excuses for yourself or demonstrate a lack of confidence. Don't undermine yourself by saying something like, "Well, I'm still pretty new at massage and don't know if it helped, but I hope it was okay. Would you like to rebook?" If you have misgivings about your work, keep them to yourself. Don't ruin their enjoyment of the moment by telling them how you could have done a better massage or any other such comments. Swallow your self-doubt, listen to their compliments, and offer them the opportunity to rebook. If they liked your work, they'll be back.

Rebooking

People will have one of three responses when you ask them to rebook. They can say "yes," "maybe," or "no." If they say "yes," you can open your calendar or fire up your PDA and figure out the next time you can get together.

If a client seems hesitant to rebook, you have a number of options. The first question is whether or not you want to rebook them. There are some people you work on that you won't want to see again, or that won't be worth it to you financially to retain, and thus you don't rebook them. However, if you want to rebook your new but hesitant clients, you will have to find out what is standing in the way.

The most common obstacles cited are lack of time and/or money. If time and money get in the way, do what you can justify your business to remove these obstacles. You can deal with the obstacle presented to you but be aware that the obstacles people bring up may or may not be the real problem. Lack of money often is an easily constructed excuse that hides a deeper issue, so before you give a discount, see if you can find out what that issue really is.

If you don't want to push and just take them at their word, you can make a number of offers. You can offer a financial incentive such as a "New Client Special" of three massages for $99, a two-for-one deal, or a prepaid package series at a lower rate. A note of warning: research in marketing has shown that the practice of giving discounts and coupons to current clients undermines the value of the service and dramatically cuts profits in the long

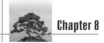

haul. You have to evaluate whether or not giving a special like a three-for-$99 offer would cement long-term relationships or diminish the value of your work. If you decide to go with a one-time special, be very clear about its purpose. Tell your clients that your regular price is X, but you are offering a onetime, special deal so they can better experience and understand the value of the cumulative effects of massage. If they still balk at that, they either don't value your work or really can't afford you, or the underlying reason for not rebooking is not financial.

If your financial incentives have not led to a rebooking, you can be up front and say, "It sounds like you're not sure about rebooking. If you don't want to, that's fine, but if I did something wrong I'd like to know about it so I can be more helpful to my future clients." Then be still and listen. If you are lucky, they will be honest and give feedback you can use the rest of your career. Once they've said what was bothering them and you've handle their dissatisfaction professionally, they actually may reconsider and rebook.

They might have liked your touch but your fingernails kept scratching them, the room was too cold, or they didn't like feeling greasy. Issues that mundane can keep a client from coming back. Another phrase to use to dig out such obstacles is, "My goal was to give you the best massage you've ever had, and if anything was less than perfect, I want to know about it. I'm here for you, so what could I have done to make it perfect for you?" Very few massage clients ever hear those words from their therapists, and if you want to be head and shoulders above your competition, the things your clients will tell you at this point will set you a world apart.

Even if you never see them again, you have done major damage control. Because they have been able to tell you what they disliked, they will be less likely to complain to others. If they were personal referrals from other clients or mutual marketers, appeasing them is even more important because they could damage your other relationships. It may not be comfortable in the moment, but the moment passes. You can either integrate what they said into your work or know that some people will be unhappy, no matter what. If they are really unhappy, insist on giving them their money back. It's one of the best investments you can make because it helps protect your reputation. After all, if someone complains about your work but concludes by saying "she gave me my money back," you at least come across as an honest professional. In addition, money is an exchange of energy, and some people's energy is better not to keep.

Your Cancellation Policy

For therapists with ongoing clients who book on a regular basis, or who book months in advance (see Figure 8–5), a rebooking issue guaranteed to show up is the one regarding cancellations. For clients who book months in advance, understand that things happen in life and sometimes clients need to change

Figure 8–5 | Booking clients far in advance can be done with a special offer as well. One of the best times to run a special is at the beginning of the year. (Image courtesy of iStock)

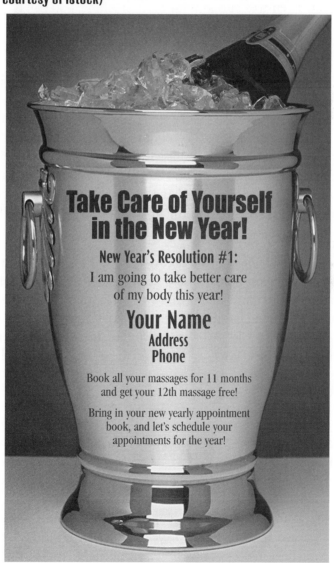

appointment times. If you have a 24-hour **cancellation policy**, let your clients know up front so they know what your rules are and that you value your time. However, if your steady clients have emergencies, which they will, don't damage your good relationship by being a boundary thug and demanding payment. Your relationship and their client net worth are too precious to risk because of an isolated incident. Instead, tell them you usually have to enforce your 24-hour cancellation policy because there are other people you could have booked and you've lost the salable hour, but you understand, are letting them off the hook since they are such a good client, and hope the business meeting, funeral, interview, or whatever goes well. Some of my clients have paid me for the canceled time anyway and others have not; they just rebooked within a few days so I really didn't lose the money.

In one case, though, I had a client who was a very wealthy businessman. The first time I showed up at his house and he wasn't there, I went ahead and billed him for that time because I had a suspicion this was going to be a trend. I was right. From then on, whenever I went to his house and he had left for some reason, his maid came to the door with a check already made out for my full fee, complete with apologies that he had to leave suddenly. I would have preferred, however, that he call ahead and not waste my time spent driving to his home. After getting paid for nothing more than the drive a number of times, I chose not to rebook him.

If you are working with clients who regularly cancel at the last minute or have to constantly rebook, do yourself a favor; take them off your client list, and stop wasting your valuable time and energy. I practice massage because I enjoy it and it is fulfilling for me. In the case of my very important client, I was genuinely disappointed not to work with him. It takes a lot of energy to prepare for my clients, and it was too hard on me when he canceled at the last minute.

Handling a Dissatisfied Client

Beyond the answers of "yes," "maybe," or other various excuses, the hardest word to hear during rescheduling is "no." If some of your clients flat-out tell you they don't want to rebook, it may hurt, but take it in stride. Massage is an art, and the odds are good that sometime during your practice, you will encounter a client who doesn't like your art. Just as some people think Picasso was a brilliant painter and some people think their four-year-old child could draw better than he did, so will you have mixed reviews to your art. Sift the reviews for ways to improve, and leave out the input from people who are perpetually negative or whose advice you think would not help your practice grow.

I once had a client who was an aesthetician seriously tell me I would get more clients if I wore peasant skirts, open-toed shoes, and painted my toenails. It took everything I had not to laugh out loud at the absurdity of her sincerely offered opinion, and while I have had many chuckles over that client suggestion, I still have not painted my toenails.

Making the Most of a Dissatisfied Client

If you are like the many successful therapists I interviewed who have a hunger for learning and growing, then losing a client can spur you to continue to work on yourself and your skills. As with the aesthetician's peasant skirt suggestion, I decided to just accept my work and be myself, even if that meant that I wouldn't draw clients who had a penchant for layered outfits. However, when I got feedback that was valuable, I would do what I could to improve. Studying anatomy, going to seminars and conventions to learn new techniques, and trading with other therapists gave me new skills and absolutely improved my client retention levels.

I love the title of a book by Janelle Barlow called *A Complaint is a Gift*. Her view is that customer and client complaints are the best source of information to improve yourself and your business, and I agree with her. If clients complain with any consistency about a certain topic, pay attention. If your room is too cold, get a better heater; if you are hard to reach, get a cell phone; and if your work is too light, get some weights, go to the gym, get stronger, or learn better body mechanics. In the case of pressure complaints, if you can't or won't increase your strength for whatever reason, have a list of other therapists who may be a better fit for your clients. Your job is to serve your clients, even if it means referring them to someone else. If you need to do this more than once, create a partnership with another therapist for a referral fee or cut of the work. You did the work of getting the client and should get some reward for it, even if it's just goodwill.

Getting Professional Feedback

Finally, if you have done all that we have covered and clients are not rebooking, get professional feedback. Call the best therapists you can access locally and ask if they will help you figure out what is keeping people from rebooking. Even if you have to pay for their time to get the chance to work on them, do so. Book appointments with as many therapists as possible, take them through your whole intake process and massage routine, do what you normally do, and see what they say. We all have our blind spots, and sometimes the only way to see ourselves clearly is to have others help us with the parts we can't see. Part of the commitment to succeed involves getting help and support, especially when it comes to an aspect as important to your business as rebooking.

Rebooking Moment 5: After the Client is Gone

Once your clients have left, there are still moments of decision they will go through. If they said "yes" to rebooking, they may question their decision or even have a touch of buyer's remorse. People are funny about doing things to take care of themselves, and what may have sounded like a good idea at the moment can be questioned later. You can help them remember why they rebooked by providing a follow-up call in the next day or two. Ask how they are feeling, remind them of the problem you were working on and what their goals were, and ask if they have any questions. Tell them you look forward to seeing them and that you enjoyed working with them. This seems so simple to do, but it can greatly help your new clients in the moments of decision they face about whether or not to keep the appointments they booked. You can even send a thank-you card as an additional follow-up.

Clients who left with a "maybe" answer to the rebooking question most likely will be harder to rebook, but you can stay in touch in numerous ways if you got the sense they would rebook at a later date. You can always call, or if you have a newsletter you make yourself or buy preprinted by someone else, send one on a regular basis, whether through snail mail or online. Promotional projects in which you are engaged, either on your own or with a marketing partner, can be announced through the mail by means of flyers, letters, or postcards. Basically, you will need to go back to the marketing methods you used for reaching new clients, only this time, your target market already has experience with your work. A satisfaction survey (which we cover later), sent off to be done in the privacy of their own home, can be a great way to stay in touch with clients and keep you a conscious part of their mental process. Be sure to include a self-addressed, stamped envelope so it is easy for them to get it back to you, or make sure you have a clear e-mail address to which they can return an electronic version.

REBOOKING TOOLS TO BUILD YOUR DREAM PRACTICE

The skills of rebooking a client can be helped a great deal with some simple rebooking tools. These tools are all designed to assist your marketing goals of creating trust, establishing value, and shaping the perception that you are a professional offering a valuable service.

TOOLS TO USE BEFORE YOUR CLIENTS ARRIVE

If you have enough time before a new client comes in for a massage, send out the rebooking tools of a welcome letter, your policy forms, and a suggestion list. These tools tell new clients about you, prepare them to make the most of their session and your time together, and let them know how you plan to comport yourself as a professional.

The Welcome Letter

Acknowledging and thanking new clients for making an appointment can reassure them that the decision to book with you was a good one. Your welcome letter can be a short card saying that you are looking forward to the appointment at the set date and time, or it can be a letter with background information about you and your practice, and what to expect from the session.

Clients who book with you over the telephone based on a referral or ad will be curious about you, and you can tell a lot about yourself in a welcoming letter. You can include your brochure and background information about yourself that you may not be able to share when you are focusing on the client upon arrival. Think about what your clients should know, what they might be curious about, and how you can set up positive expectations and anticipations for seeing you. Consider also what they might be worried about, and alleviate those worries. Let them know you keep strict privacy standards, cover them with a drape, maintain their modesty, keep them warm, or anything else that can reassure them all the way through your door.

If both you and your client are Internet savvy, you can either send your letters and forms via e-mail, or send a letter with a link to your Web site. Just don't send attachments. Many people will not open attachments for fear of computer viruses, so create your documents, and copy and paste them into an e-mail that any computer platform can open.

Policy Forms

Policy forms can be anything from a legally binding document that both you and your client sign in order to agree upon codes of conduct, to a simple list of requests such as that the client not wear perfumes. Legalistic documents can be helpful if you have a large or full practice where it matters that clients arrive on time, give 24-hour cancellation notice, or abide by other rules that let you run your practice smoothly and efficiently. Policy forms can contain requests or demands regarding client cleanliness, sexual harassment, informing you of medical conditions, giving accurate feedback during the session, or anything else that you anticipate may become an issue during or after a session.

Suggestion Lists

A suggestion list lets your clients know what they can do before, during, and after the session to make the most of their investment and experience. You can take some of the elements from the policy form and put them into a suggestion form. Suggestions for before the massage can be to shower, wear comfortable clothes, or bring a change of clothes. Suggesting places to park at your office or asking them to create a space where you can set up your table in their homes before you get there can save both of you time and frustration.

"Making-the-most-of-the-massage" suggestions can cover topics such as not needing to talk, and showing up on time so they receive all their scheduled minutes. It seems less punitive to encourage promptness for the session so they maximize their time with you than to have a legalistic-looking policy that states that the session begins and ends at the predetermined time whether the client is late or not. The end result is the same, but the tone of a suggestion is a lot friendlier and more welcoming than a statement. Suggestions for after the massage can include topics such as the value of drinking water, stretching exercises, what to expect the next day, and how to call you if they have questions later.

TOOLS TO USE DURING THE APPOINTMENT

Once you and your client are together, go over your policies and suggestion lists, either to review your points if you mailed the forms previously or to talk about them for the first time. These forms and the rebooking tools you bring out during the intake process to go over together will make up what will go into your **client files**.

Client Files

Your client files can range from a single piece of paper with basic contact information and initial session intake notes to 3-D computer graphic images of stress and compensation patterns, full medical history, fragrance and music preferences, referral source, and demographic profile. (See Figure 8–6.) If you have an office with a receptionist, you can make computerized files with backup forms in snappy folders with color-coordinated tabs. Or you can have some rumpled papers that get jammed into your portable expanding folder, left to alternately bake and freeze through the seasons in the permanent position in the trunk of your car, right beside your portable outcall table or chair. Basically, whatever you need to remember about your clients, write it down. Sophisticated or simple, your files should include at least your clients':

🌺 Contact information

🌺 Emergency contact information

🌺 Reason for getting massage

🌺 Basic medical history

🌺 Observation notes from your initial and subsequent sessions

🌺 Birth-date notation so you can send a card

Beyond that, you can add **S.O.A.P. notes** (see Figure 8–7a and Figure 8–7b), photographs of postural changes, information from their referring medical practitioners, or astrological charts, depending on the kind of work you do. Sources for standard preprinted forms showing generic bodies in various positions can provide you with whatever you need, depending on the information you want to gather on your clients. For more detailed records, consider using a software program on your computer as a way to keep track of your clients' progress. (See Figure 8–8a and Figure 8–8b.)

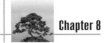

Figure 8-6 | Use an intake form to record your clients' contact information, needs, and preferences.

Client Information

Date: _____

Client ID: _____

Referred by: _____

Client Information

Name: _____

Address: _____

_____

City: _____

State: _____ Zip: _____

Phone: _____ Fax: _____

Emergency contact number: _____

E-mail address: _____

Birthday: _____

Occupation: _____

Employer: _____

Employer address: _____

Employer phone: _____

Massage Background

Approximate number of
massages received before: _____

Local therapists seen: _____

_____

_____

Type of work preferred: _____

Depth of pressure preferred: _____

Reasons for seeking massage therapy: _____

_____

_____

Problem areas (i.e. sensitive
lower back, ticklish feet, etc): _____

_____

_____

_____

Medical History

Are you under medical care now? ____ if so, for what condition(s)?: _____

Past accidents or operations: _____

List any medications being taken: _____

Please describe any physical problems or conditions which you are currently experiencing: _____

_____

Physician's name: _____

Address: _____

City: _____ State: _____ Zip: _____

Phone: _____

Figure 8–7 | **S.O.A.P. notes let you record your subjective and objective observations, assessments, and plans.**

INITIAL INFORMATION

Name_____ Date_____

S Subjective

(Symptoms, frequency, duration, intensity, how it started, aggravating/relieving activities, etc.)

Client's experience, expectations, and goals:

O Objective

Observations, tests, and results:

Treatment goals:

A Assessment & Applications

Massage treatment given:

Changes due to massage:

P Planning

Homework:

Plan for next session:

Long-range plans and goals:

(a)

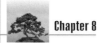

Figure 8–7 | (continued)

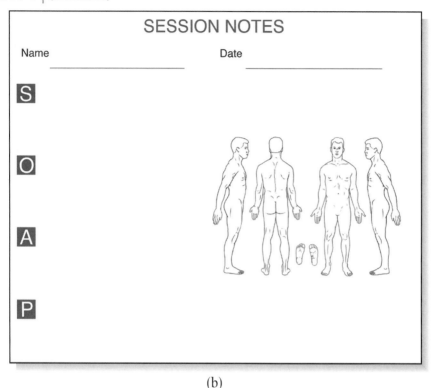

(b)

Figure 8–8 | Software for massage therapists can help you manage your information.
(Image courtesy of SOAP computer screen shot)

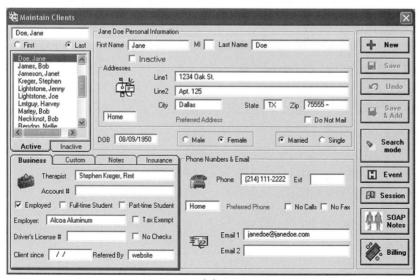

(a)

Figure 8-8 | **(continued)**

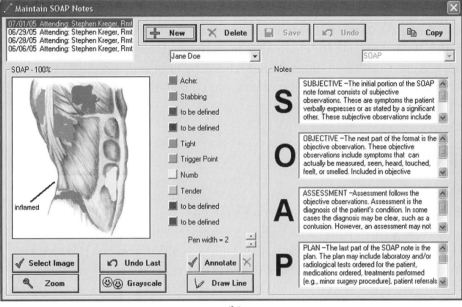

(b)

TOOLS TO USE AFTER THE MASSAGE

After the massage session is over, you face the moment where your clients let you know whether or not they are going to rebook immediately. As stated before, they can say "yes," "maybe," or "no" to rebooking. If the answer is "yes," get out your primary rebooking tool, your appointment book.

Appointment Book

If you have already filled in your calendar or PDA with preestablished time slots for massage, open up your appointment book and schedule a time that works for both of you. If you have not set up your calendar ahead of time, be careful not to overbook yourself or schedule appointments too close together. It is exciting to get a rebooking, but remember to protect your time boundaries.

Even if your new client doesn't say "yes" but gives you a "maybe," you can still use your appointment book. Look up at the person, let him or her know that you understand he or she doesn't want to rebook at the moment, and ask if you may call in a week to follow up. If the client says "yes," make a notation in your appointment book. By you writing this down, the client knows you will be calling, and he or she now expects you to since you said you would. Later, even though you may feel nervous, you still will call because you said you would. When you call, the client once again can say "yes," "maybe," or "no," and you can take it from there, either rebooking or bravely asking if the person would be willing to tell you how you could have made the massage a better experience for him or her.

Appointment Cards

Whatever happens at the moment of rebooking, be sure to have your cards close by. If you have a happy client who rebooks, you can use specialized appointment cards with blank lines to fill in the client's name and date, and the time of the next appointment. (See Figure 8–9.) Or, you can just write the information down on the back of your card, as both a reference tool and so your card can find its way, once again, to the bottom of your client's purse where it can be retrieved after she loses your first card. Really happy clients can take a stack of your cards with them to hand out to family, friends, coworkers, and others. Even your "maybe" clients can take cards with them

Figure 8–9 | Appointment cards let you give new cards to clients each session. This helps to remind them of their next appointment, and they also can give your card to a referral.

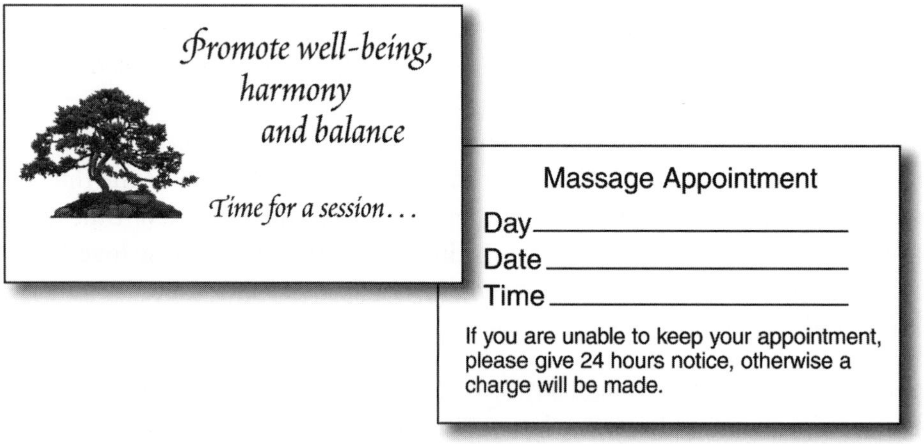

Promote well-being,
harmony
and balance

Time for a session . . .

Massage Appointment
Day_____
Date_____
Time_____
If you are unable to keep your appointment, please give 24 hours notice, otherwise a charge will be made.

as they leave. After all, they may not be rebooking because they can't afford another massage, but they probably know a lot of other people who would love your work. If that is the case, leap ahead to the section on referral and read how to help your less financially endowed clients accrue free time by referring others to you.

One-Time Specials

Trying to get an indecisive client to rebook may spur you to make a one-time deal to prove the value of your work over a number of sessions. We covered this concept earlier, but if you decide to use specials to rebook, make sure you write down the details upon which you both agree. For example, if you offer a two-for-one special, you can provide a coupon for later use, or take a check right then and book both sessions in your appointment book. If they don't want to schedule at that moment, book a deadline time to call and follow up on their decision as to whether or not they will use the special offer. (See Figure 8–10.)

Figure 8–10 | Coupons with a variety of incentives can encourage a new client to rebook another session or to try different services. (Image courtesy of Lincoln Park)

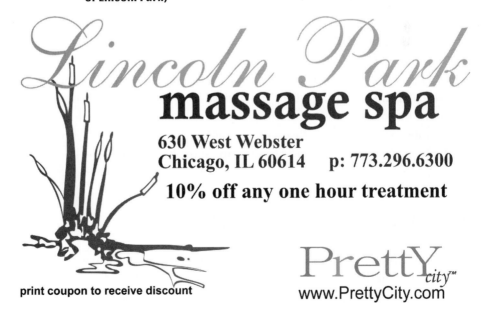

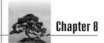

Figure 8–11 | The frequent buyer card encourages clients to consider multiple bookings.

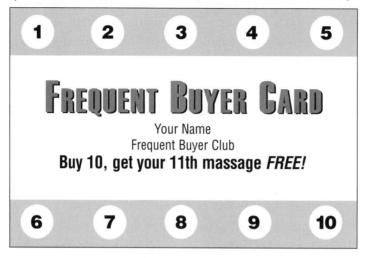

Frequent Buyer Cards

Creating customer loyalty is a big deal to a lot of big businesses, and it is to you, too. Of all the big businesses to succeed by creating customer loyalty, the airlines have one of the best records around. Smart marketers copy great ideas from other industries like these, one of which is the frequent buyer card, based on the same idea as passengers who receive frequent flyer miles from airlines with which they travel often. (See Figure 8–11.) Quite simply, you can have a card that keeps track of how many times your clients get a massage. When they reach a certain number, especially by a certain date, they get a reward. Rewards can range from extra time or a free session to a free dinner cooked in their home by your mutual marketing partner who does home meal preparations for busy people. Be creative, think outside the box, and do what you can to incite your new clients to sign up for multiple sessions.

TOOLS TO USE ONCE YOUR CLIENTS ARE GONE

After your clients have left, you can stay in touch in numerous ways. Reminders of you that show up in the mail, transmit over the Internet, or arrive by telephone keep your clients aware of you on whatever basis you choose. You can send a premade monthly newsletter (see the "Resources" section), or an electronic newsletter or e-zine, with informative articles; post e-mails announcing a seminar or class you are giving; or mail out notices about a birthday special you are offering that features an in-home gourmet meal (made by your marketing partner) and massage (by you) on their birthday.

Satisfaction surveys also are a good way to reconnect with clients. (See Figure 8–12.) You can send a form for them to fill in about what they liked or didn't like about their session, and then offer a time bonus or a gift they will receive when they come in for their next appointment, if they return the form. Thank-you notes are a great way to make thoughtful contact after a first session, and they are a rare treat in these days of impersonal e-mails.

Birthday cards are a nice touch, even for clients you have seen only once. (See Figure 8–13.) I remember sitting on my back porch by the golf course where I used to live, and, as I often did, I got into a conversation with the golfers waiting around to tee off. I was working on this book, and a golfer asked me what it was about. When I told him it was about marketing massage, he launched into an enthusiastic tale about a local therapist. As he raved about how wonderful the therapist was, I finally figured out that what brought on such a response was that the therapist had sent him a birthday card. And he had only been there once! I got a high-decibel referral, not because of a great massage but because of a card. If you are going to send a card, send a nice one, and sign it. In this day and age, a card you send through regular mail may be quite memorable.

Telephoning

If you are comfortable with the telephone, you can use it to stay in touch with clients, especially the kind who only get massage infrequently or just for special occasions. I have called clients I haven't heard from in a while only to hear, "We lost your card and wanted a massage but didn't know how to reach you," or "We were just talking about getting a massage but we got busy and forgot to call. Let me get my calendar." If new clients don't rebook but say something such as, "I should do this more often," ask permission to call them if you haven't heard from them in a while. If they say "no," then don't call them, but if they say "yes," provide good customer service and call them. Most people would love to get more massage but may have a hard time rationalizing it to themselves. One call from you, gently taking them by the hand and leading them to book an appointment, can restart your relationship.

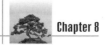

Figure 8–12 | **Follow up with new clients to constantly improve customer service . . . and your success.**

SATISFACTION SURVEY

Dear (Client):

Thank you for taking care of yourself and your health by booking a massage with me. I hope you had a good experience, and I look forward to seeing you again soon.

It is very important to me that my clients are happy with their massage experience, and I ask that you take a few minutes to complete this survey and return it in the enclosed envelope.

Thank you,
(Your Name)

What did you like about your massage? _____

_____

_____

Did you feel your needs were met? _____

_____

_____

Did you feel your expectations were met?_____

_____

_____

If you could change anything about your massage experience, what would it be?

_____

_____

What else could I have done to make your experience even better?

_____

_____

Please rate the following: Excellent   Good   Fair   Poor   Comment
    Quality of massage
    Professionalism
    Attitude
    General Atmosphere
    Environment

Figure 8-13 | Make even better use of a birthday card by including a coupon with a special offer. (Image courtesy of Getty Images)

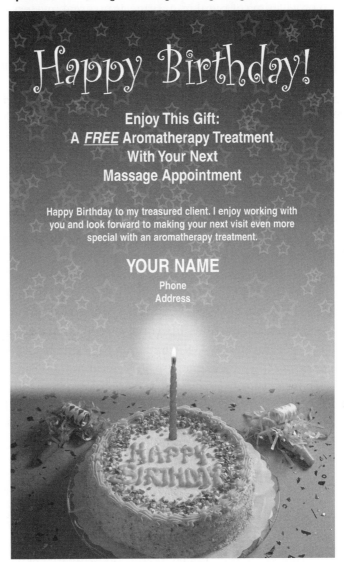

CHAPTER 8 SUMMARY

Rebooking is one of the most overlooked aspects of marketing. As you can see, it takes more than just getting a client in the door to build a practice. I have talked with hundreds of massage clients over many years about their experiences, and their tales—good and bad—are what have gone into this chapter. What makes these clients leave a therapist, or want to go back for a second session or a lifetime of regular massage, is no great mystery, at least not for you anymore. Their stories of what works and doesn't work are what you really need to know about how to market to build a dream practice. I hope the general principles and minute details they shared can help you toward success.

I encourage you to keep learning by talking to as many people as you can about massage. You may be surprised at how many people have received massage or know someone who has, and vivid stories are sure to follow if you simply ask. The best people to help you continue to learn what it really takes to rebook clients are the clients themselves, so start talking about massage to everyone, then be still and listen.

Rebooking tools can make the process of keeping a current client easier and more effective. The tools covered in this chapter are designed to get new clients to show up for their first session, and then to shape their experience so positively that they are happy to come back for other sessions. Your goal with your rebooking tools is to help people feel special, safe, and satisfied with their experience. These tools can help you create trust, shape perception, and establish value. Before a client shows up, you can send them a welcome letter, a suggestion list, your business policies, and even their intake forms to fill out ahead of time. During the intake time, use other written tools, such as S.O.A.P. notes and health history forms, to gain important information and also to establish their perception of you as a professional. After a session, the appointment book becomes an invaluable rebooking tool, and once the client is gone, cards, letters, calls, and other tools for staying in touch can remind them to come back again.

CHAPTER 8 ACTION STEPS

Based on the information in this chapter, do the following to reach new clients:

- ✳ Create a checklist of tools you can use to connect with your clients, even before their first session.
- ✳ Create a standard welcome letter to send to new clients.
- ✳ Review your work environment as if you were a new client, and make sure it makes a good impression.

❋ Practice your handshake and eye contact until you come across as confident and at ease.

❋ Practice matching and mirroring, and notice how often it happens naturally.

❋ Create a set series of questions to ask during a verbal intake.

❋ Create or purchase a standard written intake form, including a S.O.A.P. chart.

❋ Create a pre-massage conversation to guide your new clients through their first massage.

❋ Create an opening ritual to start each massage.

❋ Create a cancellation policy.

❋ Create a form for your business policies.

❋ Create a suggestion list of what clients can do to enhance their massage experience.

❋ Create a simple frequent buyer card.

CHAPTER 8 KNOWLEDGE CHECK

Check your understanding of the chapter by reviewing these questions and answers.

Q: Once a client is in the door, is marketing finished?
A: No.

Q: When is the majority of your marketing done?
A: During the session.

Q: Should you do all the talking when your new client first arrives?
A: No.

Q: What is the premise of pacing and leading?
A: Humans can lead each other more easily if they are already in step with one another.

Q: What is the purpose of your verbal intake?
A: To establish a match between what your clients want and what you offer.

Q: What is even more powerful than good word of mouth?
A: Bad word of mouth.

Q: What is the purpose of your pre-massage education?
A: To instill trust, relieve fears, and appropriately set expectations.

Q: Should you always apply deeper pressure if the client requests it?
A: No.

Q: What is one of the best forms of marketing you can do?
A: On-the-table education.

Q: What three tools can help your clients show up for their first appointment?
A: A welcome letter, policy form, and suggestion list.

Q: What are two suggestions you can make to help prepare a new client for a massage?
A: Shower, clothes, parking, creating a space to work in, talking, and promptness.

Q: What are three of the basic pieces of information your client files should contain?
A: Contact information, emergency contact information, reason for seeing you, basic medical history, observation notes, and birthday.

Q: What is one of the main benefits of the frequent buyer card?
A: It helps build customer loyalty.

Q: What are three media you can use to stay in touch with your clients?
A: Mail, Internet, and telephone.

Q: What does S.O.A.P. stand for?
A: Subjective and Objective observations and Assessments, followed by a strategic Plan.

Q: What is the purpose of a suggestion list?
A: To tell clients what to do before, during, and after the session to make the most of their investment and experience.

Q: What is the purpose of a welcome letter?

A: To thank new clients for booking an appointment and reassure them that they made a wise decision, which helps ensure that they show up for the appointment.

Q: True or False? If you want to use a newsletter to stay in touch with clients, you have to write it yourself.

A: False; you can purchase premade newsletters and articles, both electronic and hard copy.

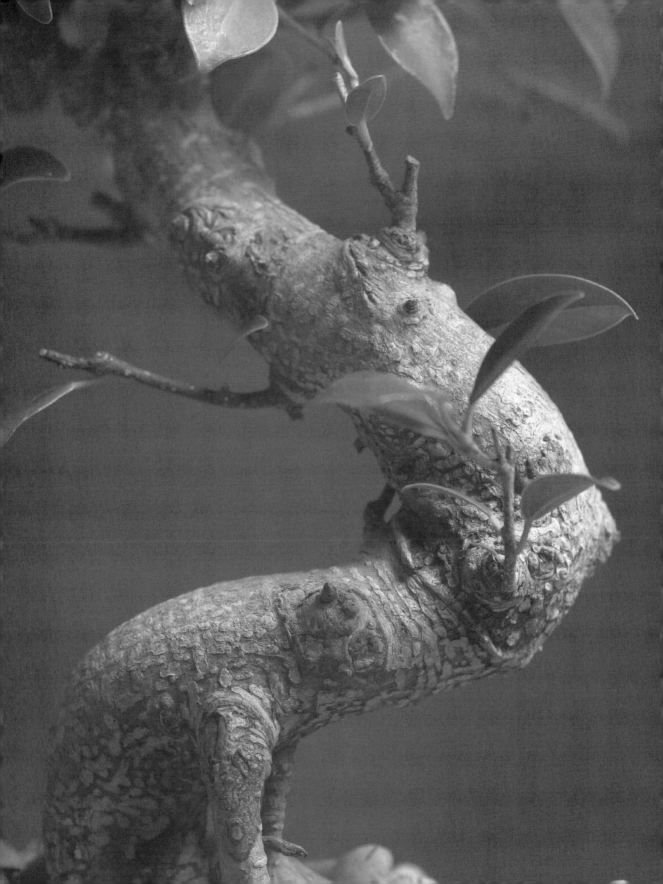

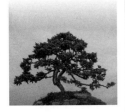

9

Referral Skills and Tools

CHAPTER OBJECTIVES

After reading this chapter, you should be able to:

- ❋ Identify communities you can target for referral marketing.

- ❋ Gain referrals from formal and informal referral sources.

- ❋ Use marketing tools for gaining referrals.

- ❋ Create incentives for those who give referrals.

- ❋ Explain the benefits and drawbacks of networking groups.

- ❋ Explain the benefits of joining professional associations for gaining referrals.

- ❋ Identify the seven basic tools for getting referrals.

- ❋ Describe the three steps for using marketing tools to get referrals.

- ❋ Explain the purpose of a **referral tracking system**.

- ❋ Describe the key elements of a referral tracking system.

REFERRAL SKILLS TO BUILD YOUR DREAM PRACTICE

Word-of-mouth referrals have been, and always will be, the best way for massage therapists to build a practice. If you have done the work covered in the prior chapters of reaching your clients, treating them like the center of the universe, and rebooking them enough times to demonstrate the value of your work, you will naturally get word-of-mouth referrals. For that reason, this chapter will be the shortest in the book because your hardest work is behind you now. To use a farming analogy, you have tilled the soil, planted the seeds, and tended to your crops, and now is the time to really harvest the fruits of your labor. You can sit back and let your happy clients do the talking, but if you love marketing, and I hope you do by now, there are a few more skills and tools you can use to build your practice with word-of-mouth referrals. Word-of-mouth or direct referrals are how most successful therapists have built their practices, so if you want a successful career in massage, pay close attention to these simple but valuable concepts.

People who refer you to others do so for a whole variety of reasons but, basically, people make referrals because it helps them in some way. If other businesses, such as your mutual marketing partners, refer you, it is because you help their businesses succeed, or they're just happy to do so. If your referral sources are your clients, they will make referrals because they like you and want you to succeed. Bonuses of time, special treatment, and thank-you gifts may motivate some clients, but most clients refer you because they have other people they care about whom you can help. Medical practitioners can be a source of referrals because they know you can help their patients with soft-tissue needs that will respond to massage. Receiving referrals in return also may be motivation for medical doctors or other professionals. Friends, family, and the checkout lady at the grocery store you go to every week just may give you referrals because, well, you asked them to.

Building Referrals Within Communities

Before you start going out and getting referrals, first think about what you want for your life and your work. Think about:

* What kind of clients you want
* Who knows them
* What you need to do to get their referrals

Go through the same mental steps that you did when working with small businesses as mutual marketing partners except, this time, think about community groups you want to serve. Community groups can be formal or informal in their composition, and while they may seem less definable than your marketing partners' customers, whole client pools are right in front of you, waiting for an introduction, if only you could see they were there.

Do you want active, living-life-to-the-fullest kinds of clients? One woman active at the local tennis club near you can be the doorway into a large enough pool of potential clients to build your whole practice. Do you enjoy the elderly and like hearing some interesting stories? One happy client in a large retirement community can be a fountain of referrals for you. Do you want more-aware people who already take care of themselves? One enthusiastic yoga student can talk about you to her classmates, teacher, friends, and coworkers. Look around at the types of communities you want to reach. If you know people in that community already, talk with them about what you can do to get yourself into the group.

If you don't know anyone in that group yet, use the material on reaching new clients. Do a marketing outreach into that community, get a client or two, and you're in. Put a flyer up at the garden club (see Figure 9–1), or teach a one-hour class on foot reflexology at the senior center, and you're on your way. If need be, join the yoga class yourself and get to know your fellow classmates. Even informal networking can be specific and strategic.

As you did with the mutual marketing material, think about what kinds of people you want to work with. Then think about where they work, play, shop, recreate, socialize, congregate, or worship. Whether they are hanging out at bowling alleys, coffee shops, bookstores, gardening clubs, city swimming pools, or gyms (see Figure 9–2), people gather because they are social animals. If you spot a herd of them that interests you, figure out your best way into the group, wander over, and introduce yourself. So many people are looking for a good massage therapist that even just introducing yourself and talking about what you do for a living can be enough to get you started. One person in that community who becomes a client can then become your leverage with the whole group.

This informal and unstructured marketing is by far the cheapest, safest, and easiest way to reach your target market directly. The successful therapists I interviewed who built their practices from one or two well-connected clients

Figure 9-1 | Look for groups who need massage and with whom you would enjoy working.

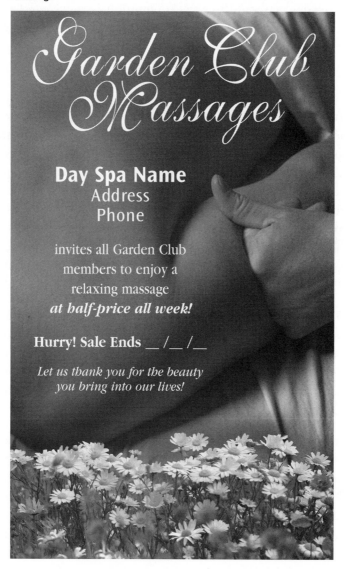

Garden Club Massages

Day Spa Name
Address
Phone

invites all Garden Club
members to enjoy a
relaxing massage
at half-price all week!

Hurry! Sale Ends __ / __ / __

*Let us thank you for the beauty
you bring into our lives!*

got started with seemingly lucky breaks, but they were out there talking to people when those breaks came. The benefit you have is that you don't have to wait for the lucky breaks or coincidental encounters to get you going. You now have the tools and skills to make your own luck, and you can be much more proactive and specific in reaching target markets.

Figure 9-2 | Some of your best referral sources will come from informal communities.

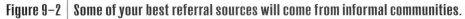

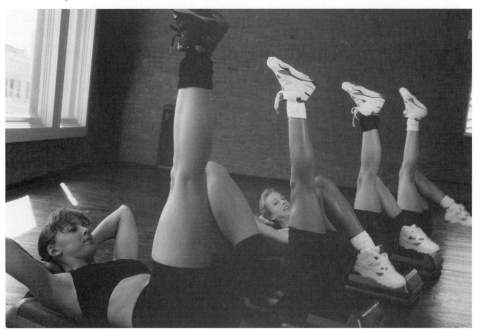

EXERCISE: IDENTIFYING COMMUNITIES YOU WANT TO WORK WITH

Think about the kinds of clients with whom you would enjoy working. You can look back at the work you did earlier in this book on describing your ideal client, or think again, with thoughts that are a little different from the ones you might have had earlier. Then write down answers to these questions about your ideal referral communities.

❋ Who is my ideal client?

❋ What five communities might my client be in?

❋ What can I do to get into those communities informally?

❋ What can I do to formally market to those communities to get my first clients?

If you are in a group, share your ideas so everyone can expand their thinking.

_____

_____

_____

_____

_____

_____

A Note About the Exercise

If you found yourself not wanting to share because someone might "steal" your ideas, take note. Scarcity will block your thinking and squelch creativity. If you find yourself viewing your classmates or colleagues as competition, you need to reread this book. There are more clients out there than you can ever reach, and there are enough methods and ideas to reach clients in this book to keep you busy for as long as you choose.

I bring up this issue because of an incident at one of my seminars. Being a golfer and having many clients who play golf, I use golf examples frequently in my seminars. During a break in a class I was giving at a massage school I was visiting, a young man stormed up to me, glaring and indignant. "Stop talking about golfers!" he scowled. "You're giving away my secret!" Then he leaned in conspiratorially, jerking his thumb at his classmates behind him. "I'm the one who thought of working with golfers first, so quit putting ideas into their heads, okay?" I could tell by looking at his face, hearing his attitude, and watching him sulk in his seat as I continued to give more golf examples that he wasn't going to last in massage for more than a couple of years. His arrogance, small-mindedness, and aggression were going to be spewed all over his clients just as they were at me, and somehow, at least from what I gathered, the all-important desire to serve just didn't seem to be present. Even if he did get a golfer or two as clients, I'd bet you a set of golf clubs they weren't going to be referring him to their golfing buddies. Getting into a community is one thing; staying in and getting referrals requires all the other things we have talked about so far.

In addition, since the massage community is often a great source of cross-referrals between therapists who collaborate instead of compete, this young man was likely to be ostracized because of his "me-first" attitude. Classmates and colleagues can be a great source of leads into communities in which they may not be interested, but which you could richly mine for new clients.

Informal Referral Sources

Many successful practices have gotten their start from the referrals of family and friends who believed in and supported the new therapist. My father kindly referred an elderly widow from his congregation to me, and though I was quaky and unconfident, and almost irritated at him for getting me a client before I felt "ready," she became an integral part of my practice and stayed with me for years. Thanks, Dad! If you are going to ask for referrals from family and friends, be prepared for them. Even if you don't feel ready, are unsure of your abilities, or don't have your cards or matching sheets yet, get started anyway. Readiness is a feeling many people only get long after they have started, so don't wait until you feel ready to take on your first clients referred by family and friends.

The clearer you know what you want, the more you can tell your friends and family how to help you reach your target market. Tell them—or better yet, show them—what your work is about so they can talk about you more enthusiastically. Then tell them what kind of clients you want, what kind of work you want to do, what days you plan to work, and other details to focus on. Being specific about what you want will help them know who to talk to and what to say in their circle of familiars. Making your dreams clear lets others help you make them a reality.

Referrals from Your Current Clients

Much advice about building a massage practice trumpets the glories of getting word-of-mouth referrals from current clients. The problem with that advice is, how do you get your first clients so that they can refer you? I hope by now you've read about many ways to reach new clients, and if you use those methods and tools, you will have a pool of clients of your own from whom to get referrals. In all likelihood, your current clients will be some of your best sources of new clients. So, why will your clients refer you? Mostly because they are pleased with you and your work, and will talk to everyone about how much better they feel.

Since a lot of people are out there looking for a good therapist, even a casual mention of you from a current client can turn into a direct referral. One of my clients found me in this manner. He was looking for a therapist, and while at a dinner table at a social function, he overheard one of my clients about four seats down say the word "massage." He immediately went over and asked her if she had a therapist she liked. She said "yes," gave him my number, and he has been a regular client now for many years.

Many of your clients will be happy to help you, and if you need more clients, let them know and ask for referrals. Be forewarned, though. One mistake I made was to talk to my clients when we were booking our appointments about how busy I had gotten and how hard it was becoming to schedule everybody. I didn't realize that this made a number of my clients protective of their staked claim to me until one client said something like, "Well, just don't get any more new clients because then you won't have time for me." Oops. If you are going to ask for referrals, realize that you are often a significant touchstone in your clients' lives, and some will have a fear of abandonment that you will leave them if you get too successful or busy. Minimize talk about how busy you are, but if they know you are busy, allay their fears of losing access to you, because that guarantees those clients won't refer you.

Make It Easy to Refer You

Give your clients and others ways that make it easy to share you. Give them your business cards to pass out, invite them to your promotional events, or, better yet, give them or sell at a deep discount gift certificates to give away to people they know who would be likely to convert to regular clients. You will gain a great deal of goodwill from your clients, and you will also gain a prescreened client, most likely in your target market, who has the trust of a personal referral with the decision to buy removed. If a full session is more than you can bear to give, offer a half-hour session instead but don't be cheap. This can be an invaluable way to safely and easily reach new clients, so make the most of it.

Making It Beneficial to Refer You

If you can't believe that clients will refer you just because you ask, come up with incentives that offer additional motivation. You can offer your clients extra time in each session or build up the minutes to a free full massage for a set number of referrals who become full-paying clients. Thank-you cards, flowers, or one of your promotional items or cross-selling bonuses are nice touches as appreciation for new referrals. Clients have different needs, so pay attention. If money is tight, give them a thank-you discount instead of extra time. If they need flexible scheduling or forgiveness for having to change their appointment times, give that instead. If they want your most coveted time slot, use it as a thank-you gift for their referrals. Some people just want gratitude, and that is easy to give. Whatever it is your referring clients want—within reason, of course—offer it. Just make sure to acknowledge their referral in some way.

Networking

In addition to your formal and informal referral sources is a well-structured source of referrals, which comes in the form of networking groups. However, since my goal is to create pinpoint-accurate, proactive marketing, I prefer mutual marketing to traditional networking, but it can be effective if used correctly. On the downside, networking groups can have time-consuming meetings, be expensive to join, may not include members who interact with your target market, and can take a long time before they are worth the investment.

On the upside, everybody has a body, and since bodies need massage, even if the group isn't directly connected to your selected market, people are still there to do business and make referrals, and you may get a lucky link into your target market.

In addition, networking groups can serve as a social group of colleagues and peers dealing with similar business matters. If you find yourself lonely in your practice, join a group for the support as well as the potential referrals. Loneliness is a big drawback to working alone, and since sleepy clients and boundary issues keep your source of human contact during your working hours at arms' length, get your needs met through structured channels upon which you can rely.

If you are going to join a formal networking group, go in knowing what you want. Tell the group you want 10 new clients or three on-site contracts with local businesses. Have specific needs people can help you with, or bring up specific problems and ask for advice. Remember, Americans are problem solvers, so use that to your best advantage. Also, stay with the group long enough for it to pay off. People I have interviewed who use networking groups have said it takes time, persistence, and showing up, as well as providing good referrals to other members. Finally, read books on how to network. This is an art and a science unto itself, and, if you're going to take the time and money to do it, you should do it right.

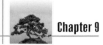

Networking with Other Massage Professionals

As a professional, you should join an association of your peers. Associations offer many benefits, including marketing opportunities. You can sign up for association referrals through printed and online directories, or through 800-number referrals. Large national organizations such as the American Massage Therapy Association (AMTA), Associated Bodywork & Massage Professionals (ABMP), or the National Certification Board for Therapeutic Massage and Bodywork (NCBTMB) offer various forms of referral.

If you are new to massage, don't be alone. Go to association meetings or have your own get-togethers with classmates or massage professionals listed in the phone book. If you want to get involved with your new profession, become active on an association committee. You will learn a lot about your profession and meet people who have already gone down the path you are walking, and you can learn a lot from them. You also can learn a lot about yourself as a practitioner and get a sense of just how broad this field is. When you are volunteering with your colleagues toward a higher mission or project, barriers come down and you can get help, advice, and a host of other rewards that only show up when you are "on the same team" together. Dreams die in solitude. If your dream is to have a successful, long-term private practice or a hundred-acre healing center, or to work with movie stars, surround yourself with others who will help you keep your dream alive. The more you know what you want and tell others about it, the more someone who knows someone who knows just the person you want to meet can make your dreams come true magically.

Colleagues also are a possible source of referrals. I have met more than my share of scarcity-minded therapists who view other therapists with suspicion and competitive animosity (probably because they don't know how to market!). However, colleagues can offer many new clients through cross-referrals. I have given away numerous client leads to other therapists I knew from my association work because I didn't work in that person's city, I was too busy, or I didn't offer the kind of work the client needed. Knowing qualified therapists to whom you can refer clients will make it easier for you to go on vacation, move, or change careers. Get to know massage professionals with other specialties or modalities. Know the benefits and limitations of your work, and if you are faced with a client who needs help beyond your abilities and training, refer him or her to the professionals you know. As often happens, what you give comes back to you. That's how cross-referrals work.

Nonpersonal Referral Sources

Massage therapists who are willing to build their practices through referrals from nonpersonal sources have a growing list of referral resources available to them. If you want to grow your practice, especially in the medical direction, you can conceivably get referrals from Internet referral services, insurance companies, HMOs, and alternative medicine networks. Check out the "Resources" section on referral sources for a sample of businesses that offer referral services, and go online and type in search terms like "massage referral" for more options.

Referrals from Health Professionals

Working in close conjunction with health professionals—whether alternative, complementary, or traditional—can be a rich source of satisfaction and referrals. Across America, medical practitioners and massage therapists are creating positive working relationships and are cross-referring patients and clients in ways that could not have been imagined even a few short years ago. Even if this form of medical mutual marketing is not common in your area yet, it is a growing trend that ultimately can be a great assistance to doctors, massage therapists, and their shared clients. Doctors, psychologists, acupuncturists, chiropractors, homoeopathists, naturopaths, and other mental or physical health professionals are all becoming viable sources of referrals.

Knowing these professionals is something you should consider, even if you don't want or expect referrals from them. Over the course of your career, it is virtually guaranteed that someone will come to you with a problem that needs medical treatment. Many people are afraid of going to the doctor and may come to you seeking help because you feel safe. It is part of your ethical duty not to take clients who need medical care and not to work beyond your scope of practice. Having a list of doctors and other practitioners to suggest to them will allow you to rest easier knowing that your client is more likely to seek additional help since the referral came from you.

REFERRAL TOOLS TO BUILD YOUR DREAM PRACTICE

The marketing function of getting referrals is crucial to the long-term success of your practice, but, in many ways, it can be the easiest function with the simplest tools. Compared to the complexities of acquiring new clients through

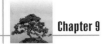

reaching skills and tools, getting referrals can be fairly straightforward, especially with the aid of personal referrals from family, friends, and clients. The primary tool you will need for getting basic referrals is your business card, because it is small, easy to carry, and a socially acceptable tool for your family, friends, clients, and others to hand out without hesitation.

That said, getting referrals can be an involved and creative undertaking, and you can use every tool you have at your disposal to get into the communities or markets you want to reach. Once you are in, you can use your tools to inform, educate, and motivate those in your target community to book with you and give you referrals. The tools you can use for getting direct referrals are the same you use for reaching clients through other means, but with some interesting twists. From earlier chapters, you are familiar with these tools, but now let's look at *new* ways to use your basic referral tools, including your:

❋ Business cards

❋ Brochures

❋ Gift certificates

❋ Coupons

❋ Flyers

❋ Special offers

❋ Promotional items

❋ Web site

As you think about the people you want to work with in your targeted communities, consider which of your tools can get you into that community quickly and easily. To make this idea more clear, let's use an example of a community of women who belong to a tennis club. Keeping these tennis players in mind, ponder how each of these tools can be used to:

1. Market to get in the door of the club

2. Reach and book a client who plays there

3. Have her refer you to her friends

First, let's look at getting in. You can ask the tennis club manager if you can put up a flyer (see Figure 9–3), do a demonstration massage class, put brochures at the cashier's counter, leave a stack of cards by the towel pile,

Figure 9–3 | Use events that are important to your community to introduce them to massage. (Image courtesy of Getty Images)

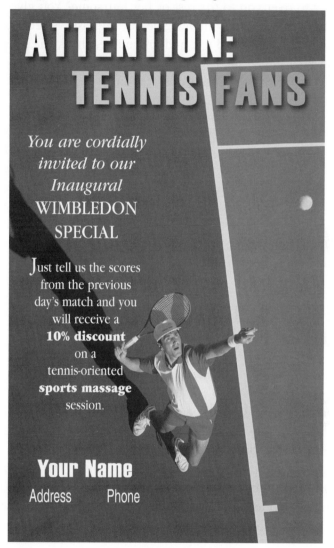

raffle off a few gift certificates at a fundraiser for new tennis nets, or leave out a basket of free wooden massage tools with your name and number on them under the tournament schedule. You can ask to include a two-for-one discount coupon in the quarterly members' dues envelopes, take out an ad in their monthly club newsletter, put up a banner on their club Web site, or write a short article for their newsletter about massage for tennis elbow. One of those ideas should get you in the door!

Second, imagine that, once you're in the door, you meet Loraine. She's got tennis elbow and decides to give you a try. How do you use your tools to get her to refer you to the rest of her foursome? You give her a great massage; help her tennis elbow; give her exercises, stretches, or recommendations for heat and ice; and, of course, check the range of motion in her neck, since she is probably chopping at the ball because she can't fully turn her neck and, therefore, turns her torso and shortens her stroke to compensate.

Thoroughly impressed, Loraine goes to her friends with great stories and a few of your tools. She has a pile of your cards, gift certificates for a free half-hour massage, and brochures that go with the gift certificates. She also has a deal for her group. If all of the other ladies come in for a free half-hour massage, or a full hour for half-price, Loraine gets a free massage. Of course, once this group of gals goes out and beats everyone's socks off, the losers will want to know how they got that spring back in their step. Surprise! The answer is you! Better get some more sheets and oil, because here they come! Any questions? Now you try it!

EXERCISE: GETTING INTO A COMMUNITY WITH A REFERRAL PROJECT

Think about a community with whom you would enjoy working. Then think about all the different ways you could get into that community to gain even one client. What marketing tools could you use? What offers could you make? How can you help them with their needs while at the same time becoming a known person in the group? Once you get one client, what can you do to get that person to refer you to other people in the group? Write down your target community and at least three ways you can get into the group. Then write a referral project plan for how to get ongoing referrals within the community.

_____

_____

_____

_____

_____

_____

_____

_____

_____

_____

_____

_____

THE REFERRAL TRACKING SYSTEM

If you are going to be doing a lot of marketing using referrals, where the incentive is more than just goodwill and gratitude, you will need a referral tracking system to keep tabs on your various promotional projects. Contact management software may be necessary if you have a lot of referrals to keep track of, but if you like systems that don't crash, pen and paper work fine, too. Basically, your system needs to record information about your:

- Client's name
- Date you started the referral project
- Terms of agreement
- Method of rewards accruement
- Referral names
- Referral usage
- Referral rebooking status
- Referral follow-up
- Deadline of the project
- Status of the project
- Termination of the project

Let's go back to Loraine and the tennis ladies as an example.

Client's name—Loraine Tennison

Date you started the referral project—10/6

Terms of agreement—one free massage for Loraine

Method of accruement—three tennis partners come in for half-price hour massages

Referral names—Susan Swing, Chris Chopper, and Nancy Netgame

Referral usage—10/9, Susan in; 10/13, Chris in; 11/1, Nancy not in yet

Referral rebooking status—Susan rebooks, Chris considering after vacation

Referral follow up—call Chris 11/1 evening

Deadline of the project—none

Status of the project—waiting for Nancy

Termination of the project—when all three have first massage and Loraine has her free hour

This is a pretty simplistic system, but you get the idea. There are so many types of projects you can undertake with both mutual marketing partners and informal communities that no one project management form would be right for all of them. However, the basics used here are what you will need most. They can help you keep track of your projects so you can keep your current clients happy, stay on top of how often they are referring, and make the most of the referrals you get. After all, the purpose of such projects is to get the referred clients to rebook, because that's how you build your dream practice.

Web Sites

While Web sites may not be the best or safest way to reach new clients, they can serve you very well in the referral stage of marketing. A strong personal referral mixed with the ability to further research you online can be a powerful combination for shaping perception, creating trust, and establishing value among new clients. If you have a professional Web presence, use your site to educate and inform those looking you up based on others' referrals.

If you have mutual marketing partners, or connections with well-known communities, put their links on your Web site, and ask them to link their sites to yours. If a person is checking you out online and sees that you have many links to other groups, a different form of referral is created that further demonstrates your value and trustworthiness.

CHAPTER 9   SUMMARY

If you have the bare-bones attributes and skills, and you use a few muscle marketing techniques to get and keep clients, you will probably find that referrals will be all you need to round out and sustain your practice over many years. In this chapter, we focused on the sources of target communities and how you can reach your ideal client through the communities and groups to which they already belong. Some referral sources can be formal, with specific projects and incentives agreed upon with networking partners, health professionals, massage colleagues, clients, and others. Informal referrals can be equally effective, with happy customers telling everyone about you because you have helped them, even if you don't give them an agreed-upon reward. As you build your practice, see the world full of opportunities and communities just waiting for the right massage therapist to come along. Know what you want, think about who you want to work with, do what it takes to get a few clients, do good work, provide excellent customer service, and watch your practice grow. In a service business such as massage, the people who want your services are looking for a personal referral, so talk with all your sources about how to help spread the good word about you and your massage practice.

Your tools are also important for gaining referrals. All of the tools you use to reach new clients can be used in other ways to gain personal referrals into and throughout your target communities. In this chapter, we took a brief look at how to use basic and advanced tools to establish your presence, broaden your reach, and enhance your reputation within the group of people you most want to serve. The simple strategy of getting in the door of some group, obtaining one client, and building referrals from there is how countless therapists have built their practices. Whether you unknowingly wander into a close group of friends or deliberately figure out a way into a members-only organization, get one person in the group to value and appreciate your work, and you are on your way to building a full practice.

CHAPTER 9   ACTION STEPS

Based on the information in this chapter, do the following to reach new clients:

❋ Think about your ideal client/target market and create a list of the different "communities" to which they belong.

❋ Give gift certificates to people with access to your target community.

* Create a strategy to network with friends and colleagues for leads into your target community.

* Create projects within your target community to gain individual clients and their referrals.

CHAPTER 9   KNOWLEDGE CHECK

Check your understanding of the chapter by reviewing these questions and answers.

Q: List three possible sources of referrals.
A: Mutual marketing partners, clients, friends, colleagues, and medical practitioners.

Q: What is the primary reason that clients will refer you?
A: You have helped them and they have people they care about whom you can help.

Q: Can informal networking be specific and strategic?
A: Yes.

Q: Should you wait until you feel ready before you start your practice?
A: No; start anyway.

Q: What is one of the best ways to make it easy for your clients to refer you?
A: Give them gift certificates to give to people they know.

Q: Can classmates or colleagues give you leads for your target community?
A: Yes!

Q: How do you make the most of networking groups?
A: Go in knowing what you want, and state your specific needs and problems.

Q: Why is a business card such a good referral tool?
A: It is small, easy to carry, and socially acceptable to hand out to others in any setting.

Q: What are the three steps of building a practice within a community?
A: Get into the community, get one first-time client, and get referrals from that one person.

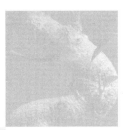

Conclusion

GOING FORWARD

When I first started giving seminars about marketing, the title I chose for the class was *Marketing: The Grand Adventure.* I named it that because I truly believe that the process of marketing, including all that we have just been through in this book, is one of the grandest adventures a human can take.

Successful marketing to get and keep clients takes knowing yourself, understanding the many facets of human nature, and being in touch with and observant of the world around you. The studies of psychology, sociology, history, philosophy, health, business, and more all go into understanding what drives human beings to have their many needs met by massage.

Grand adventures don't have any maps, road signs, or beginning and end points. An adventure is a journey, and it can begin anywhere and lead anywhere. Where you are today on your journey—with your skills, experiences, training, and goals—started a long time ago, and your road will take many twists and turns over the course of your life. My purpose for this book was to walk with you for the brief moment in time that our paths crossed, and to pass on to you the skills and tools I gleaned from countless therapists to help you build your dream practice. I hope what you have learned in this book will help to make your dreams come true, and I wish you well on your way.

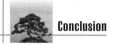
THE SKILL OF REEVALUATION

Before we part ways, though, there is one last marketing skill I want to tell you about. It is the skill of reevaluation, and it is the key to a long, happy career. Since our definition of marketing is anything that affects your ability to get and keep clients, one of the most influential elements of your marketing comes from how you grow and change over the course of your career.

Being a massage and touch professional changes you. Interactions with clients, conversations with colleagues, talking to people about yourself, touching people, learning about the body, and all that goes into your work shapes you into an ever-evolving and maturing person. Over time, you will discover that you enjoy certain skills more than others, and you will notice that you prefer certain clients. You will notice that you are really good at some things and not as good at others. Even better, you will notice that there are some things you're not good at, but it doesn't bother you anymore. Or, you may discover that there are things you're good at, but you no longer enjoy doing them.

Massage careers succeed when you pay attention and adapt to the latest terrain you are in on your adventure. They fail when you don't, leading to boredom, frustration, or burnout. It may feel secure to play it safe year after year, doing what you've always known, but over time, stagnation can ruin what was once a thriving practice. The goal of this book is to help you succeed at making a living with massage, but if you no longer enjoy your work, what's the point?

To become and stay successful and happy, conduct a regular reevaluation of yourself and your career. The more frequently you ask yourself questions of reevaluation, the sooner you can make corrections on your course, and the less time, money, and energy you will spend spinning your wheels or getting lost on bumpy side roads. At the very least, do an annual review at the beginning of each year to help you see if you are still doing the right kind of work and are still aiming for the right kind of clients.

So, what do you need to reevaluate? Yourself, your goals, your dreams, your skills, your clients, your target markets, your settings, and even your vision or mission statement. There are hundreds of questions you can ask yourself to see if you are on the right path in your journey, but included here are some key questions to ask when facing times of transition and change.

The Questions of Reevaluation

✳ How have I changed recently?

✳ Are my goals different?

✳ How am I handling success and setbacks?

✳ Am I happy and fulfilled with my work?

✳ How is my life balance? Do I need to unbalance it a while for a big growth spurt, or do I need to stop pushing myself and just recover for a while?

✳ Am I reaching my financial goals?

✳ What new skills have I learned, or would I like to learn and incorporate into my practice?

✳ Am I doing the kind of massage I want to do?

✳ Is my level of skill still serving my clients?

✳ Do I still enjoy working with my target market, or do I want a new market?

✳ Am I ready to change my work status (e.g., part time to full time, employee to owner)?

✳ Do I want to expand, get a business partner, or hire employees?

✳ Do I want to sell my practice and move?

✳ Do I want to narrow my practice and become a specialist?

✳ Do I still want to be in the massage profession?

I hope the answer to that final question is "yes" for you.

Millions of people are in need of healing and loving touch, and massage and bodywork professionals can help people around the world in ways we are just beginning to understand. You can have great success and satisfaction in this field, and if I have been able to help you learn how to reach and keep the clients you need to build your dream practice, then you can change others' lives with touch, and we all will leave this world a better place.

Glossary

Action marketing tools—written marketing tools that give the reader a specific action to take, usually within a limited period of time.

Advertising—a marketing message distributed by mass media for a price.

Attribute—a personal quality and set of characteristics demonstrated by attitude and behavior.

Bare-bones marketing—using personal and professional attributes, and basic skills and tools, to build a private practice.

Blind pitch—sending a resume to an employer who does not have a current job opening or isn't soliciting resumes through "help wanted" ads.

Cancellation policy—a statement delivered verbally or on paper saying that missing or canceling an appointment late will cause some form of repercussion.

Client expectations—what a client thinks a massage experience should be like, how a massage therapist should behave, and what kind of results they can expect from massage.

Client files—a collection of information about clients including contact and emergency contact information, reasons for getting a massage, S.O.A.P. notes, and more.

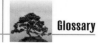

Client net worth—the sum of what a client is potentially worth to you financially over the time of your working relationship, both from their sessions and referrals.

Club spa—a facility whose primary purpose is fitness, and that offers a variety of professionally administered spa services on a day-use basis.

Commitment to succeed—a stated willingness to take the actions necessary to reach your definition of success.

Compensation package—a combination of wages, benefits, training, and other additions in exchange for your services.

Congruency—a consistent presentation between appearance and behavior, and expectations from others.

Contact list—the collection of names and contact information of your clientele.

Cross-selling bonuses—free or discounted products or services you collect from other businesses to use as promotional items or gifts for getting or keeping clients.

Cruise ship spa—a spa aboard a cruise ship providing professionally administered spa services, fitness and wellness components, and spa cuisine menu choices.

Day spa—a spa offering a variety of professionally administered spa services to clients on a day-use basis.

Desire to serve—a passionate and genuine interest in helping others, and a willingness and capacity to care.

Destination spa—a spa whose sole purpose is to provide guests with lifestyle improvement and health enhancement through professionally administered spa services, physical fitness, educational programming, and on-site accommodations. Spa cuisine is served exclusively.

FAQs (frequently asked questions)—common questions either said aloud or thought, especially on issues of trust, value, and convenience.

Fictitious business name (FBN)—a unique name you legally file at your county business registry.

Follow-up contact—getting in touch with an employer (or client) either through phone, mail, or e-mail after an interview.

Frequent buyer card—a card that indicates how many sessions a client has received. After a set number of sessions, the client receives some bonus or reward.

Hands-on interview/test massage—a massage performed on an employer where your skills, abilities, and attitudes are evaluated as part of the hiring process.

Intangible benefits—nonmonetary benefits gained on a job, including such things as social interaction.

Keeping your word—following through and fulfilling promises or agreements you make with yourself and others.

Keywords—specific terms or buzzwords used in a job, profession, or industry that make your resume attractive to computer software programs that search for those terms.

Logo—a graphic or symbolic representation of a business image.

Marketing—anything you do that affects your ability to get clients and keep them coming back.

Massage menu—a selection of massage modalities or added services at different costs and for varying lengths of time.

Matching and mirroring—copying or imitating someone else's posture, movements, expressions, words, and so forth, so that person feels that you are like him or her.

Medical spa—individuals, solo practices, groups, and institutions comprised of medical and spa professionals whose primary purpose is to provide comprehensive medical and wellness care in an environment that integrates spa services, as well as conventional and complementary therapies and treatments.

Mineral springs spa—a spa offering an on-site source of natural mineral, thermal, or seawater used in hydrotherapy treatments.

Moments of decision—times during encounters with your clients when they are most likely to evaluate and judge you and your work, and then make a decision about whether or not to rebook.

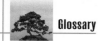

Muscle marketing—marketing skills and tools that help you reach your market with greater levels of speed and control.

Mutual marketing—a way of reaching new clients by partnering with others, especially businesses, to gain access to their customers.

Networking—a formal collection of people who share leads and access information for each others' businesses to gain new clients.

Opening ritual—a short routine repeated at the beginning of each session to demarcate the start of the massage, and to relax you and the client.

Outcall massage—a massage business where the therapist travels to the client's location.

Paper trail—business documents that detail how and where you spend your time and money.

Parallel structure—a consistent presentation of style choices, word phrasings, and punctuation on a written document such as a resume.

Partner mentality—a mindset where, as an employee, you approach every task and person as if you had a personal stake in the success and reputation of the business.

Perception Continuum—a progressive measurement of the public's different levels of understanding and acceptance of massage.

Policy form—a written form stating the rules, suggestions, or requests your clients should follow to enhance the massage experience for both of you.

Press release—a standardized submission of a newsworthy item about which you want a media outlet to do a story.

Professionalism—a way of being, including manners, courtesy, speech, dress, and behavior, that is appropriate for clients.

Promotional gifts—novelty items, premiums, or advertising specialties, such as mugs and pens, that have your name and contact information on them.

Prospect—a person who may become a paying client.

Publicity—stories told in mass media about you and something you are doing. You don't pay for it, but you also may have little control over what the report or story says.

Quality market—buyers who demand a superior service or product excellence, often regardless of cost.

Rapport—a feeling of being connected to another person, often assisted by a sense of similarity.

Rebooking—the act of getting a current client to sign up for another appointment.

Reference marketing tools—passive written materials that educate clients, enhance their perception of you and your massage, create a compelling reason to use your services, and provide contact information.

Referral tracking system—a paper or electronic record that keeps track of promotional projects.

Referrals—prospective clients recommended to you by people you know personally or professionally.

Resort/hotel spa—a spa owned by and located within a resort or hotel, providing professionally administered spa services, fitness and wellness components, and spa cuisine menu choices. In addition to the leisure guest, this is a great place for business travelers who wish to take advantage of the spa experience while away from home.

Scannable resume—a resume tailored for electronic distribution on the Internet. A scannable resume contains as many keywords as possible and uses a text-only format.

Screening interview—a phone interview or meeting with the human resources department, which often precedes an in-person interview.

Self-sabotage—behavior that undermines or blocks you from reaching your goals. It often comes from subconsciously held beliefs that run contrary to the behaviors necessary to reach your goals.

S.O.A.P. notes—a written form where you record your subjective and objective observations and assessments of the body, followed by strategic plans for one or more sessions to help with a specific need.

Spa—See Club Spa, Cruise Ship Spa, Day Spa, Destination Spa, Medical Spa, Mineral Springs Spa, Resort/Hotel Spa (all spa definitions courtesy of International SPA Association).

Target market/niche market/ideal client—a profile of the type of group or individual whose business you would enjoy and profit from.

Tax deductions—business expenses that the Internal Revenue Service allows you to subtract from your income taxes.

Testimonials—statements given by other people saying that they have been positively impacted by your work.

Time management system—a paper-based system that uses separate sections such as month-at-a-glance, daily to-do lists, contact information, expense sheets, and more.

Universal needs—the two core human needs that drive behavior and motivation: to gain pleasure and avoid pain.

Value market—buyers who put more emphasis on the cost of a product or service.

Verbal check-in—a brief questioning during the massage to find out how the client is feeling and to ask questions about pressure, comfort, temperature, and so on.

Verbal intake—a time of reviewing your clients' needs, preferences, medical issues, and contraindications, in order to establish a match between what your clients want and what you can or can't do.

Wage variances—variations or fluctuations of wages based on different circumstances.

Written intake—notes you take as your client talks to you; these can include forms they fill out and S.O.A.P. charts.

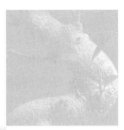

Resources

MARKETING MASSAGE RESOURCE GUIDE

The following guide is a compilation of massage-specific books, magazines, businesses, associations, organizations, and Internet connections that can help you get your first job or build your dream practice.

The topics are alphabetized and include Business and Professional Resources, Internet Connections, Massage and Bodywork Associations, Marketing Tools, Massage Products, Massage Publications, Referral Sources, Software for Massage Practices, and Spa Resources.

Business and Professional Resources

Capellini, S. (2006). *Massage therapy career guide for hands-on success* (2nd edition). Albany, NY: Thomson Delmar Learning.

Capellini, S. (2006). *Making the switch to being rich—A guide for those who care about people & the planet*. Miami, FL: Royal Treatment Enterprises.

McIntosh, N. (2005). *The educated heart: Professional guidelines for massage therapists, bodyworkers, and movement teachers*. Baltimore, MD: Lippincott Williams & Wilkins.

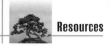

Sohnen-Moe, C. M. (1997). *Business mastery—A guide for creating a fulfilling, thriving business and keeping it successful* (3rd edition). Tucson, AZ: Sohnen-Moe Associates, Inc.

Thompson, D. L. (2001). *Hands heal: Communication, documentation, and insurance billing for manual therapists* (2nd edition). Baltimore, MD: Lippincott Williams & Wilkins.

Internet Connections

Bodywork Online
http://www.bodyworkonline.com
Online forum with help and advice from and for bodyworkers.

http://www.massageclothing.com
(800) 562-1944
A wide selection of massage clothes available online.

http://www.massagetherapy.com
Massage therapist listing, massage therapy schools, employment opportunities, products, associations, links, and so forth.

Massage Therapy Web Central
http://www.mtwc.com
Bookstore, massage school guide, training, products, and more.

My Receptionist
http://www.myreceptionist.com
Offers an answering and appointment service designed just for massage therapists, and provides Internet scheduling, messages, and more.

TimeTrade Systems, Inc.
http://www.timetrade.com/
(877) 884-9224
Web-based appointment book, home page, e-scheduling, and phone service for appointments.

Massage and Bodywork Associations

American Massage Therapy Association
500 Davis Street, Suite 900
Evanston, IL 60201-4695
(847) 864-0123
(877) 905-2700
http://www.amtamassage.org

American Organization for Bodywork Therapies of Asia
1010 Haddonfield-Berlin Road, Suite 408
Voorhees, NJ 08043-3514
(856) 782-1616
http://www.aobta.org

Associated Bodywork & Massage
Professionals, Inc.
1271 Sugarbush Dr.
Evergreen, CO 80439-9766
(303) 674-8478
(800) 458-2267
http://www.abmp.com

The IMA Group, Inc. (covers 15
wellness associations)
P.O. Drawer 421
Warrenton, VA 20188-0421
(540) 351-0800
http://www.imagroup.com
http://www.internationalmassage
.com

National Certification Board for
Therapeutic Massage and Bodywork
1901 S. Meyers Rd., Suite 240
Oakbrook Terrace, IL 60181-5243
(800) 296-0664
http://www.ncbtmb.com

The Touch Research Institutes
University of Miami School of
Medicine
P.O. Box 016820
Miami, FL 33101
(305) 243-6781
http://www.miami.edu/touch-
research

Marketing Tools

All You Knead
(800) 952-5375
http://www.allyouknead.com
Massage products, supplies, and
equipment.

Hemingway Publications
(815) 877-5590
http://www.hemingwaymassage
products.com
A full line of brochures and products
for massage therapists.

Information For People
(360) 754-9799
(800) 754-9790
http://www.info4people.com
Brochures, videos, greeting cards,
display cases, gift certificates,
postcards, and software, all designed
for helping massage therapists build
their practices.

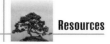
The Massage Garden
http://www.themassagegarden.com
Marketing and office products,
brochures, gift certificates, software;
offers *The Massage Kit* package with
"all the office materials you need to
run a massage business."

http://www.massageontheweb.com
Web hosting, links, newsletters and
articles to send to clients.

Massage Promos
(315) 254-4781
http://www.massagepromos.com
Marketing tools for a successful
massage practice.

Sharper Cards
(800) 561-6677
http://www.sharpercards.com
Postcards, appointment cards, and
other printed marketing tools for
massage therapists.

Staying in Touch
(877) 634-1010
http://www.stayingintouch.net
http://www.massagenewsletters.com
Massage client newsletters typeset
with your name, address, and phone
number.

Tangle Toys
(888) 829-3808
http://www.tangletoys.com
"The single greatest 3-Dimensional
Marketing Tool in history!"

WaterColors Printers
(800) 804-2019
http://www.watercolorscards.com
A full line of greeting cards, posters,
postcards, special occasion cards,
stickers, and gift certificates with a
massage theme.

Massage Products

Best of Nature
Long Branch, NJ 07740
(800) 228-6457
http://www.bestofnature.com
http://www.spabodyworkmarket
.com
A large massage supply
"superstore."

BIOTONE
San Diego, CA 92120
(619) 582-0027
(800) 445-6457
http://www.biotone.com
http://www.biotonespa.com
Massage oils, crèmes, essential oils,
books, music, videos, and spa
treatment products.

Bodywork Emporium
(800) TABLE-4-U
http://www.bodywork-emporium
.com
One of the largest retailers of
massage supplies and tables.

Bodywork Mall
Utah College of Massage Therapy
Salt Lake City, UT 84111
(888) 717-6753
http://www.bodyworkmall.com
A large selection of massage tools,
tables, and accessories.

Day Spa Warehouse, A Scrip
Company
(800) 320-7010 or (800) 747-3488
http://www.dayspawarehouse.com
Over 5,000 products for spas and
day spas.

Downeast School of Massage
Bookstore
Waldoboro, ME 04572
(207) 832-5531
http://www.dsmstore.net
A good selection of books, study
aids, charts, videos, and accessories.

Educating Hands Bookstore
Miami, FL 33130
(305) 285-0651
(800) 999-6691
http://www.educatinghands.com/
bookstore.html
A large selection of books, videos,
tables, chairs, and accessories.

Massage Warehouse, A Scrip
Company
(800) 507-3416 or (800) 747-3488
http://www.massagewarehouse.com
Thousands of products for massage
therapists and spas.

Massage Publications

*Journal of Bodywork and Movement
Therapies*
Editor: Leon K. Chaitow, ND, DO
http://www.intl.elsevierhealth.com/
journals/jbmt

Massage & Bodywork
(publications of ABMP)
BodySense Magazine
(800) 458-2267
http://www.massageandbodywork
.com
http://www.bodysensemagazine.com

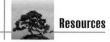
Massage Magazine
(904) 285-6020
(800) 533-4263
http://www.massagemag.com

Massage Therapy Journal
(publication of AMTA)
(877) 905-2700
http://www.amtamassage
.org/journal

Massage Today
(714) 230-3150
http://www.massagetoday.com

Referral Sources

About Massage
http://www.aboutmassage.com
Web site with referral listings and a
huge source of information.

iWantaMassage.com
(801) 497-6295
http://www.iwantamassage.com
Referral resource.

Massage Today Locator Service
(800) 359-2289
http://www.MassageToday.com
Web site on which you can list your
information in order to get referrals.

The Portable Practitioner:
Opportunities in the Healing Arts
http://www.portablepractitioner
.com
Newsletter with employment
opportunities.

Software for Massage Practices

Elite Software, Inc.
(800) 662-ELITE
http://www.elite-usa.com
Software to manage sales, inventory,
client files, marketing,
appointments, and payroll.

Island Software Co.
(877) 384-0295
http://www.islandsoftwareco.com
Business, insurance billing, and
practice-building software for
massage therapists.

Land Software
(202) 237-2733
http://www.landsw.com
Hands-on business management
software for massage therapists.
Includes client manager, session
manager, financial reports, track
referrals, session history, medical
history, and so forth.

Professional Salon from Select
Computer, Inc.
(800) 710-3879
http://www.prosalon.com
Salon, spa, and resort management
software.

Spa Associations

The American Spa Therapy
Education and Certification Council
(888) 241-2095
http://www.asteccse.com
Post-graduate spa education.

The Day Spa Association
Union City, NJ 07087
(201) 865-2065
http://www.dayspaassociation.com

International SPA Association (ISPA)
Lexington, KY 40504
(888) 651-4772
http://www.experienceispa.com

The Spa Association
Fort Collins, CO 80527
(970) 207-4293
http://www.thespaassociation.com

Spa Consultants

Preston Wynne, Inc.
Saratoga, CA
(408) 741-5936
(877) 256-3513
http://www.pwsuccesssystems.com
http://www.prestonwynne.com
Spa consulting services, seminars,
and business products for the spa
industry.

Royal Treatment Enterprises
Miami, FL
(305) 662-6674
http://www.royaltreatment.com
Steve Capellini does staff training,
spa development, and seminars on
spa services.

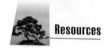 **Resources**

rational and Management
.ing
Rosa, CA
953-2202
ki@sonic.net
e Wolski offers consulting
ices for spa operations.

Tara Spa
Carmel, CA
(800) 552-0779
http://www.taraspa.com
Tara Grodjesk offers consulting
services and training for individuals
or corporations opening new spa
properties.

ja Publications

American Spa magazine
(866) 344-1315
http://www.americanspamag.com

DAYSPA magazine
(800) 442-5667
http://www.dayspamagazine.com

Healing lifestyles & spas magazine
(805) 962-7107
http://www.healingretreats.com

Premier Spas magazine
(218) 723-9200
http://www.premierspa.com

Pulse! (publication of ISPA)
(859) 226-4429
http://www.experienceispa.com/
ISPA/Pulse

Spa Finder magazine
(212) 924-6800
http://www.spafinder.com

Spa Magazine
(386) 246-3413
(866) 836-7887
http://www.spamagazine.com

Spa Management Journal
http://www.spamanagement.com

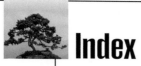

Index